Workbook and Lab Manual for Sonography:

Introduction to Normal Structure and Function

Workbook and Lab Manual for Sonography:

Introduction to Normal Structure and Function

4th Edition

Reva Arnez Curry, PhD, RT(R), RDMS
Vice-President, Instruction and Learning Services
Delta College
University Center, Michigan

Betty Bates Tempkin, BA
Ultrasound Consultant
Formerly Clinical Director of the Diagnostic Medical Sonography Program
Hillsborough Community College
Tampa, Florida

ELSEVIER

ELSEVIER

3251 Riverport Lane
St. Louis, Missouri 63043

Notices

Knowledge and best practice in this field are constantly changing. As new research and experience broaden our understanding, changes in research methods, professional practices, or medical treatment may become necessary.

Practitioners and researchers must always rely on their own experience and knowledge in evaluating and using any information, methods, compounds, or experiments described herein. In using such information or methods they should be mindful of their own safety and the safety of others, including parties for whom they have a professional responsibility.

With respect to any drug or pharmaceutical products identified, readers are advised to check the most current information provided (i) on procedures featured or (ii) by the manufacturer of each product to be administered, to verify the recommended dose or formula, the method and duration of administration, and contraindications. It is the responsibility of practitioners, relying on their own experience and knowledge of their patients, to make diagnoses, to determine dosages and the best treatment for each individual patient, and to take all appropriate safety precautions.

To the fullest extent of the law, neither the Publisher nor the authors, contributors, or editors, assume any liability for any injury and/or damage to persons or property as a matter of products liability, negligence or otherwise, or from any use or operation of any methods, products, instructions, or ideas contained in the material herein.

Library of Congress Cataloging-in-Publication Data

Workbook and lab manual for Sonography : introduction to normal structure and function /
Reva Arnez Curry, PhD, RT(R), RDMS, Vice-President, Instruction and Learning
Services, Delta College, University Center, Michigan, Betty Bates Tempkin, BA, RT(R),
RDMS, Ultrasound Consultant, Formerly Clinical Director of the Diagnostic Medical
Sonography Program, Hillsborough Community College, Tampa, Florida. -- 4th edition.
    pages cm
1. Ultrasonic imaging. I. Curry, Reva A. II. Tempkin, Betty Bates. III. Title:
Sonography : introduction to normal structure and function.
 RC78.7.U4C937 2016
 616.07'543--dc23

                                                              2015036273

Content Strategist: Sonya Seigafuse
Content Development Manager: Laurie Gower
Content Development Specialist: John Tomedi
Publishing Services Manager: Hemamalini Rajendrababu
Project Manager: Umarani Natarajan
Design Direction: Ashley Miner

Printed in United States of America

Last digit is the print number: 9 8 7 6 5 4

Contributors

Jill Beithon, RT, RDMS, RDCS, RVT
Owner
Just Wright Ultrasound Consulting, LLC
Fergus Falls, Minnesota
Fetal Echocardiography

Peggy Ann Malzi Bizjak, MBA, RDMS, RT(R)(M), CRA
Radiology Manager, Ultrasound Division
University of Virginia Health System
Charlottesville, Virginia,
Adjunct Faculty, Diagnostic Medical
   Sonography Program
Piedmont Virginia Community College
Charlottesville, Virginia
Introduction to Ergonomics and Sonographer Safety

Myka Bussey-Campbell, M.Ed., RT(R), RDMS
Program Coordinator, Diagnostic Medical
Sonography Program
Department of Therapeutic and Therapeutic Sciences
Radiologic Sciences Degree Program
Armstrong Atlantic State University
Savannah, Georgia
The Abdominal Aorta; The Inferior Vena Cava;
   The Portal Venous System

Reva Arnez Curry, PhD, RT, RDMS, FSDMS
Vice-President of Instruction and Learning Services
Delta College
University Center, Michigan
Embryology; Introduction to Laboratory Values; The
   Abdominal Aorta; The Inferior Vena Cava; The Portal
   Venous System; The Biliary System; The Pancreas;
   The Urinary and Adrenal Systems; The Spleen;
   The Neonatal Brain

Tiana V. Curry-McCoy, PhD
Assistant Professor, Medical Laboratory Science
Georgia Regents University
Augusta, Georgia
Introduction to Laboratory Values

Kacey Davis, BSRS, RDMS
Program Director, Diagnostic Medical Sonography
Darton State College
Albany, Georgia
The Spleen

Yonella Demars, MS, RDMS, RVT
Staff Sonographer/Clinical Preceptor
University of Virginia Medical Center
Charlottesville, Virginia
The Biliary System

Vivian G. Dicks, PhD, MPH, RDCS
Assistant Professor and Environmental
   Health Coordinator
Master of Public Health Program
Georgia Regents University
Augusta, Georgia
Pediatric Echocardiography

Kathryn A. Gill, MS, RT, RDMS
Program Director
Institute of Ultrasound Diagnostics
Mobile, Alabama
Before and After the Ultrasound Examination; First
   Scanning Experience

Michael J. Kammermeier, RDMS, RVT, RDCS
America's Clinical Product Specialist
Voluson Ultrasound Education Manager
GE Healthcare
Venore, Tennessee
The Male Pelvis: Prostate Gland and Seminal Vesicles
   Sonography; Scrotal and Penile Sonography

Zulfikarali H. Lalani, RDMS, RDCS, APS
Alta Bates Summit Medical Center
Department of Ultrasound
Merritt Pavilion
Oakland, California
The Male Pelvis: Prostate Gland and Seminal Vesicles
   Sonography; Scrotal and Penile Sonography

Robbi R. King, BS, RDMS, RVT
Staff Sonographer
Winn Army Community Hospital
Fort Stewart, Georgia
First Trimester Obstetrics (0 to 12 Weeks);
  Second and Third Trimester Obstetrics
  (13 to 42 Weeks)

Alexander Lane, PhD
Coordinator of Anatomy and Physiology
Triton College
River Grove, Illinois
Anatomy Layering and Sectional Anatomy

Wayne C. Leonhardt, BA, RDMS, RVT
Staff Sonographer
Mayo Clinic Hospital
Phoenix, Arizona
Clinical Instructor, Diagnostic Medical
  Sonography Program
Gurnick Medical Academy
San Mateo, California
The Thyroid and Parathyroid Glands

Vivie Miller, BA, BS, RDMS, RDCS
Ultrasound Consultant and Clinical Specialist
Hephizabah, Georgia
Pediatric Echocardiography

Marsha M. Neumyer, BS, RVT, FSVU, FAIUM, FSDMS
International Director, Vascular Diagnostic
  Educational Services
Vascular Resource Associates
Harrisburg, Pennsylvania
Abdominal Vasculature; Vascular Technology

Timothy L. Owens, RDMS, RT(R), MBA
Staff Sonographer
Fossil Creek Care
San Antonio, Texas
The Male Pelvis: Prostate Gland and Seminal
  Vesicles Sonography; Scrotal and Penile
  Sonography

J. Charles Pope III, PAC, RDCS, RVS
Echocardiology Clinical Coordinator
University Heart and Vascular Institute
Augusta, Georgia
Assistant Clinical Professor, Allied Health
  Department
Georgia Regents University
Augusta, Georgia
Adult Echocardiography

Marilyn Dickerson Prince, MPH, RDMS, RVT
Vascular Ultrasound Supervisor Technologist
Emory University Hospital
Department of Radiology
Atlanta, Georgia
The Liver, The Gastrointestinal System, The Female Pelvis

Angie Rish, RDMS
Assistant Sonography Lab Instructor, Diagnostic
  Medical Sonography Program
Department of Diagnostic and Therapeutic Sciences
Armstrong Atlantic State University
Savannah, Georgia
The Neonatal Brain

Lisa Strohl, BS, RT(R), RDMS, RVT
Master Clinical Applications Specialist
GE Healthcare Ultrasound
Wauwatosa, Wisconsin
Before and After the Ultrasound Examination;
  Ultrasound Instrumentation: "Knobology," Imaging
  Processing, and Storage; Breast Sonography

Betty Bates Tempkin, BA
Ultrasound Consultant
Formerly Clinical Director of the Diagnostic Medical
Sonography Program
Hillsborough Community College
Tampa, Florida
Before and After the Ultrasound Examination; General
  Patient Care; Interdependent Body Systems;
  Anatomy Layering and Sectional Anatomy; First
  Scanning Experience; Embryology; The Portal
  Venous System; The Biliary System; The Pancreas;
  The Urinary and Adrenal Systems, First Trimester
  Obstetrics (0 to 12 Weeks); Second and Third
  Trimester Obstetrics (13 to 42 Weeks); High-
  Risk Obstetric Sonography; The Neonatal Brain;
  Interventional and Intraoperative Ultrasound

Avian L. Tisdale, MD, FAAP
Division Director
Nemours Inpatient Pediatrics at *Inspira*
Vineland, New Jersey
Clinical Assistant Professor of Pediatrics
Rowan University School of Osteopathic Medicine
Stratford, New Jersey
Embryology

Cheryl A. Vance, MA, RT, RDMS, RVT
Chief Executive Officer
C&D Advance Consultants, LLC
San Antonio, Texas
3-D/4-D Sonography

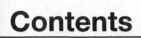

Contents

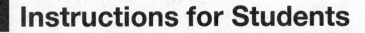

Instructions for Students

Dear Students…

The purpose of this laboratory manual is to guide you in studying concepts presented in the textbook *Sonography: Introduction to Normal Structure and Function*.

This laboratory manual:

- was written to be completed either independently during private study or with a student partner in a laboratory setting.

- is built around the six levels of cognitive learning described in Bloom's taxonomy: memorization, comprehension, application, analysis, evaluation, and synthesis.

- has been developed to help you learn sonographic anatomy, basic physiology, and image analysis through a progression from simple to complex, that is, from memorization of key words to comprehension of learning objectives, application of key concepts, analysis of images and illustrations, synthesis of chapter subheadings, and evaluation of the chapters.

Each chapter of the laboratory manual is structured to follow Bloom's taxonomy of six cognitive domains, with subsections that correlate with each cognitive level. This means that each section of the chapter "builds" on the previous one, just as each of Bloom's domains build on the previous one. The domains address memorization (knowledge), comprehension, application, analysis, evaluation, and synthesis, as shown in the chart below.

Bloom's Taxonomy Domain	Definition	Example
Memorization	Memorize facts, figures	Memorize key words, measure organs and vessels
Comprehension	Restate facts or concepts in your own words	Answer objectives in your own words

Bloom's Taxonomy Domain	Definition	Example
Application	Applying what you've learned in a new way	Draw or sketch an organ and label its parts
Analysis	Compare and contrast, note differences	Differentiate the normal appearance of organs and structures on sonographic images
Evaluation	Assess what has been learned, determine its value	Appraise the information presented and judge its value
Synthesis	Create something "new" from what has been learned	Write a technical impression

Teacher Tap is an online resource that includes a discussion of critical and creative thinking involving Bloom's taxonomy (available at http://eduscapes.com/tap/topic69.htm). For additional information, check out the detailed definition and examples on Wikipedia (https://en.wikipedia.org/wiki/Bloom%27s_taxonomy).

USING THE LABORATORY MANUAL

Before you begin each chapter, make sure you have read and studied the corresponding chapter in the *Sonography* textbook. To complete the laboratory manual chapters, you will need the following items:

- The *Sonography* textbook and notes from the reading

- Pen, colored pencils, or highlighters, and a notebook

- Anatomy and physiology notes from other previous courses may be helpful as well.

The following suggestions will help you use optimize the use of this manual:

1. Quickly skim through the chapter in the laboratory manual. Open your textbook to the corresponding chapter. Note the exercises in the laboratory manual are designed to stimulate your learning of the concepts presented in the textbook.

2. Bloom's taxonomy domains are presented in sequential order in each chapter. Only appropriate domains are included.

3. Do the exercises in sequential order.

4. Write the answers in your notebook.

5. Write in the margin questions that you may have as you work through the exercises. Make a list of your questions, answer them as best you can, then check your answers with your instructor. What additional information did your instructor provide? How was it helpful to you? (This type of reflection will help you prepare for quizzes and tests.)

6. This manual contains unlabeled images and illustrations from every chapter in the textbook to test your comfort level with sonograms and identifying anatomy. Make sure you understand the images that are presented. Can you identify structures without labels? Do you know how to describe them? If you're still confused about the images presented in the manual, go back and reread the section in the textbook. We encourage you to color the structures on the illustrations to better differentiate the anatomy.

7. Make sure you understand which things in the text are important to your instructor. Think of these as guidelines. Write down these guidelines and refer to them as you study. This technique should help you prepare for major tests on the material.

8. Allow enough time for review and reflection at the end of the laboratory chapter. What did you learn that you did not know before? How can this help you improve your learning of normal structural anatomy and physiology?

Sonography is an exciting and challenging profession. We wish you the best in your education and career.

Reva Arnez Curry and Betty Bates Tempkin

1 Before and After the Ultrasound Exam

I. MEMORIZATION EXERCISE

Directions to Students: Write the key words in your notebook or on note cards. Write the words on one side of the notepaper and then write the definitions on the opposite side of the page or on the back of the paper. If using note cards, write the key word on the front and the definition on the back. *This step should be completed before the lab session begins.*

Memorize the key word definitions silently for 5 minutes, then work with a lab partner and identify the words for which you still need help. List the words here. Add additional rows if needed.

II. COMPREHENSION EXERCISE

Directions to Students: Work with a lab partner to complete this exercise. You will need to write here or in your notebook. First, change each objective into a question.

> *Example: "Explain the roles of the sonographer and sonologist in the ultrasound procedure" becomes, "What are the roles of the sonographer and sonologist in the ultrasound procedure?"*

Next, write a short answer to the question just created.

> *Example: "A sonographer takes the patient history, explains the sonographic exam, performs the sonographic exam, and writes a technical observation of the images produced. A sonologist is a physician who assesses the images and dictates an interpretive report,*

> *which can include a definitive diagnosis or differential diagnoses."*

Highlight or circle any part of your answers about which you are unsure, and check the answers in your textbook. If you are still unsure of the answers, put a question mark next to the answer(s) for the review session of the lab.

III. APPLICATION EXERCISE

Directions to Students:

1. In your notebook, list the sources of hepatitis B virus/HIV transmission and how the transmission can occur. Ask your lab partner to critique your work. What did you miss?

2. Beneath your answers, write ways in which your exposure to hepatitis B virus/HIV can be reduced. Be as specific as possible. Ask your lab partner to check your answers. What did you miss?

3. In your opinion, what is the most important thing to remember about Standard Precautions? Write your answer and check it with your lab partner. Did your partner have the same answer?

ULTRASOUND REQUEST
THOMAS JEFFERSON UNIVERSITY HOSPITAL
DEPARTMENT OF RADIOLOGY
DIVISION OF DIAGNOSTIC ULTRASOUND

☐ STAT

☐ PORTABLE

CALL PRELIMINARY REPORT TO:

DOCTOR

LOCATION

PHONE NO

MEDICAL RECORD #
NAME

ADDRESS

AGE

BIRTH

PHONE NO.

ISOLATION PRECAUTION ☐ YES

REFERRING PHYSICIAN/CLINIC (NAME & ADDRESS) | PHONE NO.

ESSENTIAL CLINICAL FACTS • (MUST BE COMLETED BEFORE EXAM IS PERFORMED)

REASON FOR EXAMINATION

RELEVANT MEDICAL HISTORY

A 3 4 1 4 7 6

PHYSICIAN'S SIGNATURE & BEEPER#   DATE

ABDOMEN
- [ ] **ABDOMEN COMPLETE**
- [ ] LIVER
- [ ] GALLBLADDER
- [ ] SPLEEN
- [ ] ASCITES
- [ ] PALPABLE MASS
- [ ] DOPPLER

RETROPERITONEUM
- [ ] **RETROPERITONEUM COMPLETE**
- [ ] PANCREAS
- [ ] KIDNEYS
- [ ] ADRENALS
- [ ] AORTA/IVC
- [ ] LYMPH NODES
- [ ] DOPPLER

CHEST
- [ ] MEDIASTINUM
- [ ] PLEURAL EFFUSION
- [ ] THORACENTESIS

EXAM.		
TECH.		
ROOM		
DATE		

PELVIS
- [ ] **RENAL TRANSPLANT**
- [ ] URINARY BLADDER
- [ ] PROSTATE
- [ ] RECTUM
- [ ] SCROTUM
- [ ] DOPPLER

HEAD AND NECK
- [ ] BRAIN
- [ ] THYROID GLAND
- [ ] PARATHYROID GLAND

HEART
- [ ] **COMPLETE ECHOCARDIOGRAM**
- [ ] M-MODE & 2D ECHOCARDIOGRAM
- [ ] DOPPLER ECHOCARDIOGRAM

VASCULAR
- [ ] CEREBROVASCULAR COMPLETE
- [ ] PERIPHERAL VASC. (ARTERIAL)
- [ ] PERIPHERAL VASC. (VENOUS)
  - ☐ IMAGING
  - ☐ IPG

NOT LISTED
- [ ] (SPECIFY)

GYNECOLOGY
- [ ] **PELVIS COMPLETE**
- [ ] UTERUS
- [ ] OVARIES
- [ ] FOLLICLE SIZE
- [ ] IUD LOCALIZATION
- [ ] DOPPLER

OBSTETRICAL
- [ ] **FETAL COMPLETE**
- [ ] FETAL COMPLETE (INTERNAL GROWTH)
- [ ] OBSTETRIC DOPPLER
- [ ] AMNIOCENTESIS
- [ ] SPECIAL (SPECIFY)

SUPERFICIAL
- [ ] BREAST
- [ ] PALPABLE
- [ ] JOINT/TENDON/MUSCLE

INTERVENTIONAL
- [ ] BIOPSY (SPECIFY AREA BELOW)
- [ ] ASPIRATION (SPECIFY AREA BELOW)
- [ ] ABSCESS DRAINAGE
- [ ] INTRAOPERATIVE GUIDANCE

AREA:

Figure 1-1

FETAL AGE

DIAGNOSIS:

Findings compatible with complete spontaneous abortion, ectopic pregnancy, or very early intrauterine pregnancy.

COMMENT:

Real-time ultrasound of the pelvis was performed using transabdominal and endovaginal technique. No previous studies are available for review. The patient has a positive urine pregnancy test by history.

The uterus measures 10.2 x 4.2 x 5.0 cm. No intrauterine gestational sac is identified on transabdominal or endovaginal scan.

The left ovary is enlarged, measuring 4.2 x 2.9 x 3.6 cm. A cystic structure measuring less than 1 cm is seen in the left ovary.

The right ovary measures 2.6 x 1.1 x 2.8 cm. There are no right adnexal masses.

There is no free fluid in the cul de sac.

In light of the history of positive urine pregnancy test, the differential diagnosis for the above findings includes complete spontaneous abortion, ectopic pregnancy, or, less likely, very early intrauterine pregnancy. Correlation with serial beta-HCGs is advised.

Survey views of both kidneys reveal no hydronephrosis.

Figure 1-2

4. Routine Inpatient Chart Review. Briefly review the inpatient charts in Figure 1-1 and circle the diagnostic examinations. Compare and contrast inpatient chart items with items in the obstetrics, baby, rehabilitation, and psychiatry charts. What are the major similarities and differences?

IV. SYNTHESIS: DESCRIBING ABNORMAL FINDINGS EXERCISE

Review the three examples of describing abnormal findings given in your textbook. What differences do you observe between the sonographer's technical observation and the sonologist's diagnosis in Figure 1-2?

V. CHAPTER SUBHEADINGS EXERCISE

Directions to Students:
1. Convert each chapter subheading into a question; for example, change "Before the Ultrasound Examination: Understanding Standard Precautions" to, "What are Standard Precautions?" Briefly write an answer to each question in a short paragraph in your notebook.

2. Exchange answers with your lab partner and check each other's work. Refer back to the textbook for further information and explanation.

3. What questions about the chapter do you still have? Write your questions in your notebook.

VI. CHAPTER EVALUATION EXERCISE

Directions to Students: Use a fresh sheet of notebook paper. Based on your work with the chapter and its accompanying laboratory assignments, identify three concepts you believe are the most important. You may draw from any of the assignments you have already completed in the previous pages, including learning objectives, anatomy and physiology, images, or chapter subheadings. Include a detailed rationale in your answers.

Answer the questions below. Refer to page 381 for the answers.

1. List the three most important items from a patient's chart that sonographers need to review before performing an ultrasound exam.

2. Define what a sonographer can document within the parameters of a "technical observation."

3. Define what a sonographer can document within the parameters of a "technical observation" when there are abnormal findings on an exam.

4. The final interpretation of an ultrasound examination will always be the responsibility of a(n) _____.

Completion

For the following questions, assign *CH* for clinical history, *TO* for technical observation, or *IR* for interpretive report.

5. Heterogeneous liver texture ____

6. Vomiting × 3 days ____

7. Right upper quadrant pain ____

8. Hepatomegaly ____

9. 4-cm aortic aneurysm ____

10. Portal hypertension ___

2 Ultrasound Instrumentation: "Knobology," Imaging Processing, and Storage

I. MEMORIZATION EXERCISE

Directions to Students: Write the key words in your notebook or on note cards. Write the words on one side of the notepaper and then write the definitions on the opposite side of the page or on the back of the paper. If using note cards, write the key word on the front and the definition on the back. *This step should be completed before the lab session begins.*

Memorize the key word definitions silently for 5 minutes, then work with a lab partner and identify the words you still need help with. List the words here. Add additional rows if needed.

II. COMPREHENSION EXERCISE

Directions to Students: Work with a lab partner to complete this exercise. You will need to write in your notebook. First, change each objective into a question.

> *Example: "Explain why it is important to learn the 'knobology' of the ultrasound system" becomes "Why is it important to learn the 'knobology' of the ultrasound system?"*

Next, write a short answer to the question just created.

> *Example: "The sonographer has to know how each control affects the image, and how to work with all the controls to create the best image possible for the sonologist to use to render a diagnosis."*

Highlight or circle any part of your answers about which you are unsure, and check the answers in your textbook. If you are still unsure of the answers, put a question mark next to the answer(s) for the review session of the lab.

III. APPLICATION EXERCISE

Directions to Students:
1. Your instructor will distribute a section from an ultrasound systems manual for you and your partner to review.

2. Can you identify the primary imaging controls, measurement controls, and additional controls presented in Chapter 2?

3. From memory, draw the control panel illustrated in question 1 above. Label the controls. Ask your partner to check your work and suggest additional controls that should be included.

IV. IMAGE ANALYSIS EXERCISE

Directions to Students: Work on the following images with your lab partner. For each sonographic image, write an explanation in your notebook of the control settings used to render the image. How could the settings be improved? Refer to Chapter 2 in your textbook for guidance.

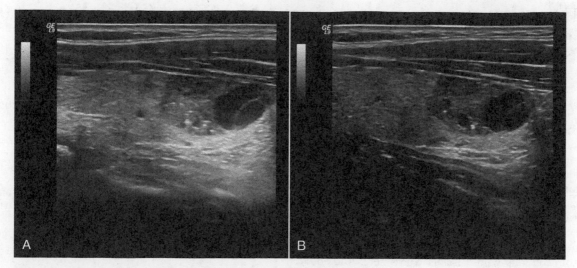

Figure 2-4A and B in the textbook

_____   _____

_____   _____

_____   _____

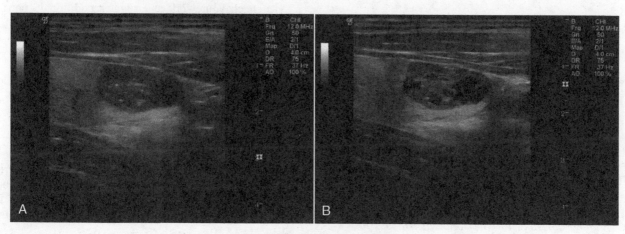

Figure 2-5A and B in the textbook

_____   _____

_____   _____

_____   _____

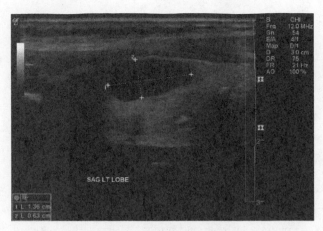

Figure 2-6 in the textbook

_____

_____

_____

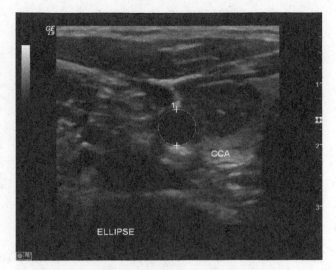

Figure 2-7 in the textbook

_____

_____

_____

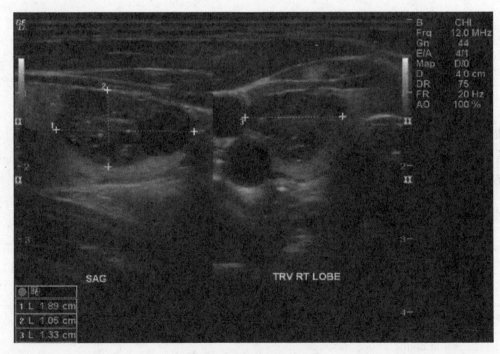

Figure 2-8 in the textbook

_____   _____

_____   _____

_____   _____

V. CHAPTER SUBHEADINGS EXERCISE

Directions to Students:

1. Convert each chapter subheading into a question. Briefly write the answer to each question in a short paragraph in your notebook.

2. Exchange answers with your lab partner and check each other's work. Refer back to the textbook for further information and explanation.

3. What questions do you still have about the chapter? Write your questions in your notebook.

VI. CHAPTER EVALUATION EXERCISE

Directions to Students: Use a fresh sheet of notebook paper. Based on your work with the chapter and its accompanying laboratory assignments, identify three concepts you believe are the most important. You may draw from any of the assignments you've already completed in the previous pages, including learning objectives, anatomy and physiology, images, or chapter subheadings. Include a detailed rationale in your answers.

Answer the questions below. Refer to page 381 for the answers.

Multiple Choice

1. The clinical applications specialist serves all the following roles except:
   a. Customizes imaging settings
   b. Demonstrates the proper use of the ultrasound system
   c. Performs the initial configuration during installation of the ultrasound system
   d. Customizes imaging measurements

2. If you want to erase all user-entered text from where the cursor is located, you would use:
   a. Annotation On/Off
   b. Backspace
   c. Erase/Clear/Clear Screen
   d. Comments On/Off

3. Which of the following increases the amplification in the far field of the image?
   a. Moving the bottom TGC pods to the right
   b. Moving the bottom TGC pods to the left
   c. Moving the top TGC pods to the right
   d. Moving the top TGC pods to the left

4. What primary imaging control or function would you use when imaging a crying infant, which resulted in a blurred, frozen image of his kidney?
   a. Depth
   b. Time-gain compensation
   c. Focal number
   d. Cine loop

5. You place the transducer on the patient's abdomen to begin your scan and notice the image is backward. You check to make sure you have your transducer oriented correctly. What primary imaging control or function would you use to correct this issue?
   a. Image direction
   b. Freeze key
   c. Track ball
   d. Dual image

6. When imaging the left and right testicles for comparison of echotexture and color flow at the same time, what primary imaging control or function would you use?
   a. Cine loop
   b. Dual image
   c. Freeze key
   d. Image direction

7. Which of the following measurement keys would you use to obtain the circumference of a fetal head?
   a. Distance
   b. Measure
   c. Off
   d. Trace/Ellipse

8. While scanning a patient's liver you notice a mass in the anterior portion of the right lobe about 3 cm below the skin. To accurately assess this mass, the focal zone should be placed:
   a. Above the level of the mass
   b. At the level of the mass
   c. At the deepest part of the liver
   d. Any level is fine but zoom the image

9. Which of the following functions does the trackball perform while scanning with the color Doppler application active?
   a. Guides cursor on the screen
   b. Positions measurement cursors
   c. Changes the scan area for the color box size
   d. Trackball has no function in color Doppler application

10. After ensuring the correct preset and placing the transducer on the patient you should:
    a. Adjust the TGC until the desire imaged is obtained
    b. Adjust the focal zones to cover the area of interest
    c. Adjust the number of focal zones
    d. Adjust the image size using the depth control

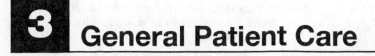

3 General Patient Care

I. MEMORIZATION EXERCISE

Directions to Students: Write the key words in your notebook or on note cards. Write the words on one side of the notepaper and then write the definitions on the opposite side of the page or on the back of the paper. If using note cards, write the key word on the front and the definition on the back. *This step should be completed before the lab session begins.*

Memorize the key word definitions silently for 5 minutes, then work with a lab partner and identify the words you still need help with. List the words here. Add additional rows if needed.

II. COMPREHENSION EXERCISE

Directions to Students: Work with a lab partner to complete this exercise. You will need to write in your notebook. First, change each objective into a question.

> *Example: "Describe the sonographer's responsibilities regarding patient care" becomes "What are the sonographer's responsibilities regarding patient care?"*

Next, write a short answer to the question just created.

> *Example: "The sonographer should be aware of the institution's Standard Precautions and isolation policies and 'Code' procedures for incidences of heart failure. He or she should also check patient identification, assist patients who need help changing or positioning themselves, and instruct the patient in a slow, clear, and concise manner."*

Highlight or circle any part of your answers about which you are unsure, and check the answers in your textbook. If you are still unsure of the answers, put a question mark next to the answer(s) for the review session of the lab.

III. APPLICATION EXERCISE

Directions to Students:
1. Your instructor will provide mission statements from health care providers for you and your partner to review.

2. Can you identify the patient care elements of the statement? In your opinion, does it clearly convey patient care standards to patients? How can the statement be "measured"? What types of outcomes would help measure the statement's validity?

3. Check your answers with your lab partner. Is there anything else you can add?

IV. CHAPTER SUBHEADINGS EXERCISE

Directions to Students:
1. Convert each chapter subheading into a question; for example, change "Interpersonal Skills" to, "What are the interpersonal skills used by sonographers in general patient care?" Write a brief answer to each question in a short paragraph in your notebook.

2. Exchange answers with your lab partner and check each other's work. Refer back to the textbook for further information and explanation.

3. What questions do you still have about the chapter? Write your questions in your notebook.

VI. CHAPTER EVALUATION EXERCISE

Directions to Students: Use a fresh sheet of notebook paper. Based on your work with the chapter and its accompanying laboratory assignments, identify three concepts you believe are the most important. You may draw from any of the assignments you've already completed in the previous pages, including learning objectives, anatomy and physiology, images, or chapter subheadings. Include a detailed rationale in your answers.

Answer the questions below. Refer to page 381 for the answers.

Multiple Choice

1. Conversations with patients should be restricted to
   a. small talk.
   b. informal but respectful and professional topics.
   c. obtaining a medical history.
   d. discussing your opinion of the ultrasound findings.

2. When a sonographer asks a patient the details about his or her medical history, questions should
   a. be the type that require only a yes or no answer.
   b. be limited to the patient's knowledge and understanding of their lab test results.
   c. be open-ended to obtain more accurate and specific details.
   d. use proper medical terminology.

3. When asking a patient from the lobby to follow you to the ultrasound exam room, what would be the proper way to address him?
   a. Mr. James Smith
   b. Mr. Smith
   c. James
   d. Jim

4. Arrange the tasks in the correct order to safely assist a patient from a wheelchair to an exam table.
   1. Lock the wheelchair brakes
   2. Move the leg and footrests out of the way
   3. Have a handled step-stool available
   4. Lock the examination table brakes
      a. 1, 2, 4, 3
      b. 4, 1, 2, 3
      c. 1,3 2, 3, 4
      d. 4, 3, 1, 2

5. You are performing a pelvic ultrasound and are measuring an ovarian mass on the right side. The patient asks you, "What is that?" The appropriate response to the patient is:
   a. "I'm measuring your ovarian mass."
   b. "I am not allowed to tell you anything about what I see."
   c. "I'm looking at your right ovary and getting some measurements for the doctor."
   d. "I'm measuring your ovarian mass but don't worry, it is probably not cancer."

True/False

6. It is standard practice to obtain a brief medical history from patients before an ultrasound examination.

7. Patients readily admit when they do not comprehend a question.

8. During an ultrasound examination, the well-being of the patient is the physician's responsibility.

9. It is the responsibility of the hospital or outpatient office nurses to obtain a brief medical history from the patient and present that information before an ultrasound examination.

10. A sonographer should never insist that patients discuss details about themselves if they are uncomfortable or appear anxious.

4 Introduction to Ergonomics and Sonographer Safety

I. MEMORIZATION EXERCISE

Directions to Students: Write the key words in your notebook or on note cards. Write the words on one side of the notepaper and then write the definitions on the opposite side of the page or on the back of the paper. If using note cards, write the key word on the front and the definition on the back. *This step should be completed before the lab session begins.*

Memorize the key word definitions silently for 5 minutes, then work with a lab partner and identify the words you still need help with. List the words here. Add additional rows if needed.

II. COMPREHENSION EXERCISE

Directions to Students: Work with a lab partner to complete this exercise. You will need to write in your notebook. First, change each objective into a question.

> *Example: "List the types of patient injuries most likely to occur while scanning."*

Next, write a short answer to the question just created.

> *Example: "The types of injuries that can occur while scanning include bursitis, carpal tunnel syndrome, De Quervain's disease, tendon inflammation, plantar fasciitis, rotator cuff injury, and spinal degeneration."*

Highlight or circle any part of your answers about which you are unsure, and check the answers in your textbook. If you are still unsure of the answers, put a question mark next to the answer(s) for the review session of the lab.

III. APPLICATION EXERCISE

Directions to Students:
1. For each workplace activity or condition listed below, discuss proactive approaches to reduce work-related musculoskeletal disorders and musculoskeletal injuries:
   * Workspace design
   * Infrequent breaks or rest periods
   * Incentives for overtime and being on-call
   * Delayed injury reporting
   * Improper cable management
   * Improper sitting height of chair
   * Monitor too low, causing flexion of the neck
   * "Pinch grip" of the transducer
   * Air quality factors such as heat, cold, humidity
   * Poor posture
   * Increase in the number of portable exams
   * Sustained shoulder abduction
   * Aging workforce
   * Staffing shortages
   * Higher workloads due to advancement in technology

2. What are the most important strategies sonographers can use to reduce injuries? Provide a rationale for your answers.

IV. CHAPTER SUBHEADINGS EXERCISE

Directions to Students:
1. Convert each chapter subheading into a question; for example, change "Work-Related Musculoskeletal Disorders" to, "What are the work-related musculoskeletal disorders?" Write a brief answer to each question in a short paragraph in your notebook.

2. Exchange answers with your lab partner and check each other's work. Refer back to the textbook for further information and explanation.

3. What questions do you still have about the chapter? Write your questions in your notebook.

V. CHAPTER EVALUATION EXERCISE

Directions to Students: Use a fresh sheet of notebook paper. Based on your work with the chapter and its accompanying laboratory assignments, identify three concepts you believe are the most important. You may draw from any of the assignments you've already completed in the previous pages, including learning objectives, anatomy and physiology, images, or chapter subheadings. Include a detailed rationale in your answers.

Answer the questions below. Refer to page 381 for the answers.

Multiple Choice

1. Work-related musculoskeletal disorders (WRMSDs) are defined as injuries that involve musculoskeletal symptoms that remain for
   a. 1 month or longer.
   b. 7 weeks or longer.
   c. 2 weeks or longer.
   d. 7 days or longer.

2. Repeated gripping of the transducer during scanning is associated mostly with
   a. thoracic outlet syndrome.
   b. cubital tunnel syndrome.
   c. carpal tunnel syndrome.
   d. De Quervain's disease.

3. Carpal tunnel syndrome is caused by:
   a. Inflammation of the bursa
   b. Entrapment of the median nerve
   c. Muscle weakness
   d. Intervertebral disc degeneration

4. As a sonographer, you can reduce your exposure for injury by
   a. avoiding awkward positions.
   b. using support cushions for your arms.
   c. taking mini-breaks during the procedure.
   d. maintaining good physical fitness.
   e. All of the above.

5. WRMSDs are
   a. injuries with a sudden onset.
   b. injuries that result in restricted work.
   c. the result of short-term exposure to risk factors.
   d. usually mild.

6. Which of the following regarding stress is NOT true?
   a. Stress has physical symptoms such as fatigue, headaches, and insomnia.
   b. Stress can lead to illness and injury.
   c. Stress relief requires complex strategies that are not easy to implement in the workplace.
   d. A symptom of stress is low self-esteem.

True/False

7. More than 80% of the sonographers in the workforce scan while they are in pain.

8. One of the most frequent causes of a WRMSD is awkward scanning postures such as bending or twisting.

9. Sonographers should be aware of body positions while scanning and avoid lengthy static postures.

10. Most sonographer injuries involve the lower back.

5 Interdependent Body Systems

I. MEMORIZATION EXERCISE

Directions to Students: Write the key words in your notebook or on note cards. Write the words on one side of the notepaper and then write the definitions on the opposite side of the page or on the back of the paper. If using note cards, write the key word on the front and the definition on the back. *This step should be completed before the lab session begins.*

Memorize the key word definitions silently for 5 minutes, then work with a lab partner and identify the words you still need help with. List the words here. Add additional rows if needed.

II. COMPREHENSION EXERCISE

Directions to Students: Work with a lab partner to complete this exercise. You will need to write in your notebook. Select one of the body systems discussed in the chapter and describe its function(s).

Highlight or circle any part of your answers about which you are unsure, and check the answers in your textbook. If you are still unsure of the answers, put a question mark next to the answer(s) for the review session of the lab.

III. ANATOMY APPLICATION EXERCISE

Directions to Students: Work on the following with your lab partner.

1. After reviewing the illustrations of these systems in your textbook, draw the major components of the endocrine, circulatory, musculoskeletal, reproductive, urinary, digestive, and respiratory systems. (Do this with the textbook closed.) How many structures were you able to include in your drawing? Review your diagrams with your partner. What did you miss?

2. Check your drawing using the sketches in your textbook and complete any structures missing from your drawing.

3. Below your drawing, write two or three summary sentences for each system. Ask your lab partner to check your work. Now check your work against the explanations in the textbook. What else can you add to your description?

IV. CHAPTER SUBHEADINGS EXERCISE

Directions to Students:

1. Convert each chapter subheading into a question; for example, change "Digestive System" to "What is the digestive system and how does it relate to other body systems?" Write a brief answer to each question in a short paragraph in your notebook.

2. Exchange answers with your lab partner and check each other's work. Refer back to the textbook for further information and explanation.

3. What questions do you still have about the chapter? Write your questions in your notebook.

V. CHAPTER EVALUATION EXERCISE

Directions to Students: Use a fresh sheet of notebook paper. Based on your work with the chapter and its accompanying laboratory assignments, identify three concepts you believe are the most important. You may draw from any of the assignments you've already completed in the previous pages, including learning objectives, anatomy and physiology, images, or chapter subheadings. Include a detailed rationale in your answers.

Answer the questions below. Refer to page 381 for the answers.

Multiple Choice

1. The _____ is the muscular partition between the thoracic and abdominal cavities.
   a. visceral pleural
   b. parietal peritoneum
   c. diaphragm
   d. visceral peritoneum

2. The _____ regulates blood volume and composition by filtering waste from the blood that passes through the _____.
   a. endocrine system; kidneys
   b. urinary system; kidneys
   c. respiratory system; lungs
   d. spleen; portal vein

3. _____ is defined as the chemical reactions that occur in the body to maintain life.
   a. Metabolism
   b. Homogeneous
   c. Hematopoiesis
   d. Histogenesis

4. The _____ secretes hormones directly into the bloodstream to regulate reproduction, growth and development, metabolism, blood glucose concentrations, stress response, and ovulation.
   a. thyroid
   b. reproductive system
   c. pineal gland
   d. endocrine system

5. All body systems are assisted by the _____ either directly or indirectly.
   a. endocrine system
   b. urinary system
   c. respiratory system
   d. digestive system

6. _____ is defined as the equilibrium of the body's normal physiologic condition.
   a. Metabolism
   b. Homogeneous
   c. Hematopoiesis
   d. Homeostasis

7. The _____ monitors and controls almost every organ in the body.
   a. thymus gland
   b. endocrine system
   c. pineal gland
   d. nervous system

True/False

8. Because of its location in the neck, the thyroid gland is considered part of the respiratory system.

9. The liver is an accessory organ to the excretory system.

10. The pancreas is an accessory organ to the digestive system.

Anatomy Layering and Sectional Anatomy

I. MEMORIZATION EXERCISE

Directions to Students: Write the key words in your notebook or on note cards. Write the words on one side of the notepaper and then write the definitions on the opposite side of the page or on the back of the paper. If using note cards, write the key word on the front and the definition on the back. *This step should be completed before the lab session begins.*

Memorize the key word definitions silently for 5 minutes and then work with a lab partner and identify the words you still need help with. List the words here. Add rows if needed.

II. COMPREHENSION EXERCISE

Directions to Students: Work with a lab partner to complete this exercise. You will need to write in your notebook. First, change each objective into a question.

> *Example: "Explain the importance of using two different scanning planes" becomes "Why is it important to use two different scanning planes?"*

Next, write a short answer to the question just created.

> *Example: "Multiple scanning planes are used in ultrasound imaging because single plane views do not provide enough confirmation to make definitive judgments."*

Highlight or circle any part of your answers about which you are unsure, and check the answers in your textbook. If you are still unsure of the answers, put a question mark next to the answer(s) for the review session of the lab.

III. ANATOMY APPLICATION EXERCISE

Directions to Students: Using clay or any other product that is easy to shape, re-create Figures 6-14 to 6-23 (in the textbook), the abdominal layers, and Figures 6-24 to 6-29 (in the textbook), the pelvic layers, building the anatomy in layers from posterior (back) to anterior (front). Label each structure, taping the label to toothpicks, before inserting into the structure. When the layers are complete, use a knife to cut out various axial and longitudinal sections; identify the anatomy in these cross-sections.

IV. STRUCTURAL ORIENTATION EXERCISE

Directions to Students: On the following page, identify each numbered structure in Figure 6-3 (in the textbook) and its orientation (or lie) within the body.

15

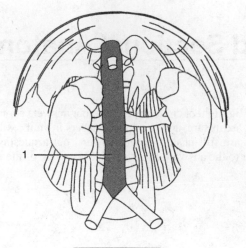

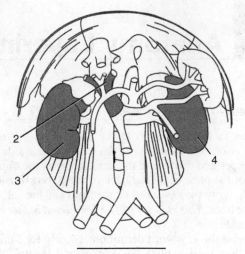

1 _____

1 _____   3 _____
2 _____   4 _____

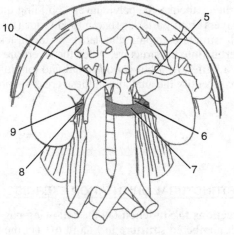

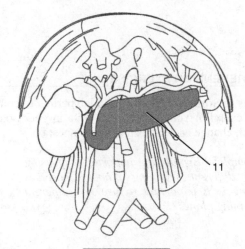

_____

(the lateral end of the pancreas is slightly more
superior than the medial end)

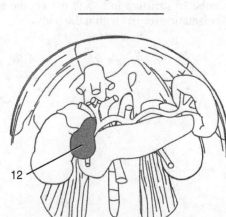

_____

5 _____
6 _____
7 _____
8 _____
9 _____
10 _____
11 _____
12 _____

Figure 6-3 in the textbook

V. BODY STRUCTURE RELATIONSHIPS EXERCISE

Directions to Students: Use directional terms—anterior, posterior, superior, inferior, and medial, right or left lateral—as they apply to describe the location of adjacent structures to a designated area of interest.

1. Transabdominal sagittal scanning plane image taken just to the left of the midline of the body. The pancreas body is the area of interest. Identify the directional relationship of the adjacent anatomy.

Example: Liver: anterior.

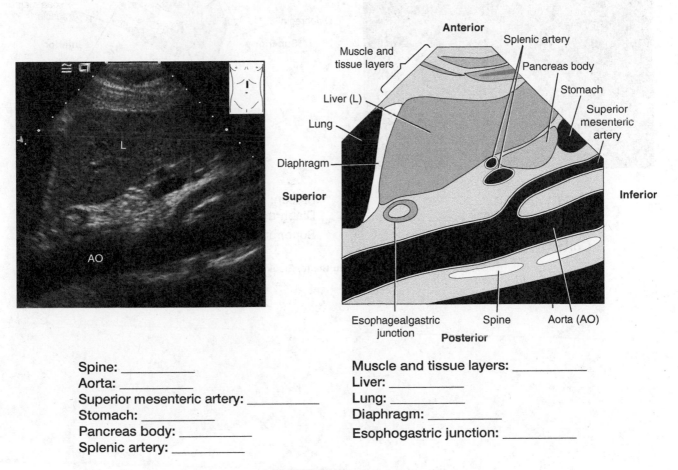

Spine: _____
Aorta: _____
Superior mesenteric artery: _____
Stomach: _____
Pancreas body: _____
Splenic artery: _____

Muscle and tissue layers: _____
Liver: _____
Lung: _____
Diaphragm: _____
Esophogastric junction: _____

Figure 6-5 in the textbook

2. Transabdominal coronal scanning plane image from a left lateral approach. The superior pole of the left kidney is the area of interest. Identify the directional relationship of the adjacent anatomy.

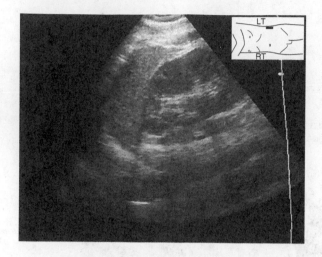

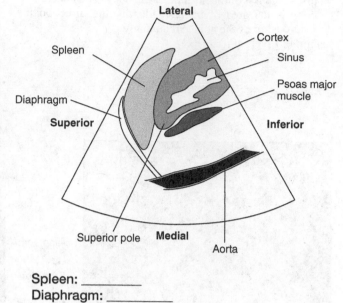

Aorta: _____
Psoas major muscle: _____
Sinus: _____
Cortex: _____

Spleen: _____
Diaphragm: _____
Superior pole: _____

Figure 6-6 in the textbook

3. Transabdominal transverse scanning plane image taken at the level of the midepigastrium. The pancreas neck is the area of interest. Identify the directional relationship of the adjacent anatomy.

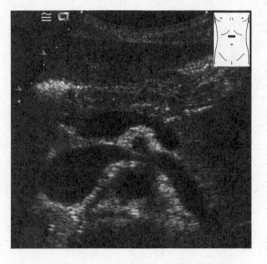

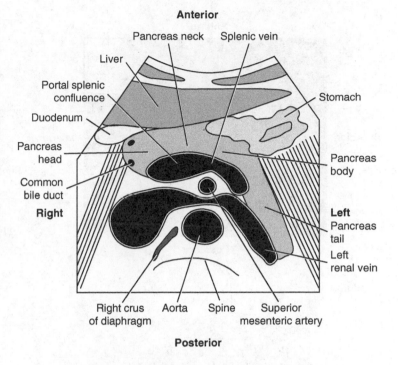

Aorta: _____
Spine: _____
Superior mesenteric artery: _____
Left renal vein: _____
Pancreas tail: _____
Pancreas body: _____
Stomach: _____
Splenic vein: _____

Pancreas neck: _____
Liver: _____
Portal splenic confluence: _____
Duodenum: _____
Pancreas head: _____
Common bile duct: _____
Right crus of diaphragm: _____

Figure 6-7 in the textbook

VI. COMPARING ULTRASOUND IMAGE SECTIONS WITH CORRESPONDING GROSS ANATOMY LAYERS EXERCISE

Directions to Students:
Identify the labeled anatomy in the image on the corresponding gross anatomy layers.

1. Transabdominal sagittal scanning plane image taken just to the right of the midline of the body (represented by the solid line on the layering illustrations).

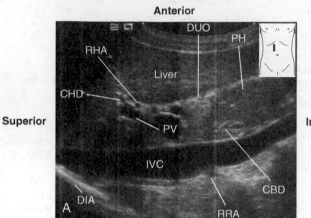

A

Figure 6-8A in the textbook DIA (diaphragm), RRA (right renal artery), IVC (inferior vena cava), PV (portal vein), CBD (common bile duct), PH (pancreas head), CHD (common hepatic duct), RHA (right hepatic artery), DUO (duodenum)

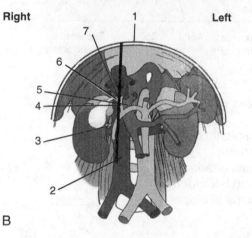

B

Figure 6-8B in the textbook

1 _____

2 _____

3 _____

4 _____

5 _____

6 _____

7 _____

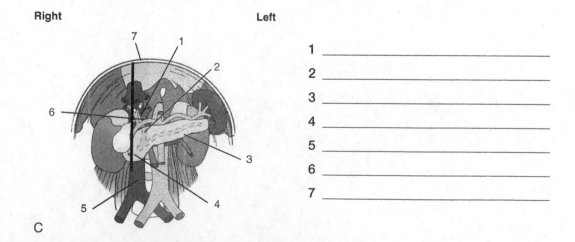

C

Figure 6-8C in the textbook

1 _____

2 _____

3 _____

4 _____

5 _____

6 _____

7 _____

2. Transabdominal transverse scanning plane image of the mid to lower epigastrium (represented by the dotted line on the layering illustrations).

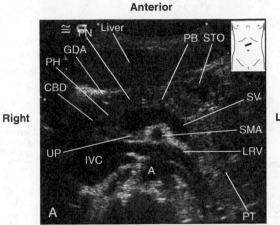

Figure 6-9A in the textbook A (aorta), IVC (inferior vena cava), LRV (left renal vein), SMA (superior mesenteric artery), UP (uncinate process of the pancreas), PT (pancreas tail), SV (splenic vein), SMA (superior mesenteric artery), PH (pancreas head), CBD (common bile duct), PN (pancreas neck), GDA (gastroduodenal artery), PB (pancreas body), STO (stomach)

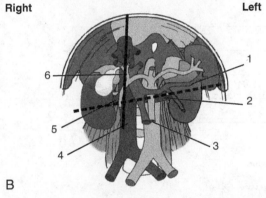

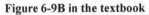

1 _____

2 _____

3 _____

4 _____

5 _____

6 _____

Figure 6-9B in the textbook

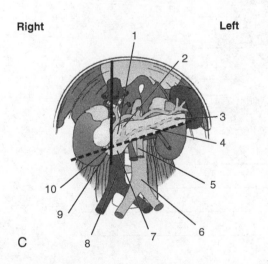

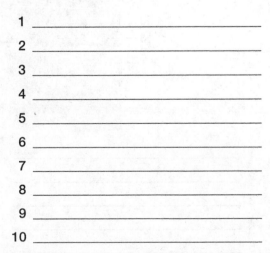

1 _____

2 _____

3 _____

4 _____

5 _____

6 _____

7 _____

8 _____

9 _____

10 _____

Figure 6-9C in the textbook

VII. COMPARING CADAVER SECTIONS WITH ULTRASOUND IMAGE SECTIONS EXERCISE

Directions to Students:
1. Identify the anatomy on the image and accompanying sketch and the corresponding cadaver section.

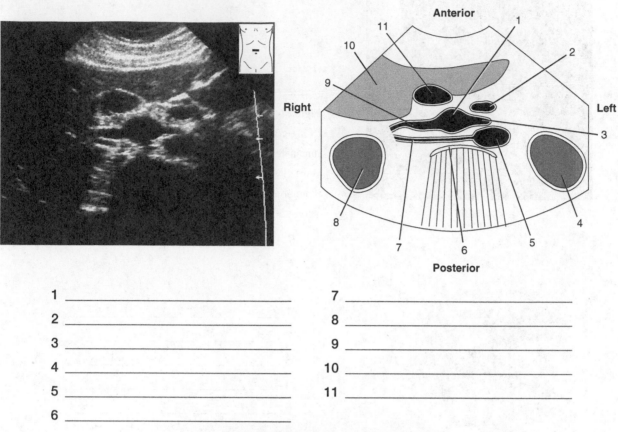

1 _____	7 _____
2 _____	8 _____
3 _____	9 _____
4 _____	10 _____
5 _____	11 _____
6 _____	

Figure 6-12, top, in the textbook

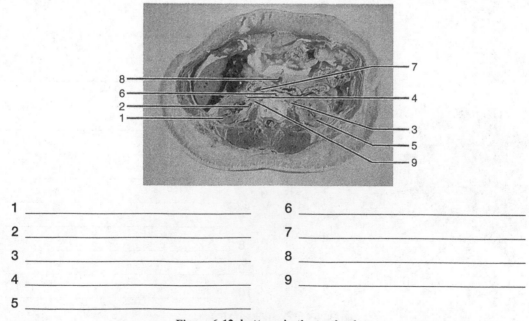

1 _____	6 _____
2 _____	7 _____
3 _____	8 _____
4 _____	9 _____
5 _____	

Figure 6-12, bottom, in the textbook

2. Identify the anatomy on the image and accompanying sketch and the corresponding cadaver section.

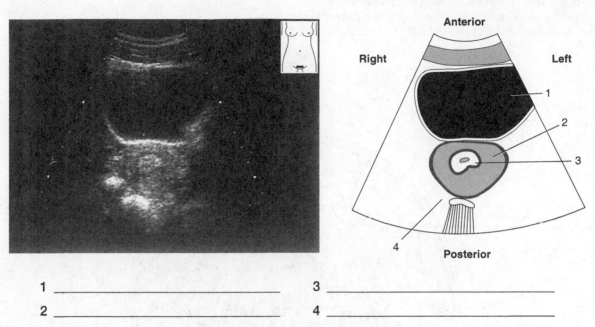

1 _____ 3 _____

2 _____ 4 _____

Figure 6-13, top, in the textbook

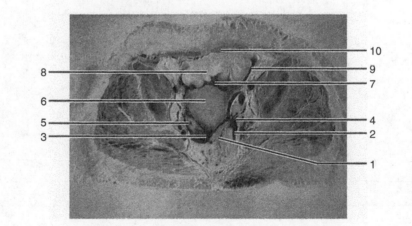

1 _____ 6 _____

2 _____ 7 _____

3 _____ 8 _____

4 _____ 9 _____

5 _____ 10 _____

Figure 6-13, bottom, in the textbook

VIII. ANATOMY SYNTHESIS EXERCISE: ANATOMY LAYERS AND ILLUSTRATIONS

Directions to Students: Work on the following with your lab partner. Label all abdominal sketches at once and then go back and work with each figure with your lab partner to check your answers. The goal is to label all of the sketches correctly.

1.

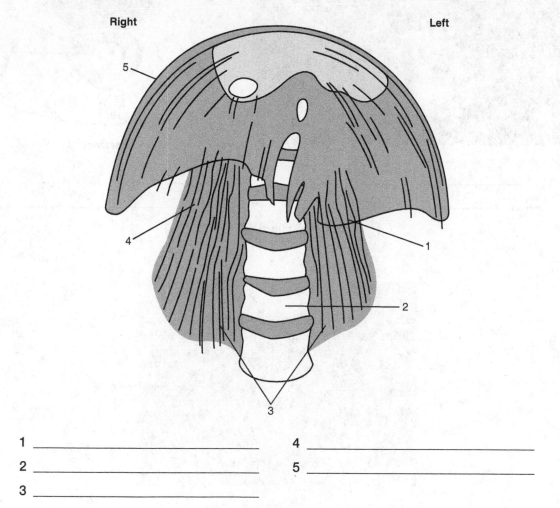

Right   Left

1 _____   4 _____

2 _____   5 _____

3 _____

Figure 6-14 in the textbook

2.

Right   Left

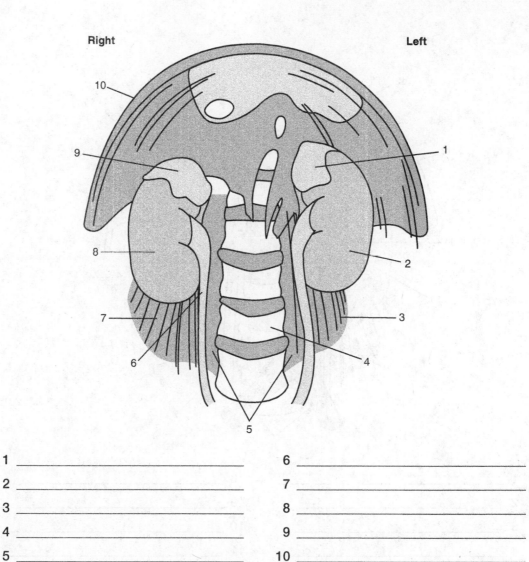

1 _____	6 _____
2 _____	7 _____
3 _____	8 _____
4 _____	9 _____
5 _____	10 _____

Figure 6-15 in the textbook

3.

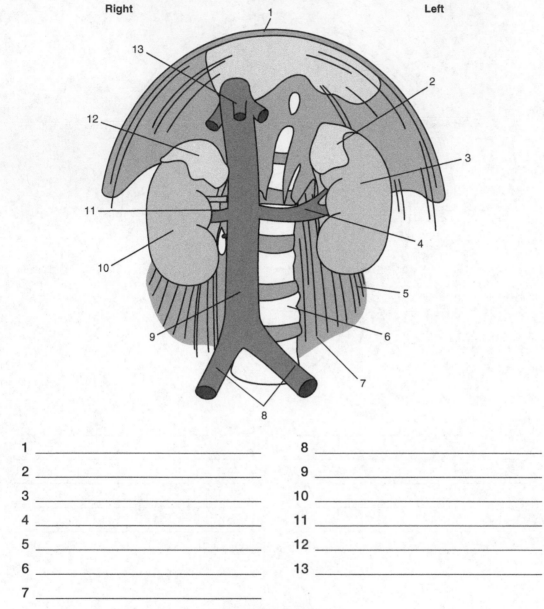

Right   Left

Figure 6-16 in the textbook

1 _____	8 _____
2 _____	9 _____
3 _____	10 _____
4 _____	11 _____
5 _____	12 _____
6 _____	13 _____
7 _____	

4.

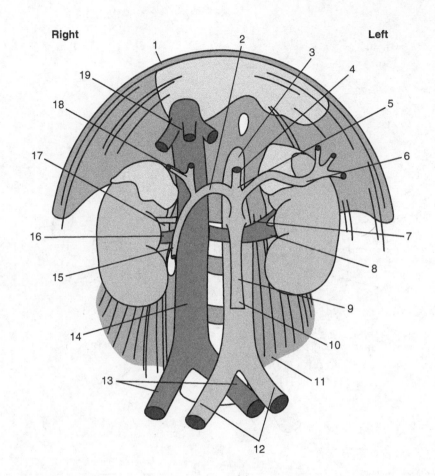

Right   Left

Figure 6-17 in the textbook

1 _____   11 _____
2 _____   12 _____
3 _____   13 _____
4 _____   14 _____
5 _____   15 _____
6 _____   16 _____
7 _____   17 _____
8 _____   18 _____
9 _____   19 _____
10 _____

5.

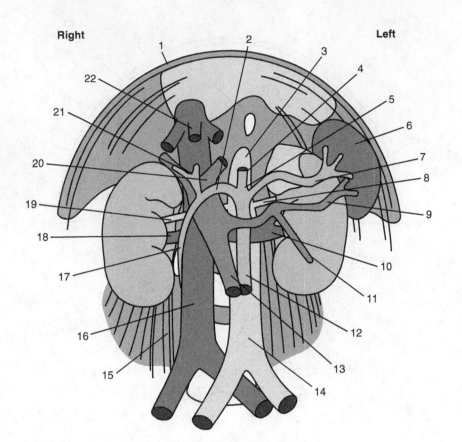

Right   Left

1	_____	12	_____
2	_____	13	_____
3	_____	14	_____
4	_____	15	_____
5	_____	16	_____
6	_____	17	_____
7	_____	18	_____
8	_____	19	_____
9	_____	20	_____
10	_____	21	_____
11	_____	22	_____

Figure 6-18 in the textbook

6.

Right   Left

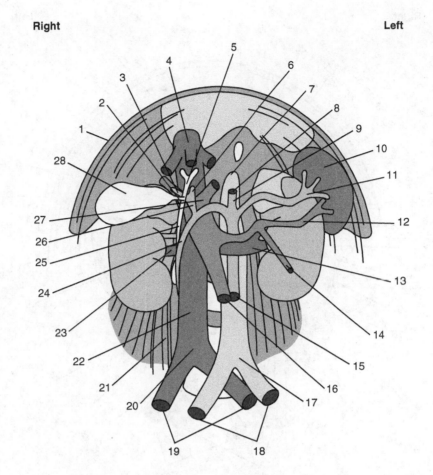

Figure 6-19 in the textbook

1 _____   15 _____
2 _____   16 _____
3 _____   17 _____
4 _____   18 _____
5 _____   19 _____
6 _____   20 _____
7 _____   21 _____
8 _____   22 _____
9 _____   23 _____
10 _____   24 _____
11 _____   25 _____
12 _____   26 _____
13 _____   27 _____
14 _____   28 _____

7.

Right   Left

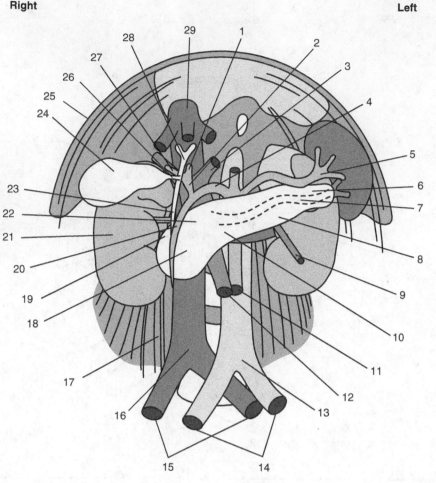

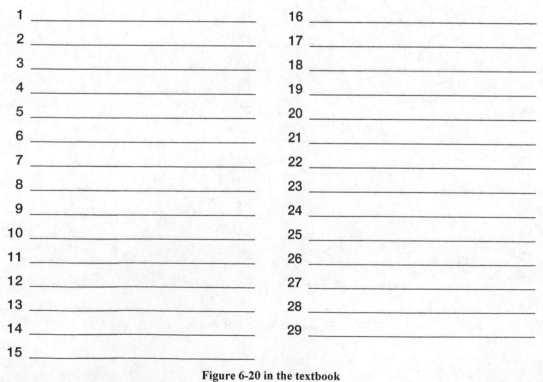

1	_____	16	_____
2	_____	17	_____
3	_____	18	_____
4	_____	19	_____
5	_____	20	_____
6	_____	21	_____
7	_____	22	_____
8	_____	23	_____
9	_____	24	_____
10	_____	25	_____
11	_____	26	_____
12	_____	27	_____
13	_____	28	_____
14	_____	29	_____
15	_____		

Figure 6-20 in the textbook

8.

Right   **Left**

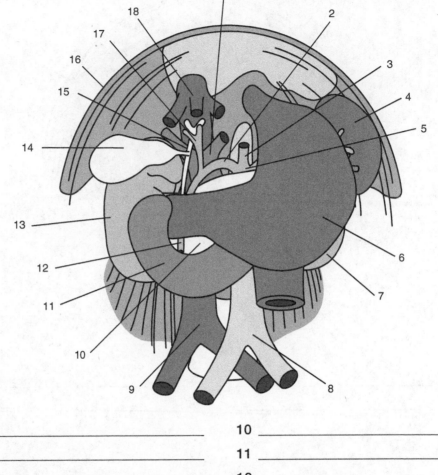

1	_____	10	_____
2	_____	11	_____
3	_____	12	_____
4	_____	13	_____
5	_____	14	_____
6	_____	15	_____
7	_____	16	_____
8	_____	17	_____
9	_____	18	_____

Figure 6-21 in the textbook

9.

Right   Left

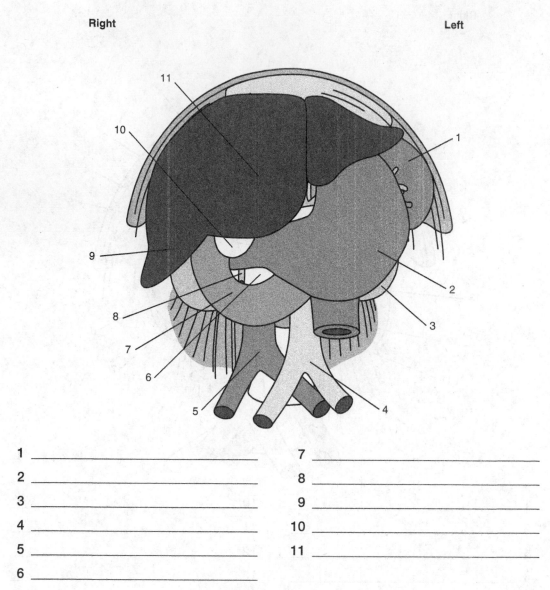

1	_____	7	_____
2	_____	8	_____
3	_____	9	_____
4	_____	10	_____
5	_____	11	_____
6	_____		

Figure 6-22 in the textbook

10.

Right   **Left**

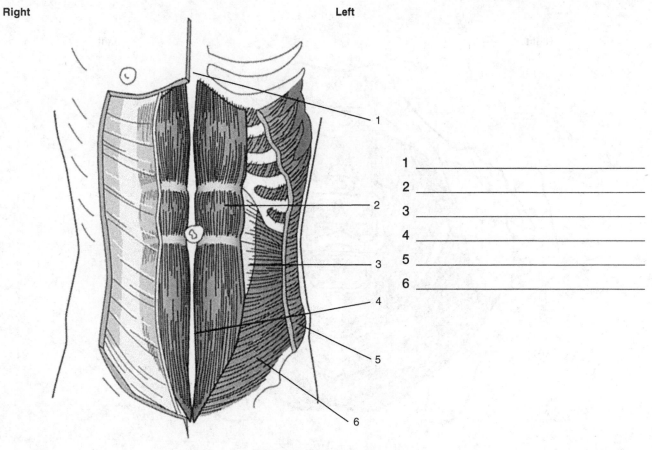

1 _____

2 _____

3 _____

4 _____

5 _____

6 _____

Figure 6-23 in the textbook

Do you have any questions about the abdominal anatomy? Write your questions and share them with your lab partner and instructor.

Label all of the pelvic images (1–6) at once and then
go back and work with each figure with your lab partner.
The goal is to label all of the sketches correctly.

1.

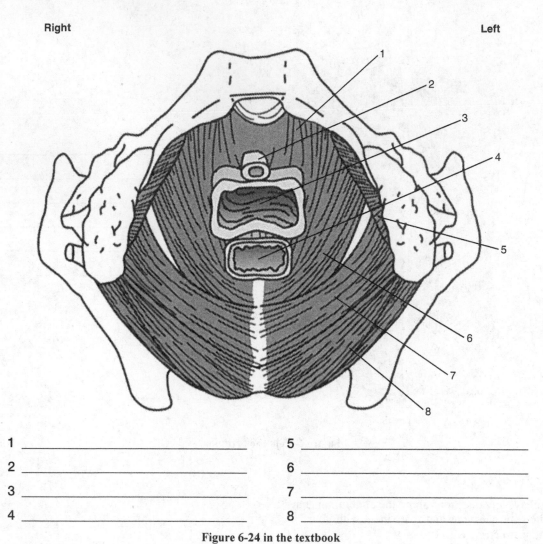

Right   **Left**

1 _____   5 _____

2 _____   6 _____

3 _____   7 _____

4 _____   8 _____

Figure 6-24 in the textbook

2.

Right   Left

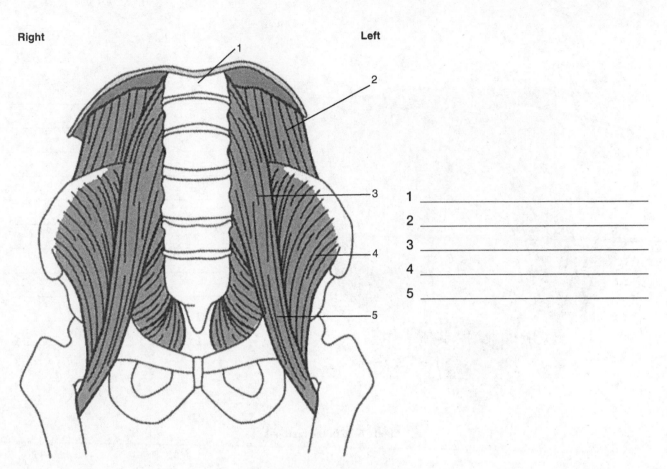

1 _____

2 _____

3 _____

4 _____

5 _____

Figure 6-25 in the textbook

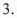

3.

Right   **Left**

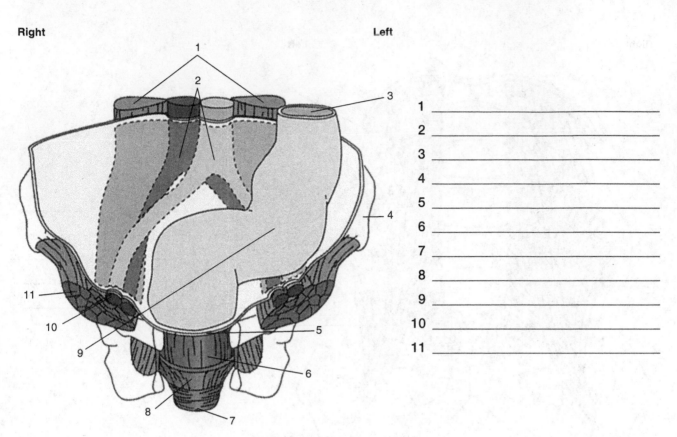

1 _____
2 _____
3 _____
4 _____
5 _____
6 _____
7 _____
8 _____
9 _____
10 _____
11 _____

Figure 6-26 in the textbook

4.

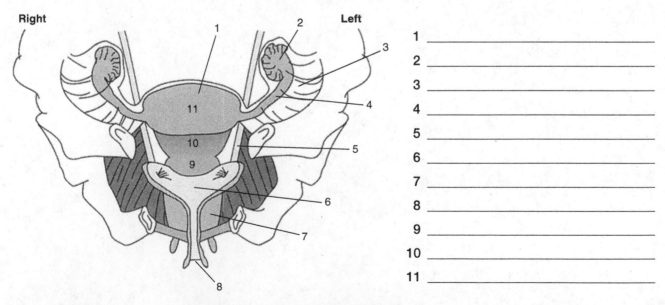

1 _____
2 _____
3 _____
4 _____
5 _____
6 _____
7 _____
8 _____
9 _____
10 _____
11 _____

Figure 6-27 in the textbook

5.

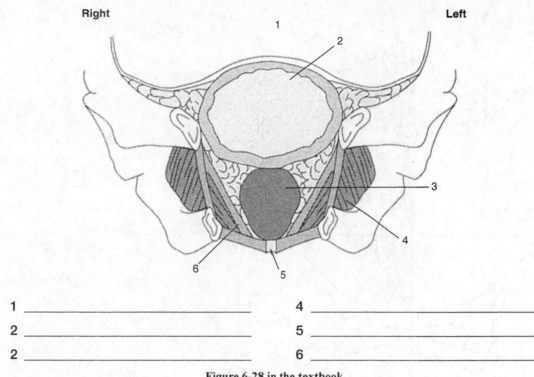

Right   **Left**

1	_____	4	_____
2	_____	5	_____
2	_____	6	_____

Figure 6-28 in the textbook

6.

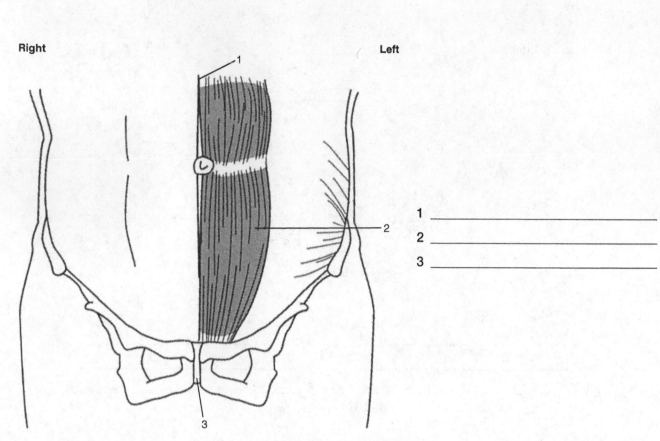

Right   **Left**

1 _____

2 _____

3 _____

Figure 6-29 in the textbook

IX. CHAPTER EVALUATION EXERCISE

Directions to Students: Use a fresh sheet of notebook paper. Based on your work with the chapter and its accompanying laboratory assignments, identify three concepts you believe are most important. You may draw from any of the assignments you have already completed in the previous pages, including learning objectives, anatomy and physiology, images, or chapter subheadings. Include a detailed rationale in your answers.

Answer to the questions below. Refer to page 381 for the answers.

True/False

1. The pancreas is a retroperitoneal organ.

2. The spleen is a retroperitoneal organ.

3. The gallbladder is a retroperitoneal organ.

4. The liver is a retroperitoneal organ.

5. The splenic vein is oriented horizontally in the body.

6. The long axis of the kidneys is in a vertical oblique orientation.

7. The inferior vena cava has a variable orientation.

8. The gallbladder has a variable orientation.

9. The pancreas has a horizontal oblique orientation.

10. The splenic artery might be tortuous but it is vertically oriented.

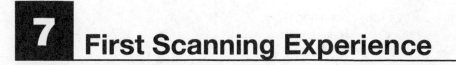

7 First Scanning Experience

I. MEMORIZATION EXERCISE

Directions to Students:

1. For each view shown in Figures 7-3A, B, and C from the textbook, identify on the pie shape the appropriate directional terms (e.g., posterior/anterior, superior/inferior, lateral/medial, right/left, right or left lateral) as indicated by numbers 1, 2, 3, and 4 on each wedge.

Saggital Scanning Plane
2 sound wave approaches are possible
Anterior or Posterior

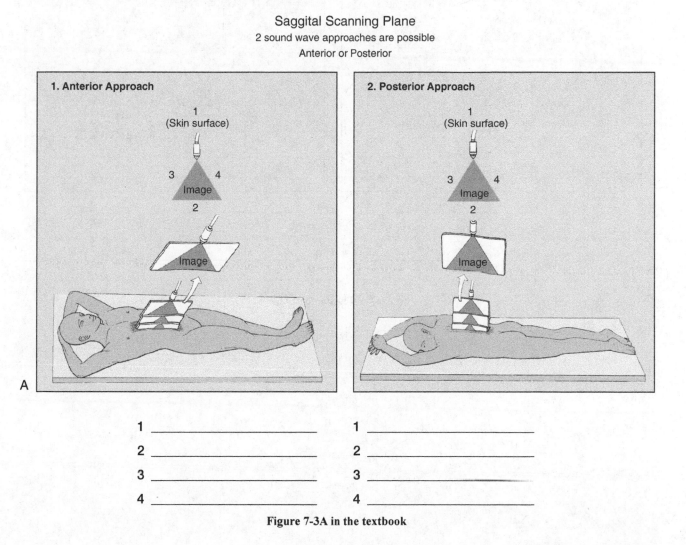

1 _____	1 _____
2 _____	2 _____
3 _____	3 _____
4 _____	4 _____

Figure 7-3A in the textbook

Coronal Scanning Plane

2 sound wave approaches are possible

Left lateral or Right lateral

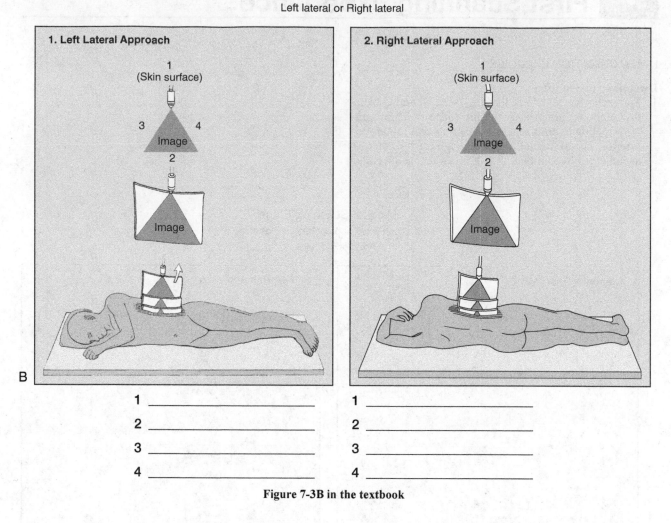

1. Left Lateral Approach	2. Right Lateral Approach
1 (Skin surface)	1 (Skin surface)
3 4	3 4
Image	Image
2	2
Image	Image

1 _____   1 _____

2 _____   2 _____

3 _____   3 _____

4 _____   4 _____

Figure 7-3B in the textbook

Transverse Scanning Plane
4 sound wave approaches are possible
Anterior, Posterior,
Left lateral, or Right lateral

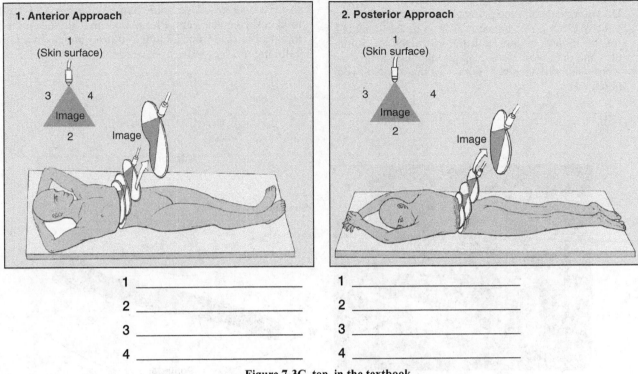

1. Anterior Approach

1
(Skin surface)

3   4

Image

2   Image

1 _____

2 _____

3 _____

4 _____

2. Posterior Approach

1
(Skin surface)

3   4

Image

2

Image

1 _____

2 _____

3 _____

4 _____

Figure 7-3C, top, in the textbook

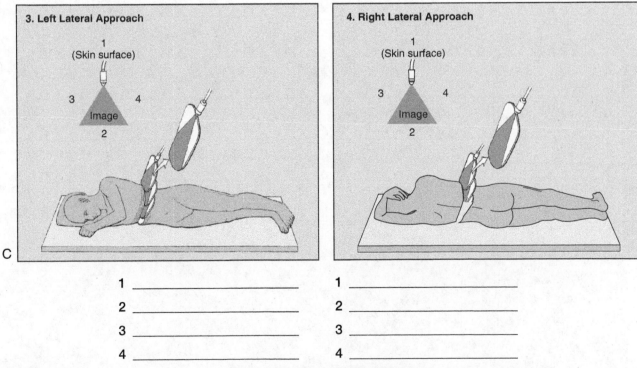

3. Left Lateral Approach

1
(Skin surface)

3   4

Image

2

C

1 _____

2 _____

3 _____

4 _____

4. Right Lateral Approach

1
(Skin surface)

3   4

Image

2

1 _____

2 _____

3 _____

4 _____

Figure 7-3C, bottom, in the textbook

41

2. Review the patient positions in your textbook and write them in your notebook. Take turns correctly identifying the patient positions as demonstrated by you and your lab partner. (You may need a floor mat and wear casual clothes to do this exercise.)

3. Do you understand the patient positions? If not, write your question(s) or concern(s) in your lab notebook for the review session with the instructor for 5 minutes and then work with a lab partner and identify the words you still need help with. List the words in your notebook.

II. COMPREHENSION EXERCISE

Directions to Students:
Longitudinal Images—Abdominal Aorta: Sagittal Plane/Transabdominal Anterior Approach. Identify the anatomy. Use your textbook (pages 105-109) to check your answers. Please note that the numbered images below do not include required images without calipers.

1.

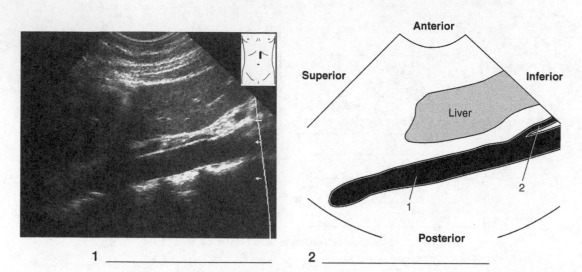

1 _____   2 _____

Page 105, top, in the textbook

2.

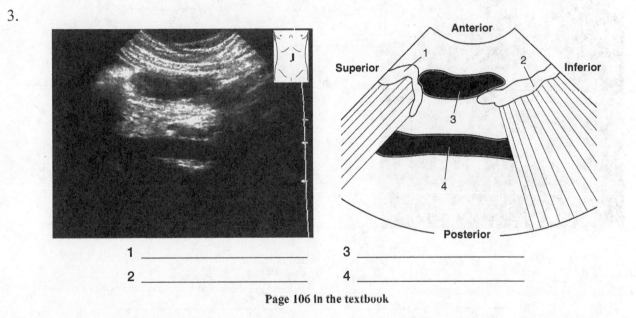

1 _____ 5 _____

2 _____ 6 _____

3 _____ 7 _____

4 _____

Page 105, bottom, in the textbook

3.

1 _____ 3 _____

2 _____ 4 _____

Page 106 in the textbook

Using the eraser end of your pencil to simulate the transducer, practice transducer placement on yourself for the longitudinal images. If your instructor has old transducers, you may use them for this exercise. Ask your partner to critique your placement. In the textbook, refer to figures on pages 98-101 and 103 in Chapter 7 in the textbook for additional guidance on transducer placement.

Note: It is advisable to wear comfortable, casual clothing while practicing this exercise, although coats and heavy outerwear will need to be removed.

4.

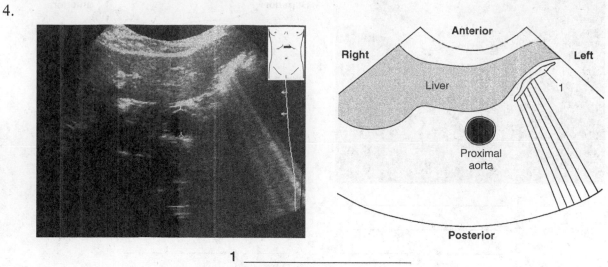

1 _____

Page 107 in the textbook

5.

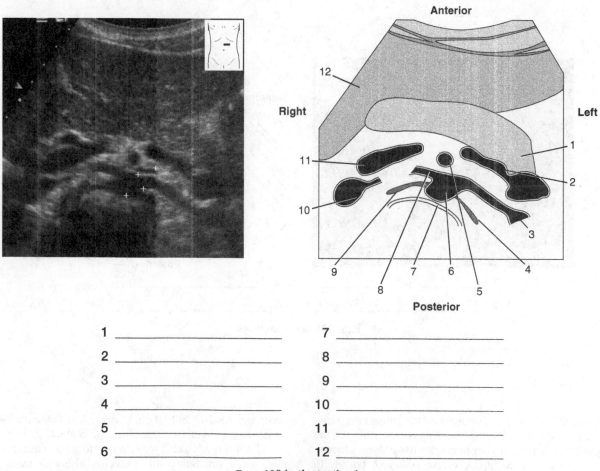

1 _____	7 _____
2 _____	8 _____
3 _____	9 _____
4 _____	10 _____
5 _____	11 _____
6 _____	12 _____

Page 108 in the textbook

6.

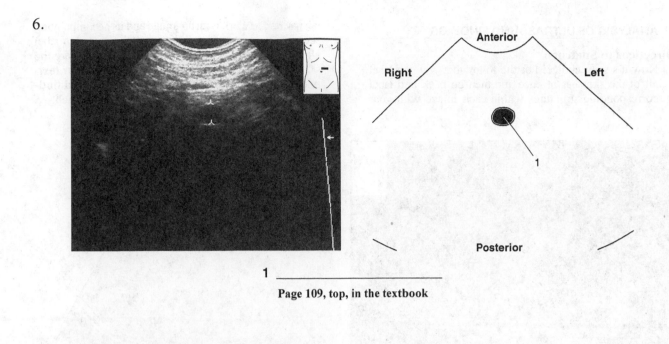

1 _____

Page 109, top, in the textbook

7.

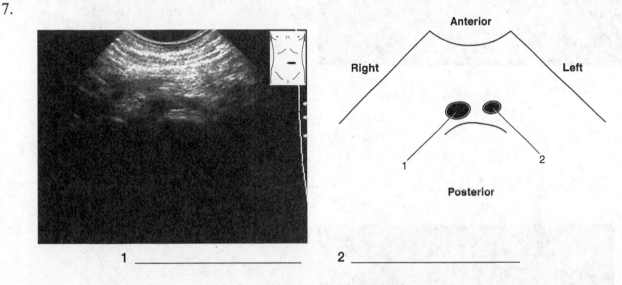

1 _____   2 _____

Page 109, bottom, in the textbook

Using the eraser end of your pencil to simulate the transducer, practice transducer placement on yourself for the transverse images. (remember to rotate the transducer to simulate changing from longitudinal to transverse planes). You can also use old transducers if available. Ask your partner to critique your placement.

In the textbook, refer to figures on pages 93-101 and 103 in Chapter 7 in the textbook for additional guidance on transducer placement. Note: It is advisable to wear comfortable, casual clothing while practicing this exercise, although coats and heavy outerwear will need to be removed.

Chapter **7   First Scanning Experience**

III. ANALYSIS OF ULTRASOUND FINDINGS

Directions to Students:

1. Now it's your choice! For the following, you can label all of the sketches at once and then go back and label corresponding structures within each image with your lab partner, or work with an image and its accompanying sketch at the same time. Either way, the goal is to label all of the sketches correctly and carefully compare the sketch with the sonographic image. **Also, use your textbook and write a description of the ultrasound findings below each image and accompanying sketch.**

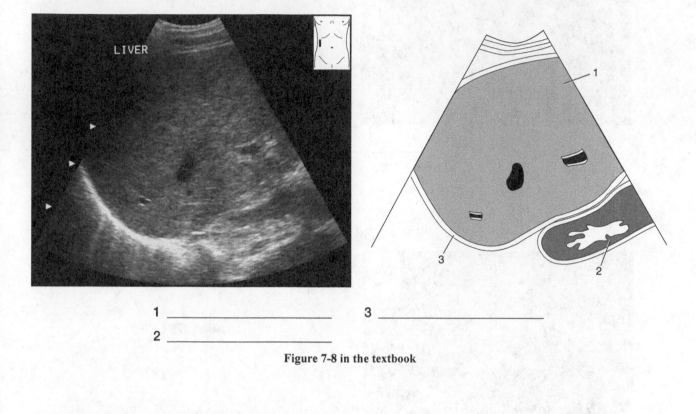

1 _____ 3 _____

2 _____

Figure 7-8 in the textbook

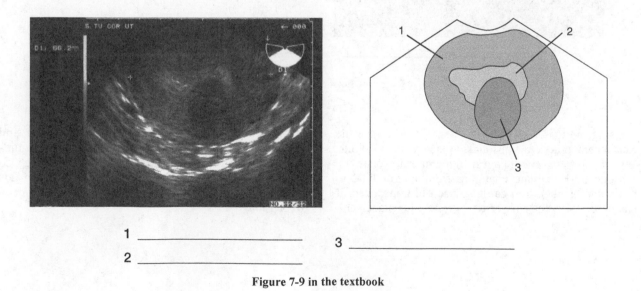

1 _____ 3 _____

2 _____

Figure 7-9 in the textbook

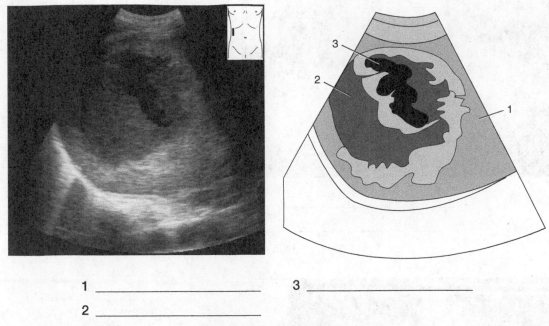

1 _____ 3 _____
2 _____

Figure 7-10 in the textbook

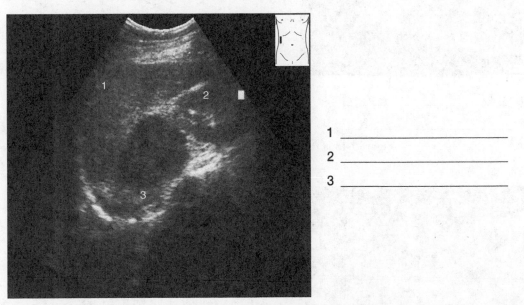

1 _____
2 _____
3 _____

Figure 7-11 in the textbook

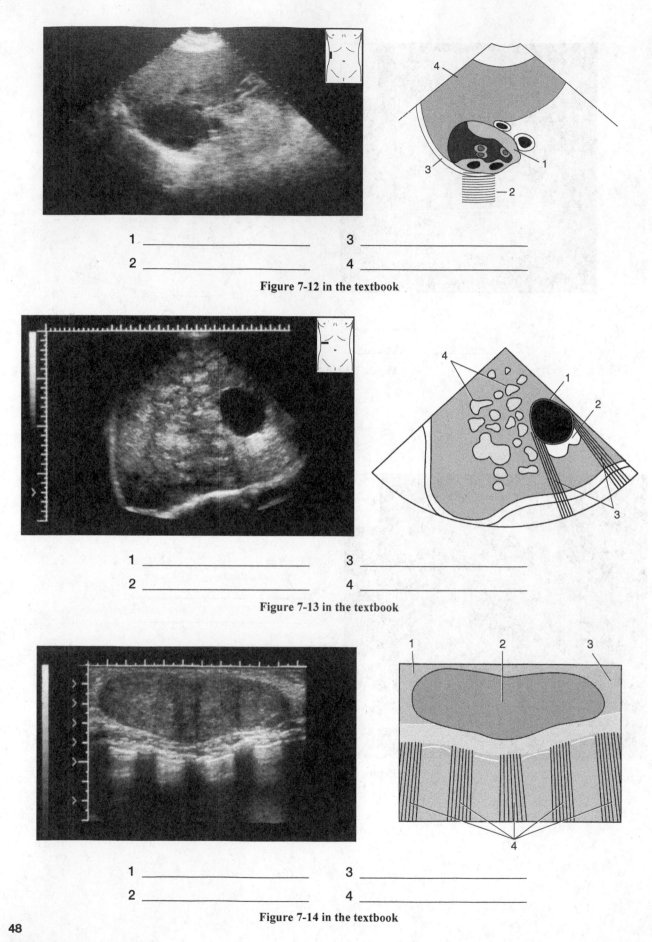

Figure 7-12 in the textbook

1 _____   3 _____
2 _____   4 _____

Figure 7-13 in the textbook

1 _____   3 _____
2 _____   4 _____

Figure 7-14 in the textbook

1 _____   3 _____
2 _____   4 _____

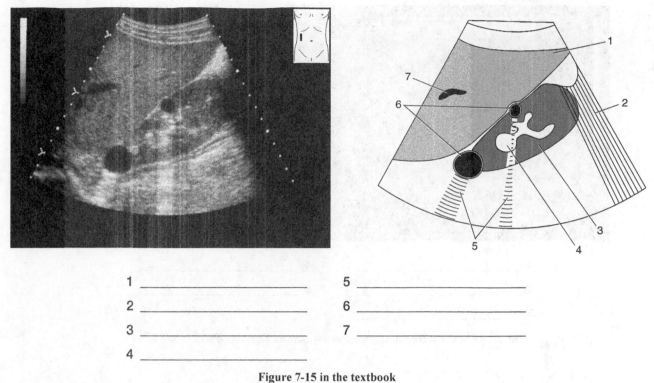

1 _____	5 _____
2 _____	6 _____
3 _____	7 _____
4 _____	

Figure 7-15 in the textbook

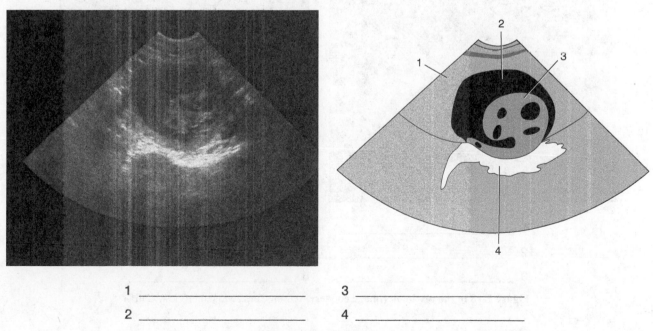

| 1 _____ | 3 _____ |
| 2 _____ | 4 _____ |

Figure 7-16 in the textbook

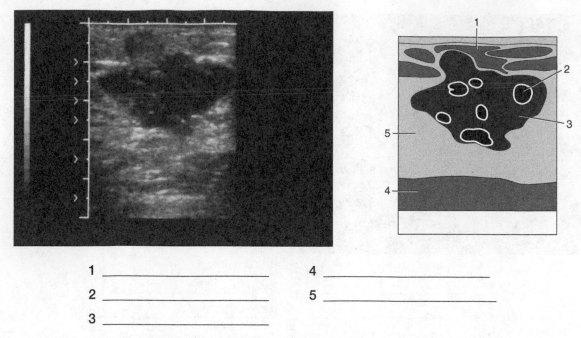

1 _____   4 _____

2 _____   5 _____

3 _____

Figure 7-17 in the textbook (Image courtesy Sentara Norfolk Genera, Norfolk, Va.)

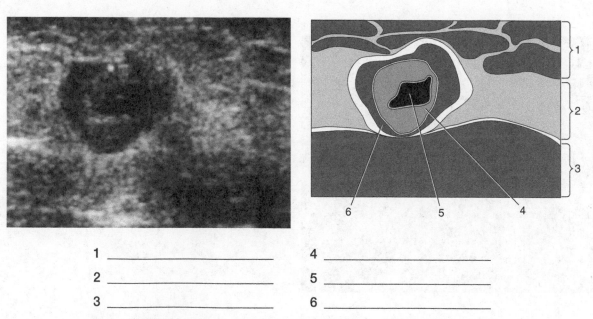

1 _____   4 _____

2 _____   5 _____

3 _____   6 _____

Figure 7-18 in the textbook (Image courtesy Acuson Corp., Mountain View, Calif.)

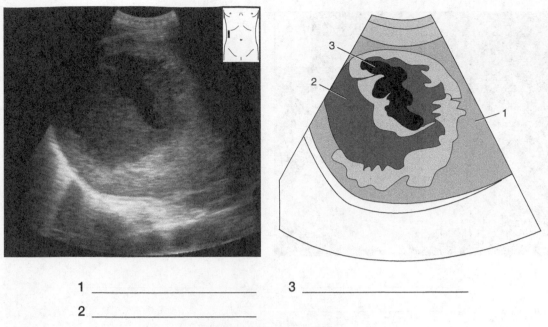

1 _____   3 _____

2 _____

Figure 7-19 in the textbook

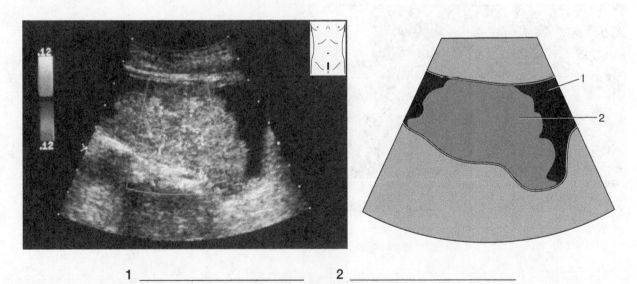

1 _____   2 _____

Figure 7-20 in the textbook (Image courtesy Acuson Corp., Mountain View, Calif.)

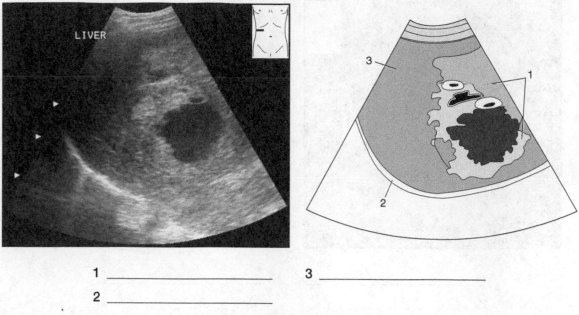

1 _____   3 _____
2 _____

Figure 7-21 in the textbook

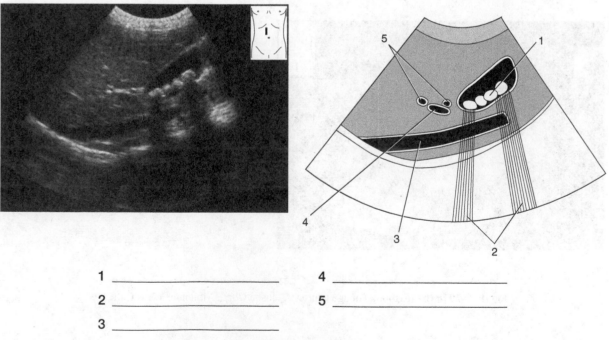

1 _____   4 _____
2 _____   5 _____
3 _____

Figure 7-22 in the textbook

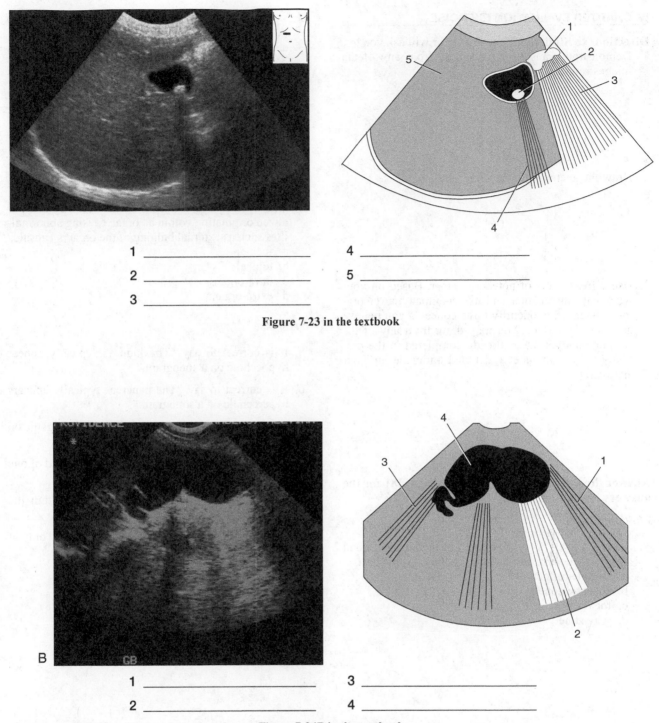

1 _____   4 _____

2 _____   5 _____

3 _____

Figure 7-23 in the textbook

B

1 _____   3 _____

2 _____   4 _____

Figure 7-24B in the textbook

2. For all of the previous images, write a description of the ultrasound findings that could be presented to your instructor, a clinical sonographer, or a sonologist. Your description will be based on information in this chapter, which describes how to write a technical observation. Please use your textbook to correlate and check your answers.

IV. CHAPTER EVALUATION EXERCISE

Directions to Students: Your instructor will ask you to:

1. Demonstrate transducer placement from any of the images reviewed so far.

2. Draw the anatomy for the view announced.

3. Use a fresh sheet of notebook paper. Based on your work with the chapter and its accompanying laboratory assignments, identify three concepts you believe are most important. You may draw from any of the assignments you have already completed in the previous pages. Include a detailed rationale in your answers.

Answer the questions below. Refer to page 381 for the answers.

Multiple Choice

1. The _____ is the point at which the sound beam is the narrowest and the resolution is the best.
   a. Doppler effect
   b. acoustic zone
   c. focal zone
   d. gray zone

2. _____ describes an irregular or mixed echo pattern on an ultrasound image.
   a. Doppler effect
   b. Heterogeneous
   c. Homogeneous
   d. Gray scale

3. _____ describes uniform or similar echo patterns on an ultrasound image.
   a. Doppler effect
   b. Heterogeneous
   c. Homogeneous
   d. Gray scale

4. A(n) _____ disease process may be visualized originating within an organ causing abnormalities such as external bulging of the organ's capsule.
   a. focal
   b. topical
   c. intra-organ
   d. extra-organ

True/False

5. It is correct to say "The kidneys typically appear hypoechoic on a sonogram."

6. It is correct to say "The pancreas typically appears hyperechoic on a sonogram."

7. It is correct to say "Body structures are echogenic on a sonogram."

8. An abnormal mass within the body composed of one thing, tissue, is called a complex mass.

9. A complex mass is an abnormal mass within the body composed of both tissue and fluid.

10. An abnormal mass within the body composed only of fluid is described as a neoplasm.

8 Embryology

I. MEMORIZATION EXERCISE

Directions to Students: Write the key words in your notebook or on note cards. Write the words on one side of the notepaper and then write the definitions on the opposite side of the page or on the back of the paper. If using note cards, write the key word on the front and the definition on the back. *This step should be completed before the lab session begins.*

Memorize the key word definitions silently for 5 minutes, then work with a lab partner and identify the words you still need help with. List the words here. Add additional rows if needed.

II. COMPREHENSION EXERCISE

Directions to Students: Work with a lab partner to complete this exercise. You will need to write in your notebook. First, change each objective into a question.

Example: "Describe the three layers of the embryo and the organs formed from each layer" becomes "What are the three layers of the embryo and which organs are formed from each layer?"

Next, write a short answer to the question just created.

Example: "The embryo consists of three layers; the most external is the ectoderm (brain and spinal cord); the middle mesoderm (heart, circulatory, kidneys, and reproductive systems); and the inner layer, endoderm (lungs, intestines, and urinary bladder)."

Highlight or circle any part of your answers about which you are unsure, and check the answers in your textbook. If you are still unsure of the answers, put a question mark next to the answer(s) for the review session of the lab.

III. APPLICATION OF ANATOMY AND PHYSIOLOGY EXERCISE

Directions to Students:
1. Layers: Label the figure. In your notebook, write a brief description of the function of the layers described in the figure.

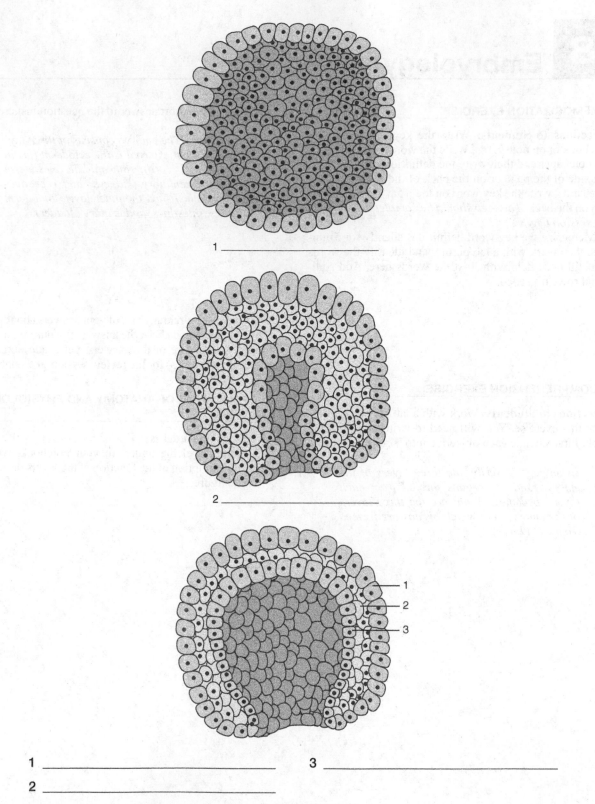

1 _____

2 _____

1 _____ 1
2 _____ 2
3 _____ 3

1 _____   3 _____

2 _____

Figure 8-1 in the textbook

2. Vessels: Label the figure. In your notebook, write
   a brief description of the function of the vessels
   described in the figure.

Superior   Inferior

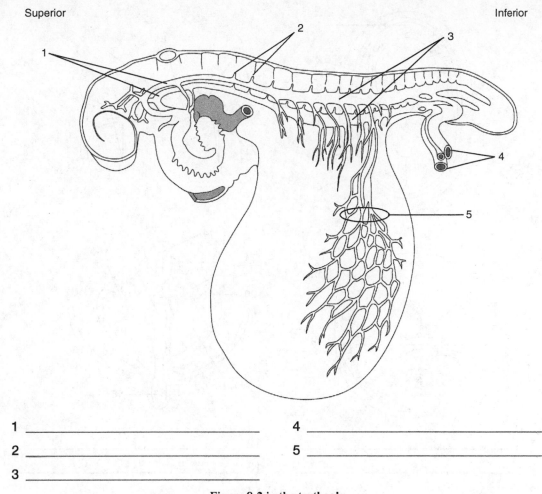

1 _____   4 _____

2 _____   5 _____

3 _____

Figure 8-2 in the textbook

3. Organs: Label the figures. In your notebook, write a brief description of the function of each organ represented in the figures.

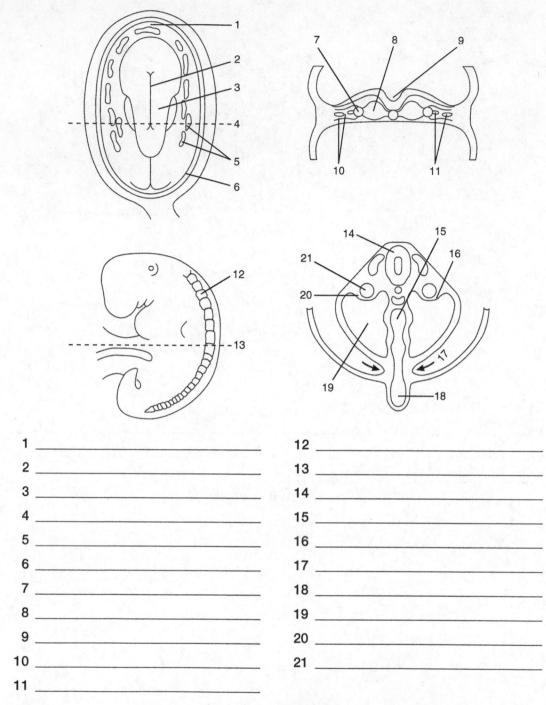

1 _____
2 _____
3 _____
4 _____
5 _____
6 _____
7 _____
8 _____
9 _____
10 _____
11 _____

12 _____
13 _____
14 _____
15 _____
16 _____
17 _____
18 _____
19 _____
20 _____
21 _____

Figure 8-6 in the textbook

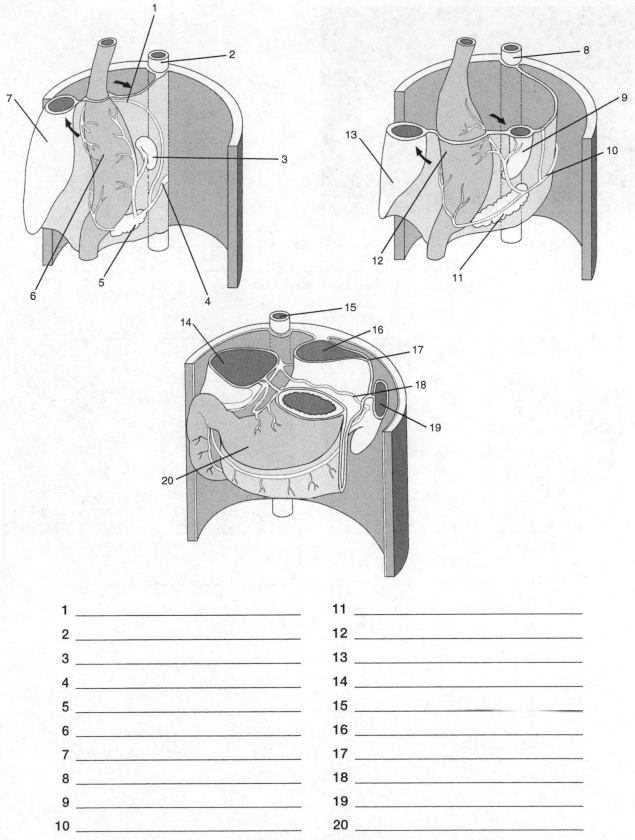

Figure 8-8 in the textbook

1 _____   11 _____

2 _____   12 _____

3 _____   13 _____

4 _____   14 _____

5 _____   15 _____

6 _____   16 _____

7 _____   17 _____

8 _____   18 _____

9 _____   19 _____

10 _____   20 _____

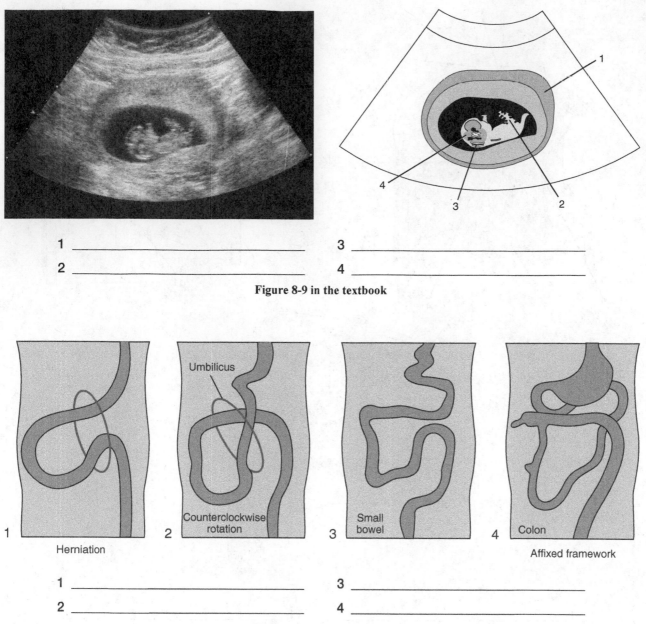

1 _____   3 _____

2 _____   4 _____

Figure 8-9 in the textbook

1 _____   3 _____

2 _____   4 _____

Figure 8-10 in the textbook

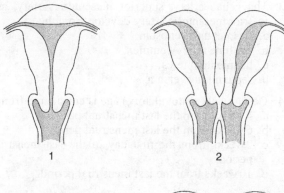

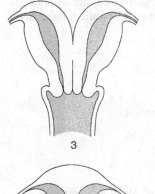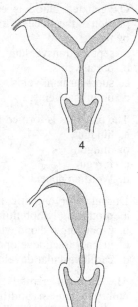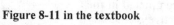

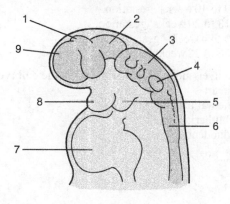

Figure 8-11 in the textbook

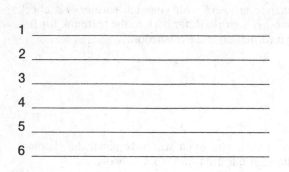

1 _____
2 _____
3 _____
4 _____
5 _____
6 _____

3. Brain and neck: Label of the figure. In your notebook, write a brief description of the function of each organ represented in the figure.

1 _____
2 _____
3 _____
4 _____
5 _____
6 _____
7 _____
8 _____
9 _____

Figure 8-19 in the textbook

IV. CHAPTER SUBHEADINGS EXERCISE

Directions to Students:

1. Convert each chapter subheading into a question; for example, change "Liver Development" to "What is the embryological development of the liver?" Briefly answer each question in a short paragraph in your notebook.

2. Exchange answers with your lab partner and check each other's work. Refer back to the textbook for further information and explanation.

3. What questions do you still have about the chapter? Write your questions in your notebook.

V. CHAPTER EVALUATION EXERCISE

Directions to Students: Use a fresh sheet of notebook paper. Based on your work with the chapter and its accompanying laboratory assignments, identify three concepts you believe are the most important. You may draw from any of the assignments you've already completed in the previous pages, including learning objectives, anatomy and physiology, images, or chapter subheadings. Include a detailed rationale in your answers.

Answer the questions below. Refer to page 381 for the answers.

Multiple Choice

1. The ductus venosus
   a. shunts deoxygenated blood away from the heart.
   b. is nonfunctional in the embryo.
   c. persists functionally into adulthood.
   d. shunts oxygenated blood past the liver into the inferior vena cava.

2. The first system to become functional in the embryo is the
   a. gastrointestinal system.
   b. neurologic system.
   c. cardiovascular system.
   d. pulmonary system.

3. The celiac artery, superior mesenteric artery, and inferior mesenteric artery develop from the
   a. ligamentum venosum.
   b. vitelline artery complex.
   c. ligamentum teres.
   d. septum transversum.

4. Gestational (postovulatory) age is considered from
   a. 4 weeks from the last menstrual period.
   b. 6 weeks from the last menstrual period.
   c. 2 weeks from the first day of the last menstrual period.
   d. 10 weeks from the last menstrual period.

5. Oxygenated blood is carried from the embryonic portion of the placenta to the embryonic tubular heart by the
   a. septum transversum.
   b. portal veins.
   c. supracardinal veins.
   d. umbilical veins.

6. The pancreas is formed from the
   a. hindgut.
   b. midgut.
   c. foregut.
   d. Wolffian ducts.

7. During embryonic life, the spleen is responsible for
   a. producing lymph fluid.
   b. producing red and white blood cells.
   c. urinary tract development.
   d. cardiovascular development.

8. The external genitals of both male and female embryos remain undifferentiated until the eighth week of gestation; before that, all embryos have a region known as the
   a. genital tubercle.
   b. mesonephros.
   c. pronephros.
   d. umbilical veins.

9. Neural tube formation takes place at
   a. 9 to 10 weeks' gestation.
   b. 18 to 20 weeks' gestation.
   c. 3 to 4 weeks' gestation.
   d. 26 to 28 weeks' gestation.

10. The liver and pancreas originate in the embryonic
    a. heart.
    b. neural tube.
    c. Müllerian ducts.
    d. duodenum.

Introduction to Laboratory Values

I. MEMORIZATION EXERCISE

Directions to Students: Write the key words in your notebook or on note cards. Write the words on one side of the notepaper and then write the definitions on the opposite side of the page or on the back of the paper. If using note cards, write the key word on the front and the definition on the back. *This step should be completed before the lab session begins.*

Memorize the key word definitions silently for 5 minutes, then work with a lab partner and identify the words you still need help with. List the words here. Add additional rows if needed.

II. COMPREHENSION EXERCISE

Directions to Students: Work with a lab partner to complete this exercise. For each laboratory value presented in the text, work with your partner to memorize the normal range for adults, two implications for low values, and two implications for high values.

Alanine aminotransferase (ALT)
Alpha fetoprotein
Aspartate aminotransferase (AST)
Amylase
Bilirubin
Blood urea nitrogen
Cholesterol
Creatine
Creatine phosphokinase
Estrogen
Glucose
Hematocrit
Human chorionic gonadotropin (hCG)
Lactate dehydrogenase (LD)
Lipase
Prostate-specific antigen (PSA)
Thyroid-stimulating hormone (TSH)

III. APPLICATION OF ANATOMY AND PHYSIOLOGY EXERCISE

Directions to Students: Work on the following with your lab partner.
1. Using the table below, describe the location of each organ. What body system is it a part of? Use Chapter 5 if additional help is needed. What did you miss?

Review Table

Organ	Laboratory Test
Abdominal aorta	Hematocrit
Neonatal brain	
Liver	Bilirubin
Liver	ALT
Pancreas	AST
	ALP
	Total protein levels
Liver	LDL
Heart	HDL
	VLDL
	Total proteins
Liver	BUN
Kidney	Creatinine
Pancreas	Amylase
	Lipase
	Glucose
Heart	LD
	CPK
Male pelvis	PSA
Female pelvis	Estrogen (E1, E2, E3)
Obstetrics	hCG
	AFP
Thyroid gland	THS
Parathyroid gland	T3
	T4

2. Write two or three summary sentences for each system listed in question 1. Ask your lab partner to check your work. Now check your work against the explanations in the textbook. What else can you add to your description?

IV. CHAPTER EVALUATION EXERCISE

Directions to Students: Use a fresh sheet of notebook paper. Based on your work with the chapter and its accompanying laboratory assignments, identify three concepts you believe are the most important. You may draw from any of the assignments you've already completed in the previous pages. Include a detailed rationale in your answers.

Answer the questions below. Refer to page 382 for the answers.

Multiple Choice

1. Agencies such as CLIA and CAP-LAP require laboratories to participate in external proficiency testing in addition to
   a. daily cleaning.
   b. daily QC.
   c. daily reports.
   d. daily Levey-Jennings plots.

2. Bilirubin can be tested by
   a. venipuncture.
   b. urine collection.
   c. stool collection.
   d. all of the above.
   e. a and b.

3. The three major types of cholesterol are
   a. LDL, HDL, IDL.
   b. LDL, VLDL, ADL.
   c. VLDL, HDL, IDL.
   d. VLDL, LDL, HDL.

4. Creatine phosphokinase is found in
   a. heart muscle.
   b. brain muscle.
   c. skeletal muscle.
   d. all of the above.

5. Which test uses AFP?
   a. Liver enzyme
   b. Triple screen
   c. Quadruple screen
   d. Cardiac function

6. Which hormones are used to measure TSH? **Select all that apply.**
   a. T1
   b. T2
   c. T3
   d. T4
   e. T5

7. CLIA is an abbreviation for
   a. Clinical Laboratory Institutional Amendments.
   b. Clinical Laboratory Institutional Association.
   c. Clinical Laboratory Improvement Amendments.
   d. Clinical Laboratory Improvement Association.

Completion.

8. PSA is used to detect _____ cancer.

9. Normal PSA screening occurs between the ages of _____ in patients with no risk factors. Screening for patients with risk factors occurs between the ages of _____.

10. Creatinine is a byproduct of _____.

10   The Abdominal Aorta

I. MEMORIZATION EXERCISE

Directions to Students: Write the key words in your notebook or on note cards. Write the words on one side of the notepaper and then write the definitions on the opposite side of the page or on the back of the paper. If using note cards, write the key word on the front and the definition on the back. *This step should be completed before the lab session begins.*

Memorize the key word definitions silently for 5 minutes, then work with a lab partner and identify the words you still need help with. List the words here. Add additional rows if needed.

II. COMPREHENSION EXERCISE

Directions to Students: Work with a lab partner to complete this exercise. You will need to write in your notebook. First, change each objective into a question.

> *Example: "Describe the normal location, course, and size of the aorta" becomes, "What are the normal location, course, and size of the aorta?"*

Next, write a short answer to the question just created.

> *Example: "The aorta is a retroperitoneal vessel located slightly to the left of the spine. It leaves the heart and courses to the common iliac arteries in the pelvis. Its diameter should be no more than 3 cm at its widest point."*

Highlight or circle any part of your answers about which you are unsure, and check the answers in your textbook. If you are still unsure of the answers, put a question mark next to the answer(s) for the review session of the lab.

III. ANATOMY APPLICATION EXERCISE

Directions to Students: Work on the following with your lab partner.
1. In your notebook, draw the aorta and as many branches as you can from memory.

2. Label the aorta and its branches. Include each structure's orientation in the body (either vertical, horizontal, vertical oblique, or horizontal oblique). Ask your lab partner to critique your work. What did you miss? Check your drawing using the sketches in your textbook and complete any structures missing from your drawing.

3. Below your drawing, write two or three summary sentences of the physiology of the aorta. Ask your lab partner to check your work. Then, check your work against the physiology section in the textbook. What else can you add to your description?

IV. IMAGE ANALYSIS EXERCISE

Directions to Students: Work on the following figures with your lab partner. You can label all the sketches at once, then go back and label each image with your lab partner, or you can label an image and its accompanying sketch at the same time. It's your choice! Either way, the goal is to label correctly all of the sketches and carefully compare the sketch with the sonographic image.

For each sonographic image, write a brief observation that could be "presented" to your instructor, a clinical sonographer, or a sonologist. Your observation should be based on Chapter 7 in the textbook, which describes how to write a technical observation. Please go back and review that chapter if necessary.

For each image, your assessment should include (1) the view of each major structure (axial or longitudinal; note: these are not the scanning planes) and (2) structures identified in the image with correct sonographic appearance description and measurements if shown (see Chapter 7 in the textbook for information on how to write a technical observation).

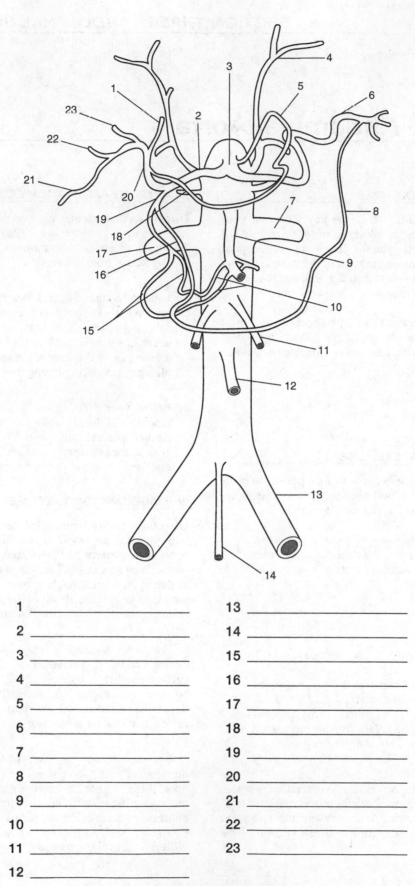

Figure 10-3 in the textbook

1	_____	13	_____
2	_____	14	_____
3	_____	15	_____
4	_____	16	_____
5	_____	17	_____
6	_____	18	_____
7	_____	19	_____
8	_____	20	_____
9	_____	21	_____
10	_____	22	_____
11	_____	23	_____
12	_____		

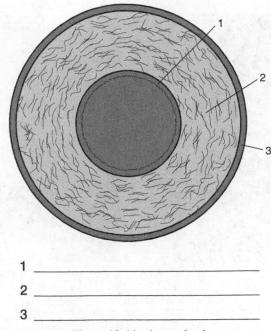

1 _____

2 _____

3 _____

Figure 10-4 in the textbook

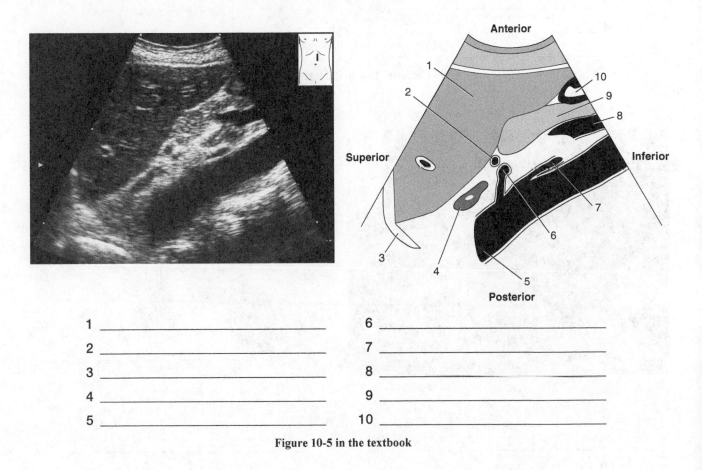

1 _____   6 _____

2 _____   7 _____

3 _____   8 _____

4 _____   9 _____

5 _____   10 _____

Figure 10-5 in the textbook

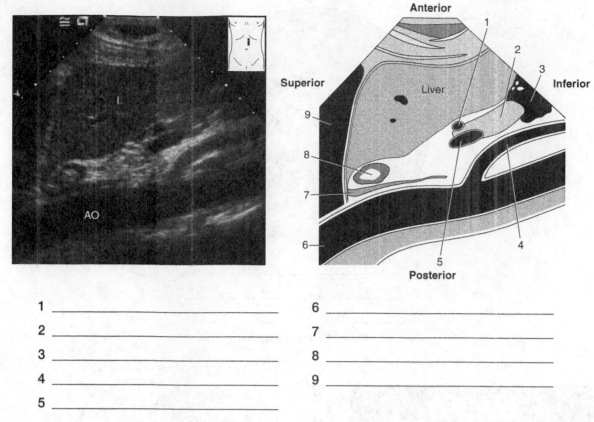

1	_____	6	_____
2	_____	7	_____
3	_____	8	_____
4	_____	9	_____
5	_____		

Figure 10-6 in the textbook

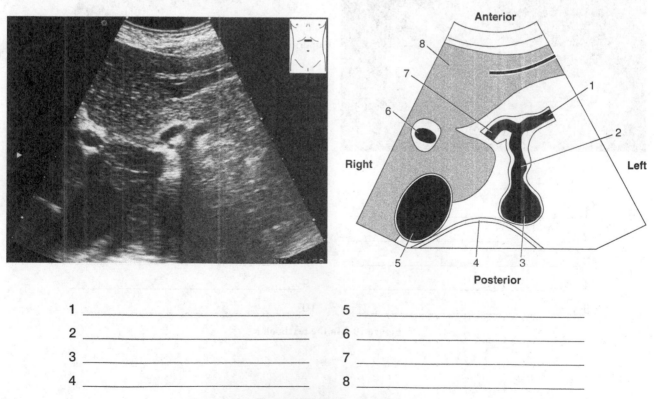

1	_____	5	_____
2	_____	6	_____
3	_____	7	_____
4	_____	8	_____

Figure 10-7 in the textbook

Chapter 10   The Abdominal Aorta

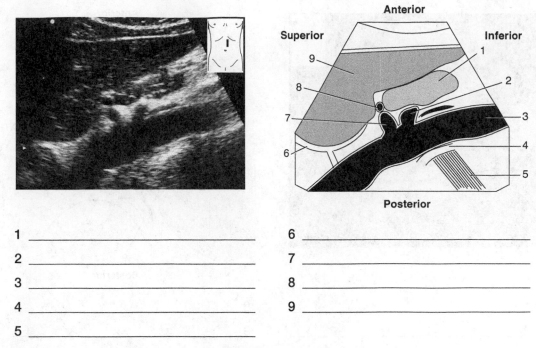

1 _____   6 _____

2 _____   7 _____

3 _____   8 _____

4 _____   9 _____

5 _____

Figure 10-8 in the textbook

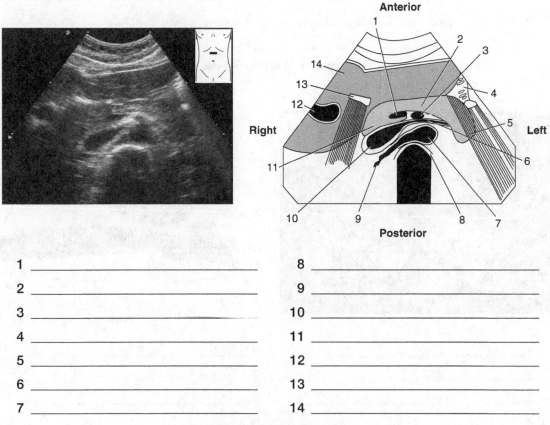

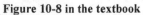

1 _____   8 _____

2 _____   9 _____

3 _____   10 _____

4 _____   11 _____

5 _____   12 _____

6 _____   13 _____

7 _____   14 _____

Figure 10-9 in the textbook

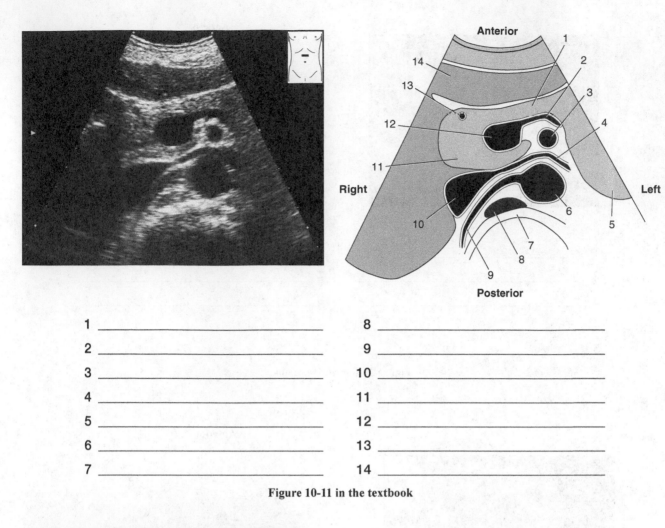

Figure 10-11 in the textbook

1	_____	8	_____
2	_____	9	_____
3	_____	10	_____
4	_____	11	_____
5	_____	12	_____
6	_____	13	_____
7	_____	14	_____

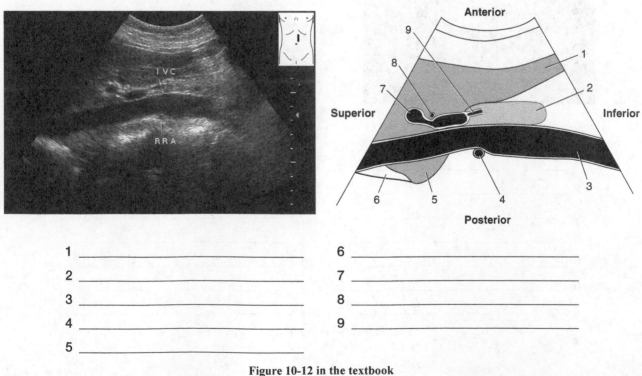

1	_____	6	_____
2	_____	7	_____
3	_____	8	_____
4	_____	9	_____
5	_____		

Figure 10-12 in the textbook

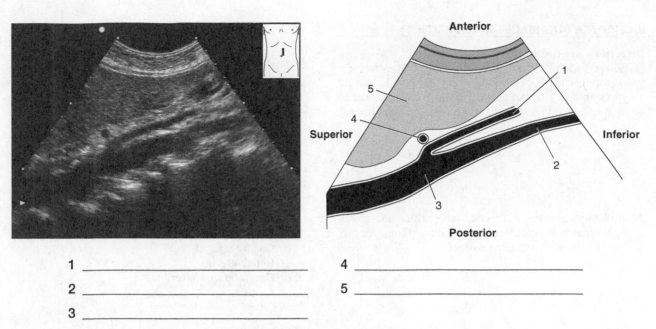

1 _____

2 _____

3 _____

4 _____

5 _____

Figure 10-13 in the textbook

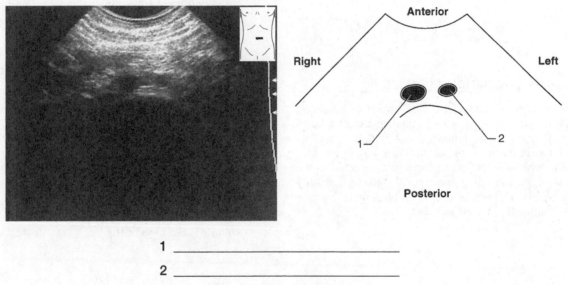

1 _____

2 _____

Figure 10-15 in the textbook

V. CHAPTER SUBHEADINGS EXERCISE

Directions to Students:

1. Convert each chapter subheading into a question; for example, change "Gross Anatomy" to, "What is the gross anatomy of the aorta?" Write a brief answer to each question in a short paragraph in your notebook.

2. Exchange answers with your lab partner and check each other's work. Refer back to the textbook for further information and explanation.

3. What questions about the chapter do you still have? Write your questions in your notebook.

VI. CHAPTER EVALUATION EXERCISE

Directions to Students: Use a fresh sheet of notebook paper. Based on your work with the chapter and its accompanying laboratory assignments, identify three concepts you believe are the most important. You may draw from any of the assignments you've already completed in the previous pages, including learning objectives, anatomy and physiology, images, or chapter subheadings. Include a detailed rationale in your answers.

Answer the questions below. Refer to page 382 for the answers.

Multiple Choice

1. Which of the following vessels is seen sonographically as a linear structure that courses inferior and parallel to the aorta?
   a. Celiac artery
   b. Superior mesenteric artery
   c. Renal arteries
   d. Inferior mesenteric artery

2. Which of the following vessels are seen in a longitudinal course when the transducer is oriented in a transverse scanning plane?
   a. Hepatic arteries
   b. Gastric arteries
   c. Renal arteries
   d. Common iliac arteries

True/False

3. The celiac artery (CA) cannot be seen with reasonable consistency on ultrasound.

4. The anteroposterior measurement of the aorta should be obtained in an axial section to decrease variation among different sonographers.

5. The SMA demonstrates a high-resistance waveform in a patient who has not eaten.

6. The right gastric artery can originate from the proper hepatic artery, the gastroduodenal artery, or the common hepatic artery.

7. The right renal artery is longer than the left renal artery.

8. Longitudinal sections of the proximal portion of the abdominal aorta appear linear in configuration, and the mid and distal portions appear curvilinear.

9. The most inferior branch of the aorta is the inferior mesenteric artery.

10. Hematocrit measures how much of the total blood volume is red blood cells.

11 The Inferior Vena Cava

I. MEMORIZATION EXERCISE

Directions to Students: Write the key words in your notebook or on note cards. Write the words on one side of the notepaper and then write the definitions on the opposite side of the page or on the back of the paper. If using note cards, write the key word on the front and the definition on the back. *This step should be completed before the lab session begins.*

Memorize the key word definitions silently for 5 minutes, then work with a lab partner and identify the words you still need help with. List the words here. Add additional rows if needed.

II. COMPREHENSION EXERCISE

Directions to Students: Work with a lab partner to complete this exercise. You will need to write in your notebook. First, change each objective into a question.

> *Example: "Describe the normal location and course of the inferior vena cava" becomes "What are the normal location and course of the inferior vena cava?"*

Next, write a short answer to the question just created.

> *Example: "The inferior vena cava is a retroperitoneal vessel located slightly to the right of the spine. It begins at the union of the common iliac veins and empties into the right atrium of the heart."*

Highlight or circle any part of your answers about which you are unsure, and check the answers in your textbook. If you are still unsure of the answers, put a question mark next to the answer(s) for the review session of the lab.

III. ANATOMY APPLICATION EXERCISE

Directions to Students: Work on the following with your lab partner.

1. In your notebook, draw the inferior vena cava (IVC) and as many branches as you can from memory.

2. Label the IVC and its branches. Include each structure's orientation in the body (either vertical, horizontal, vertical oblique, or horizontal oblique). Ask your lab partner to critique your work. What did you miss? Check your drawing using the sketches in your textbook and complete any structures missing from your drawing.

3. Below your drawing, write two or three summary sentences of the physiology of the IVC. Ask your lab partner to check your work. Now check your work against the physiology section in the textbook. What else can you add to your description?

IV. IMAGE ANALYSIS EXERCISE

Directions to Students: Work on the following figures with your lab partner. It's your choice! You can label all the sketches at once, then go back and label each image with your lab partner, or you can label an image and its accompanying sketch at the same time. Either way, the goal is to correctly label all of the sketches and carefully compare the sketch with the sonographic image.

For each image, your assessment should include (1) the view of each major structure (axial or longitudinal; note: these are not the scanning planes) and (2) structures identified in the image with correct sonographic appearance description and measurements if shown (see Chapter 7 in the textbook for information on how to write a technical observation).

For each sonographic image, write a brief observation that could be "presented" to your instructor, a clinical sonographer, or a sonologist. Your observation should be based on Chapter 7 in the textbook, which describes how to write a technical observation. Please go back and review that chapter if necessary.

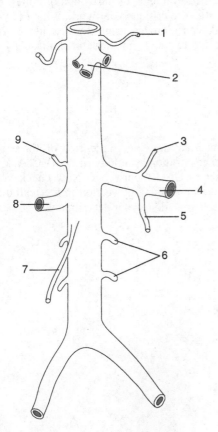

Figure 11-2 in the textbook

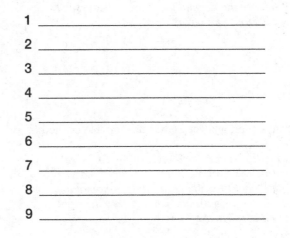

1 _____

2 _____

3 _____

4 _____

5 _____

6 _____

7 _____

8 _____

9 _____

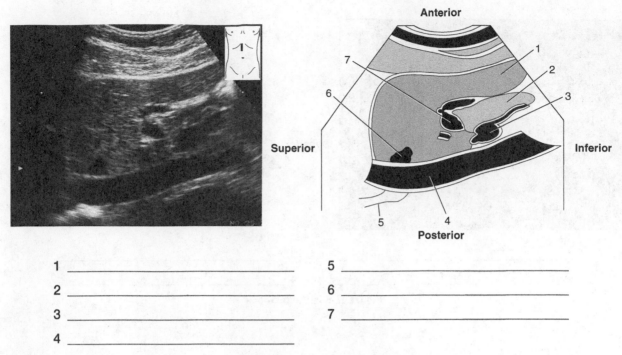

1	_____	5	_____
2	_____	6	_____
3	_____	7	_____
4	_____		

Figure 11-3 in the textbook

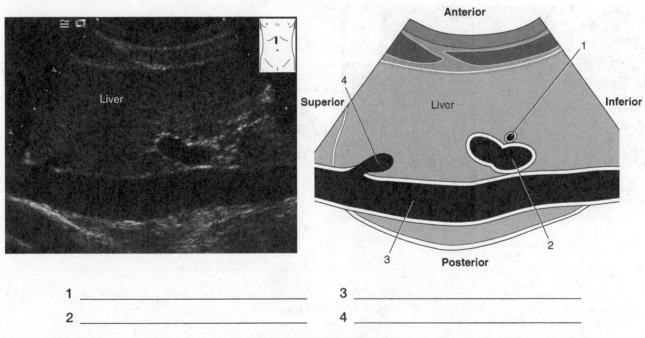

| 1 | _____ | 3 | _____ |
| 2 | _____ | 4 | _____ |

Figure 11-4 in the textbook

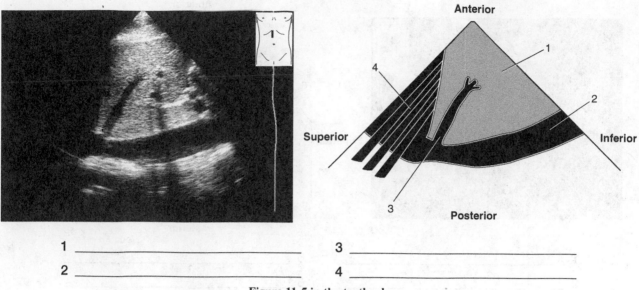

1 _____   3 _____

2 _____   4 _____

Figure 11-5 in the textbook

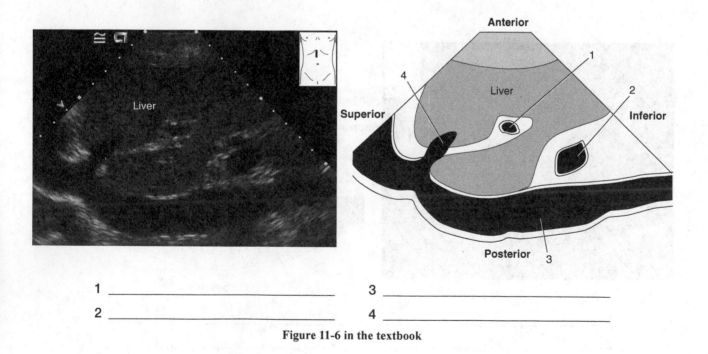

1 _____   3 _____

2 _____   4 _____

Figure 11-6 in the textbook

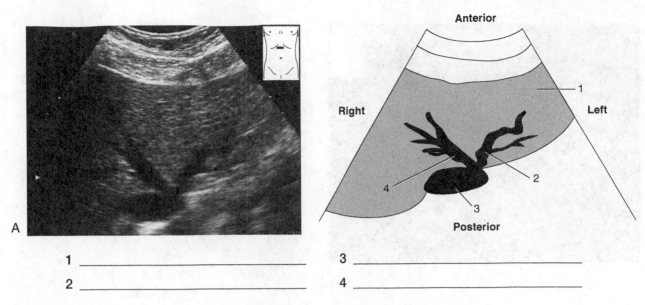

1 _____   3 _____

2 _____   4 _____

Figure 11-7A in the textbook

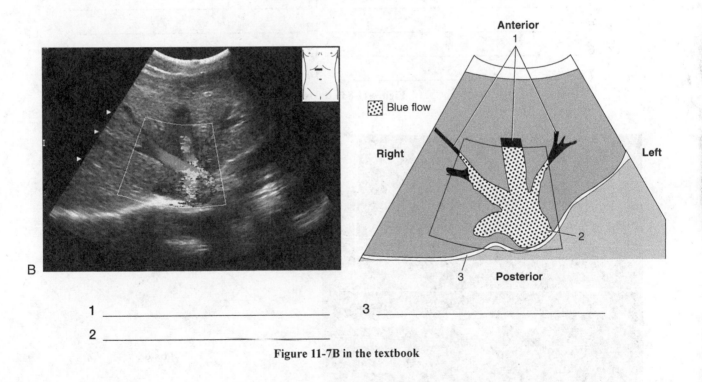

1 _____   3 _____

2 _____

Figure 11-7B in the textbook

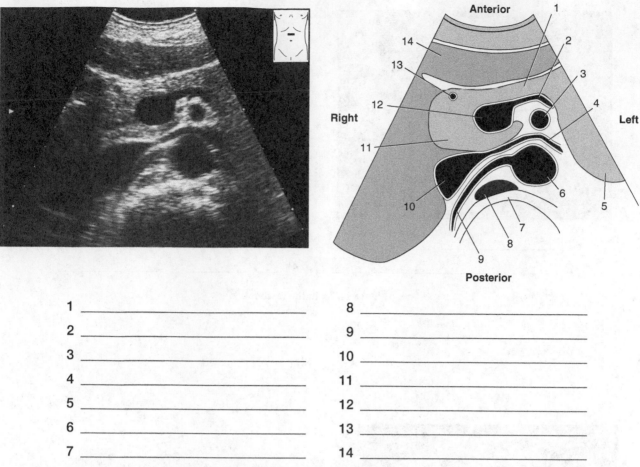

1 _____	8 _____
2 _____	9 _____
3 _____	10 _____
4 _____	11 _____
5 _____	12 _____
6 _____	13 _____
7 _____	14 _____

Figure 11-8 in the textbook

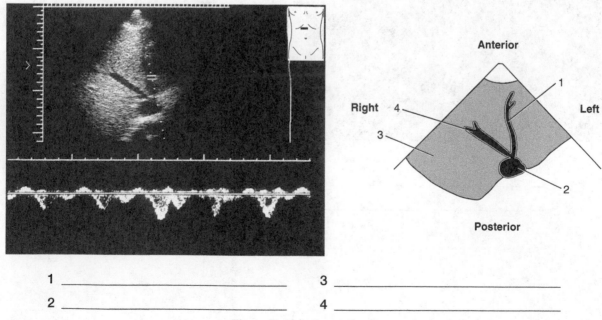

1 _____	3 _____
2 _____	4 _____

Figure 11-10 in the textbook

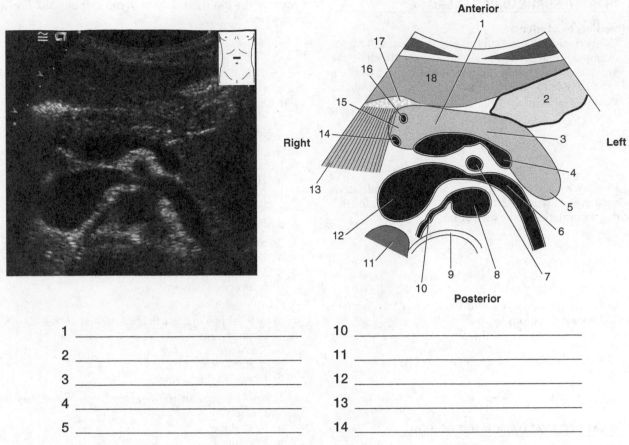

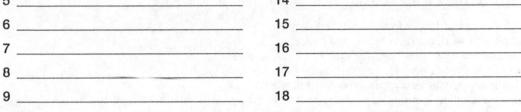

1	_____	10	_____
2	_____	11	_____
3	_____	12	_____
4	_____	13	_____
5	_____	14	_____
6	_____	15	_____
7	_____	16	_____
8	_____	17	_____
9	_____	18	_____

Figure 11-9 in the textbook

V. CHAPTER SUBHEADINGS EXERCISE

Directions to Students:

1. Convert each chapter subheading into a question; for example, change "Gross Anatomy" to "What is the gross anatomy of the inferior vena cava?" Write a brief answer to each question in a short paragraph in your notebook.

2. Exchange answers with your lab partner and check each other's work. Refer back to the textbook for further information and explanation.

3. What questions do you still have about the chapter? Write your questions in your notebook.

VI. CHAPTER EVALUATION EXERCISE

Directions to Students: Use a fresh sheet of notebook paper. Based on your work with the chapter and its accompanying laboratory assignments, identify three concepts you believe are the most important. You may draw from any of the assignments you've already completed in the previous pages, including learning objectives, anatomy and physiology, images, or chapter subheadings. Include a detailed rationale in your answers.

Answer the questions below. Refer to page 382 for the answers.

Multiple Choice

1. The IVC travels through the diaphragm and empties into the
   a. right atrium.
   b. left atrium.
   c. right ventricle.
   d. left ventricle.

2. Which portion of the IVC extends inferior to the hepatic veins and superior to the renal veins?
   a. Hepatic section
   b. Prerenal section
   c. Renal section
   d. Postrenal section

3. The left gonadal vein empties into the
   a. IVC.
   b. left renal vein.
   c. left suprarenal vein.
   d. left iliac vein.

4. Which is not a major tributary of the IVC?
   a. Hepatic veins
   b. Renal veins
   c. Portal veins
   d. Common iliac veins

5. Into which lobe of the liver does the middle hepatic vein empty?
   a. Right lobe
   b. Left lobe
   c. Caudate lobe
   d. Quadrate lobe

True/False

6. The renal section is the most inferiorly located portion of the IVC.

7. The right gonadal vein empties into the IVC.

8. The left common iliac vein is longer than the right common iliac vein.

9. The hepatic veins decrease in diameter as they approach the IVC.

10. Small, moving echoes visualized in the lumen of the IVC are a normal finding.

12 The Portal Venous System

I. MEMORIZATION EXERCISE

Directions to students: Write the key words in your notebook or on note cards. Write the words on one side of the notepaper and then write the definitions on the opposite side of the page or on the back of the paper. If using note cards, write the key word on the front and the definition on the back. *This step should be completed before the lab session begins*.

Memorize the key word definitions silently for 5 minutes, then work with a lab partner and identify the words you still need help with. List the words here. Add additional rows if needed.

II. COMPREHENSION EXERCISE

Directions to students: Work with a lab partner to complete this exercise. You will need to write in your notebook. First, change each objective into a question.

> *Example: "Describe the normal location, course, and size of the portal vein" becomes "What is the normal location, course, and size of the portal vein?"*

Next, write a short answer to the question just created.

> *Example: "The portal vein is an intraabdominal structure that drains the gastrointestinal tract. It courses from left to right and is formed near the head of the pancreas before entering the liver at the liver hilus. Its diameter is up to 13 mm, and its length is 5 to 6 cm."*

Highlight or circle any part of your answers about which you are unsure, and check the answers in your textbook. If you are still unsure of the answers, put a question mark next to the answer(s) for the review session of the lab.

III. APPLICATION OF ANATOMY AND PHYSIOLOGY EXERCISE

Directions to students: Work on the following with your lab partner.
1. In your notebook, draw the portal vein, the tributaries that form it, and the branches that lead off the portal vein, as much as you can from memory.

2. Label the portal vein and its branches. Include each structure's orientation in the body (either vertical, horizontal, vertical oblique, or horizontal oblique). Ask your lab partner to critique your work. What did you miss? Check your drawing using the sketches in your textbook and complete any missing structures from your drawing.

3. Below your drawing, write two or three summary sentences of the physiology of the portal vein. Ask your lab partner to check your work. Now check your work against the physiology section in the textbook. What else can you add to your description?

IV. IMAGE ANALYSIS EXERCISE

Directions to students: Work on the following figures with your lab partner. It's your choice! You can label all the sketches at once, then go back and label each image with your lab partner, or label an image and its accompanying sketch at the same time. Either way, the goal is to correctly label all of the sketches and carefully compare the sketch with the sonographic image.

For each sonographic image, write a very brief observation that could be "presented" to your instructor, the clinical sonographer, or the sonologist. Your observation will be based on Chapter 7 in the textbook, which describes how to write a technical observation. Please go back and review that chapter if needed.

For each image, your assessment should include: (1) a view of each major structure (axial or longitudinal; note: these are not the scanning planes) and (2) structures identified in the image with correct sonographic appearance description and measurements if shown (see Chapter 7 in the textbook for information on how to write a technical observation).

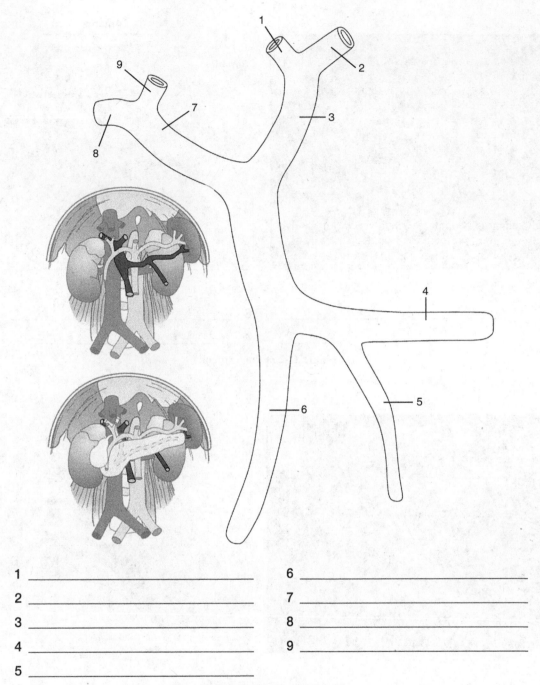

Figure 12-1 in the textbook

1	_____	6	_____
2	_____	7	_____
3	_____	8	_____
4	_____	9	_____
5	_____		

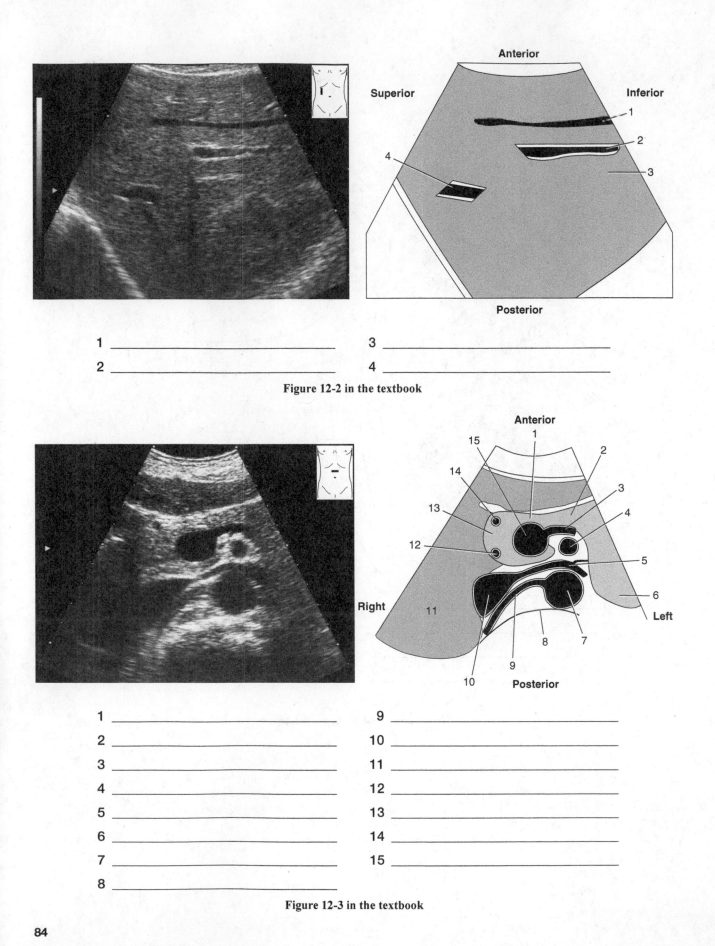

1 _____ 3 _____
2 _____ 4 _____

Figure 12-2 in the textbook

1 _____ 9 _____
2 _____ 10 _____
3 _____ 11 _____
4 _____ 12 _____
5 _____ 13 _____
6 _____ 14 _____
7 _____ 15 _____
8 _____

Figure 12-3 in the textbook

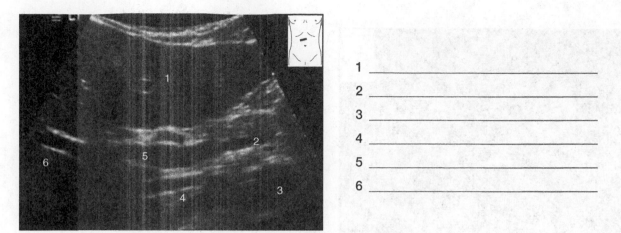

1 _____
2 _____
3 _____
4 _____
5 _____
6 _____

Figure 12-4 in the textbook

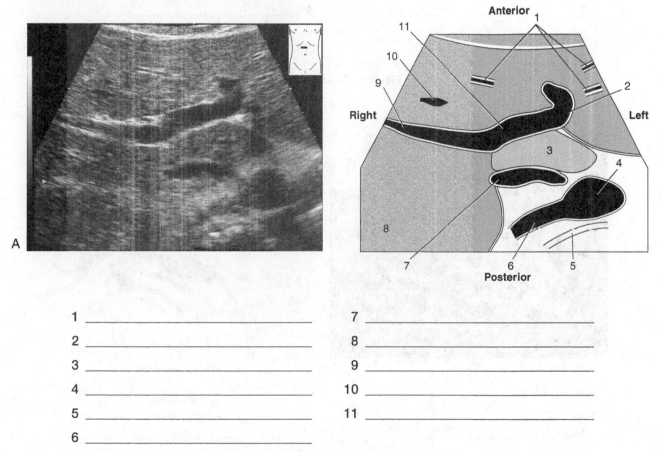

1 _____ 7 _____
2 _____ 8 _____
3 _____ 9 _____
4 _____ 10 _____
5 _____ 11 _____
6 _____

Figure 12-5A in the textbook

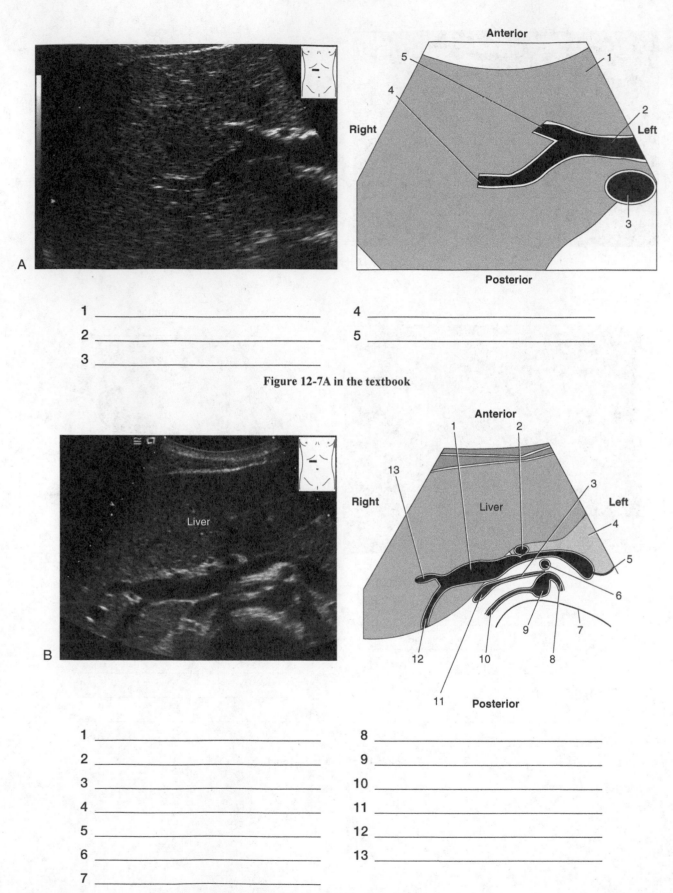

Figure 12-7A in the textbook

1 _____ 4 _____
2 _____ 5 _____
3 _____

1 _____ 8 _____
2 _____ 9 _____
3 _____ 10 _____
4 _____ 11 _____
5 _____ 12 _____
6 _____ 13 _____
7 _____

Figure 12-7B in the textbook

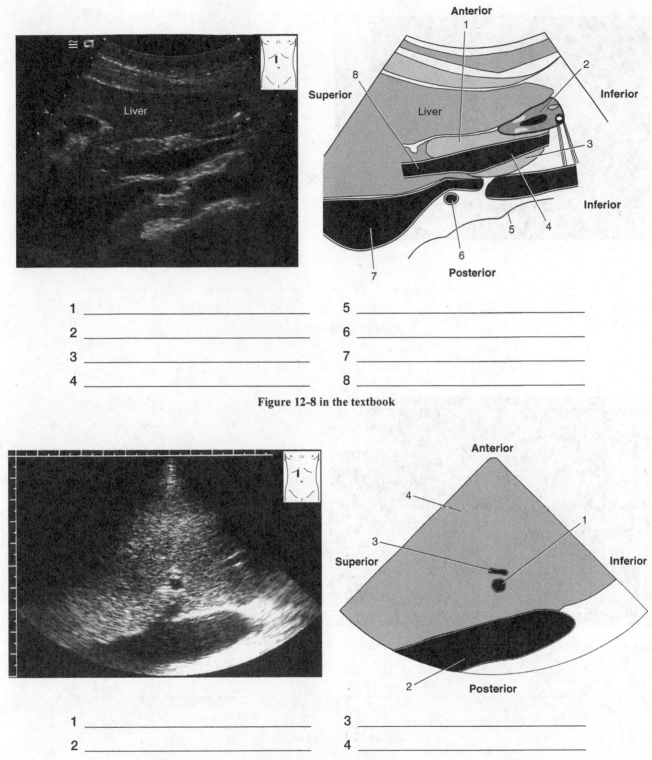

1	_____	5	_____
2	_____	6	_____
3	_____	7	_____
4	_____	8	_____

Figure 12-8 in the textbook

| 1 | _____ | 3 | _____ |
| 2 | _____ | 4 | _____ |

Figure 12-9 in the textbook

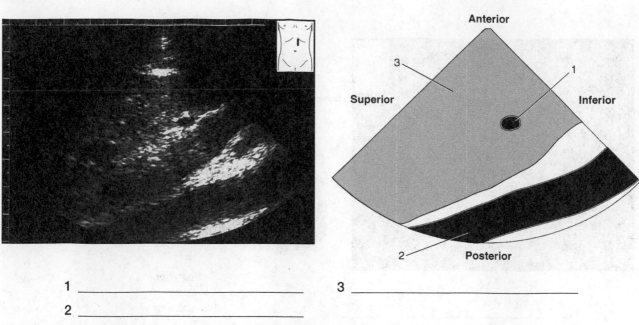

1 _____ 3 _____

2 _____

Figure 12-10 in the textbook

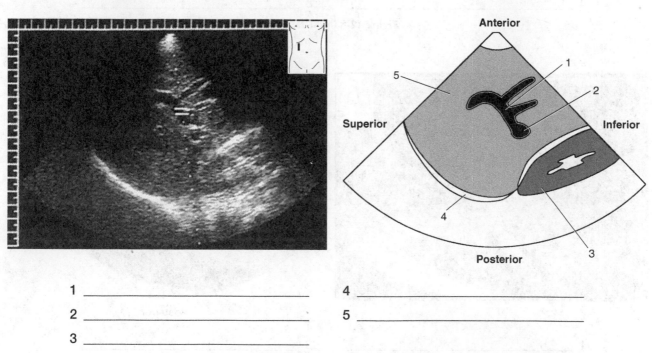

1 _____ 4 _____

2 _____ 5 _____

3 _____

Figure 12-11 in the textbook

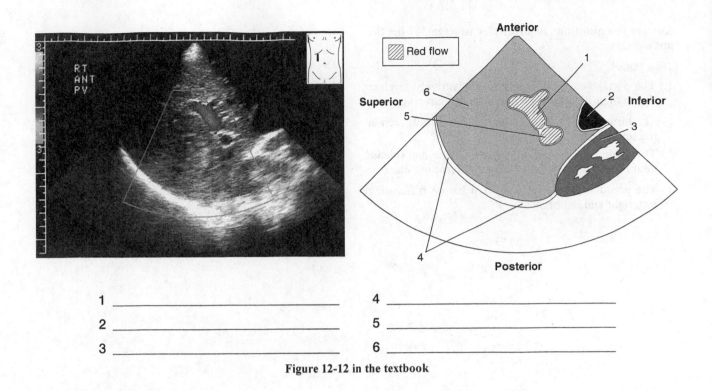

1	_____	4	_____
2	_____	5	_____
3	_____	6	_____

Figure 12-12 in the textbook

V. CHAPTER SUBHEADINGS EXERCISE

Directions to students:

1. Convert each chapter subheading into a question; for example, change "Gross Anatomy" to "What is the gross anatomy of the portal venous system?" Briefly write the answer to each question in a short paragraph in your notebook.

2. Exchange answers with your lab partner and check each other's work. Refer back to the textbook for further information and explanation.

3. What questions do you still have about the chapter? Write your questions in your notebook.

VI. CHAPTER EVALUATION EXERCISE

Directions to students: Use a fresh sheet of notebook paper. Based on your work with the chapter and its accompanying laboratory assignments, identify three concepts you believe are the most important. You may draw from any of the assignments you have already completed in the previous pages including learning objectives, anatomy and physiology, images, or chapter subheadings. Include a detailed rationale in your answers.

Answer the questions below. Refer to page 382 for the answers.

True/False

1. The portal vein's walls appear distinctively brighter due to their high fat content and sheath covering.

2. The bifurcation of the right portal vein is best seen in the transverse scanning plane.

3. The union of the superior mesenteric vein and splenic vein is best appreciated in a sagittal scanning plane.

4. The portal vein courses 6 to 8 cm before bifurcating into right and left branches.

Completion

Indicate the primary path of the vessel as S (superior), IS (inferior to superior), LM (lateral to medial), R (to the right), or L (to the left).

5. Superior mesenteric vein _____

6. Inferior mesenteric vein _____

7. Splenic vein _____

8. Right portal vein _____

9. Left portal vein _____

10. Portal vein _____

13 Abdominal Vasculature

I. MEMORIZATION EXERCISE

Directions to students: Write the key words in your notebook or on note cards. Write the words on one side of the notepaper and then write the definitions on the opposite side of the page or on the back of the paper. If using note cards, write the key word on the front and the definition on the back. *This step should be completed before the lab session begins.*

Memorize the key word definitions silently for 5 minutes, then work with a lab partner and identify the words you still need help with. List the words here. Add additional rows if needed.

II. COMPREHENSION EXERCISE

Directions to students: Work with a lab partner to complete this exercise. You will need to write in your notebook. First, change each objective into a question.

> *Example: "Describe the anatomy of the vasculature of the liver, spleen, mesenteric, and renal system" becomes "What is the anatomy of the vasculature of the liver, spleen, mesenteric, and renal system?"*

Next, write a short answer to the question just created.

> *Example: "The anatomy of the vasculature consists of the abdominal arterial system: the aorta with its main branches, the celiac axis, the common hepatic, splenic, superior mesenteric, inferior mesenteric, and renal arteries."*

Highlight or circle any part of your answers about which you are unsure, and check the answers in your textbook. If you are still unsure of the answers, put a question mark next to the answer(s) for the review session of the lab.

III. APPLICATION OF ANATOMY AND PHYSIOLOGY EXERCISE

Directions to students: Work on the following with your lab partner.
1. In your notebook, draw the abdominal vasculature and as many branches as you can from memory.

2. Label the vasculature. Include each structure's orientation in the body (either vertical, horizontal, vertical oblique, or horizontal oblique). Ask your lab partner to critique your work. What did you miss? Check your drawing using the sketches in your textbook and complete any missing structures from your drawing.

3. Below your drawing, write two or three summary sentences of the physiology of the arterial and venous vasculature. Ask your lab partner to check your work. Now check your work against the physiology section in the textbook. What else can you add to your description?

IV. IMAGE ANALYSIS EXERCISE

Directions to students: Work on the following figures with your lab partner. It's your choice! You can label all the sketches at once, then go back and label each image with your lab partner, or label an image and its accompanying sketch at the same time. Either way, the goal is to correctly label all of the sketches and carefully compare the sketch with the sonographic image.

For each sonographic image, write a very brief observation that could be "presented" to your instructor, the clinical sonographer, or the sonologist. Your observation will be based on Chapter 7 in the textbook, which describes how to write a technical observation. Please go back and review that chapter if needed.

For each image, your assessment should include: (1) a view of each major structure (axial or longitudinal; note: these are not the scanning planes) and (2) structures identified in the image with correct sonographic appearance description and measurements if shown (see Chapter 7 in the textbook for information on how to write a technical observation).

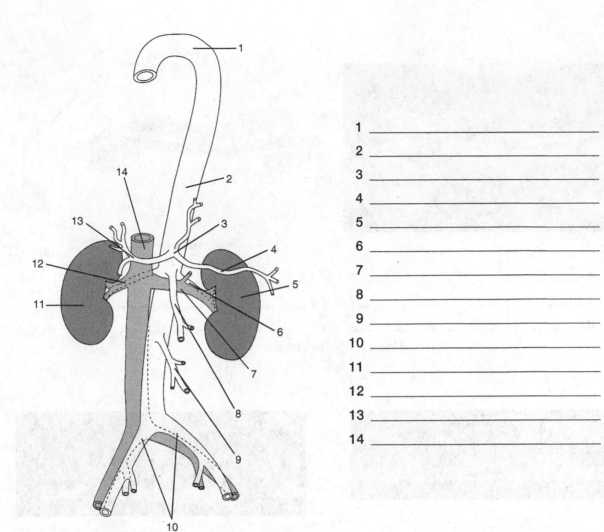

1 _____
2 _____
3 _____
4 _____
5 _____
6 _____
7 _____
8 _____
9 _____
10 _____
11 _____
12 _____
13 _____
14 _____

Figure 13-1 in the textbook

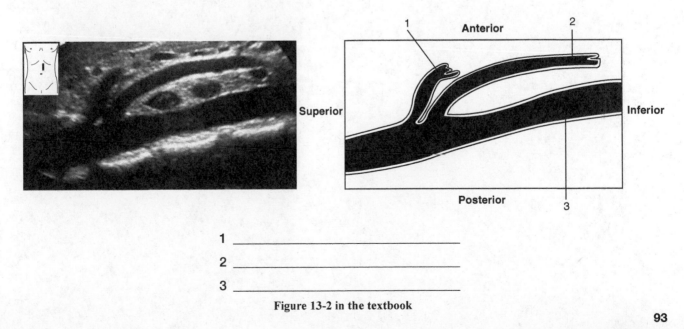

1 _____
2 _____
3 _____

Figure 13-2 in the textbook

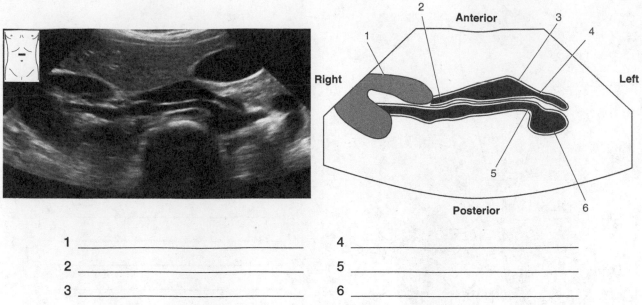

Right

Anterior

Left

Posterior

1 _____	4 _____
2 _____	5 _____
3 _____	6 _____

Figure 13-3 in the textbook

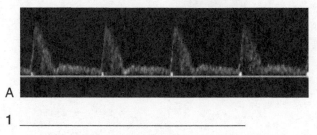

A

1 _____

Figure 13-5A in the textbook

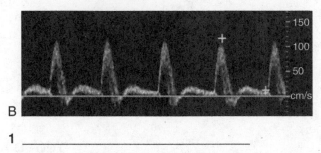

B

1 _____

Figure 13-5B in the textbook

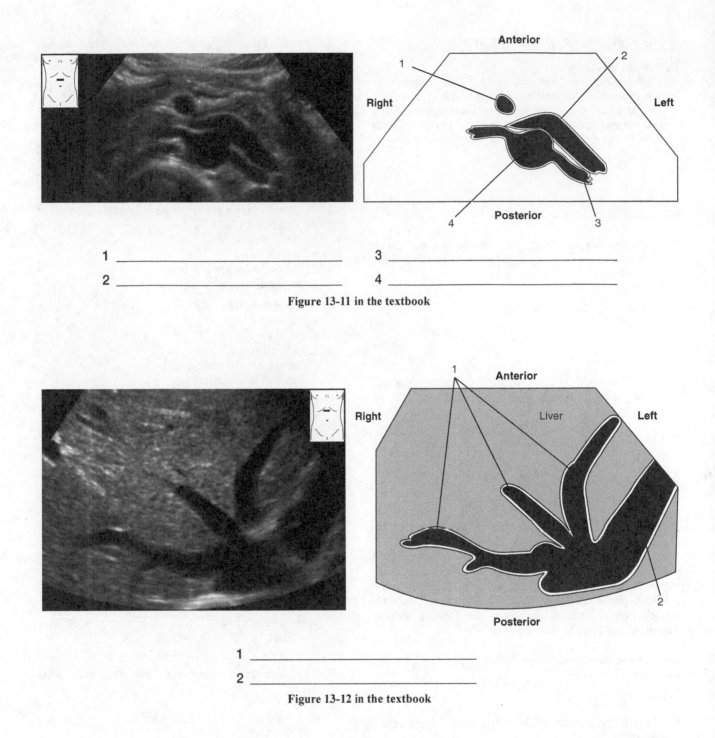

1 _____ 3 _____

2 _____ 4 _____

Figure 13-11 in the textbook

1 _____

2 _____

Figure 13-12 in the textbook

V. CHAPTER SUBHEADINGS EXERCISE

Directions to students:

1. Convert each chapter subheading into a question; for example, change "Sonographic Appearance" to "What is the sonographic appearance of the arterial and venous vessels?" Briefly write the answer to each question in a short paragraph in your notebook.

2. Exchange answers with your lab partner and check each other's work. Refer back to the textbook for further information and explanation.

3. What questions do you still have about the chapter? Write your questions in your notebook.

VI. CHAPTER EVALUATION EXERCISE

Directions to students: Use a fresh sheet of notebook paper. Based on your work with the chapter and its accompanying laboratory assignments, identify three concepts you believe are the most important. You may draw from any of the assignments you have already completed in the previous pages including learning objectives, anatomy and physiology, images, or chapter subheadings. Include a detailed rationale in your answers.

Answer the questions below. Refer to page 382 for the answers.

Multiple Choice

1. Which of the following is NOT a branch of the celiac artery?
   a. Splenic artery
   b. Gastroduodenal artery
   c. Common hepatic artery
   d. Left gastric artery

2. The low resistance Doppler spectral waveform pattern associated with the proximal abdominal aorta reflects
   a. the flow demands of the organs supplied by the aortic branches.
   b. the variations in intraabdominal pressure associated with respiration.
   c. changes in right atrial and ventricular contractions and compliance.
   d. difference in diameter of the aortic branches compared to the aortic diameter.

3. The abdominal aorta is bordered anteriorly by all of the following EXCEPT the
   a. celiac axis.
   b. splenic vein.
   c. inferior mesenteric artery.
   d. superior mesenteric artery.

4. In the fasting state, the _____ is a high resistance vessel.
   a. renal artery
   b. celiac artery
   c. superior mesenteric artery
   d. proper hepatic artery

5. Organs with high metabolic demands are normally supplied by arteries with
   a. low diastolic flow.
   b. reversed diastolic flow.
   c. phasic diastolic flow
   d. high diastolic flow.

6. The peak systolic velocity in the abdominal aorta averages
   a. 30-60 cm/s.
   b. 40-100 cm/s.
   c. 60-120 cm/s.
   d. 80-140 cm/s.

7. The superior mesenteric artery supplies blood to the
   a. caudate lobe.
   b. transverse colon.
   c. spleen.
   d. rectum.

8. The diameter of the normal adult abdominal aorta averages
   a. 1.0-1.5 cm.
   b. 2.0-2.5 cm.
   c. 3.0-3.5 cm.
   d. 4.0-4.5 cm.

9. When vascular resistance increases, diastolic flow
   a. decreases.
   b. reverses.
   c. does not change.
   d. goes to zero.

10. The caudate lobe of the liver is drained by the
    a. inferior vena cava.
    b. right hepatic vein.
    c. middle hepatic vein.
    d. left hepatic vein.

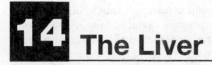

14 The Liver

I. MEMORIZATION EXERCISE

Directions to students: Write the key words in your notebook or on note cards. Write the words on one side of the notepaper and then write the definitions on the opposite side of the page or on the back of the paper. If using note cards, write the key word on the front and the definition on the back. *This step should be completed before the lab session begins.*

Memorize the key word definitions silently for 5 minutes, then work with a lab partner and identify the words you still need help with. List the words here. Add additional rows if needed.

II. COMPREHENSION EXERCISE

Directions to students: Work with a lab partner to complete this exercise. You will need to write in your notebook. First, change each objective into a question.

> *Example: "Describe the location of the liver" becomes "What is the location of the liver?"*

Next, write a short answer to the question just created.

> *Example: "The liver lies in the right hypochondrium. It extends inferiorly to the epigastrium and laterally to the left hypochondrium. Its superior portion reaches the diaphragm."*

Highlight or circle any part of your answers about which you are unsure, and check the answers in your textbook. If you are still unsure of the answers, put a question mark next to the answer(s) for the review session of the lab.

III. APPLICATION OF ANATOMY AND PHYSIOLOGY EXERCISE

Directions to students: Work on the following with your lab partner.
1. In your notebook, draw the liver from memory.

2. Label the liver and its lobes. Include each structure's orientation in the body (either vertical, horizontal, vertical oblique, or horizontal oblique). Ask your lab partner to critique your work. What did you miss? Check your drawing using the sketches in your textbook and complete any missing structures from your drawing.

3. Below your drawing, write two or three summary sentences of the physiology of the liver. Ask your lab partner to check your work. Now check your work against the physiology section in the textbook. What else can you add to your description?

IV. IMAGE ANALYSIS EXERCISE

Directions to students: Work on the following figures with your lab partner. It's your choice! You can label all the sketches at once, then go back and label each image with your lab partner, or label an image and its accompanying sketch at the same time. Either way, the goal is to correctly label all of the sketches and carefully compare the sketch with the sonographic image.

For each sonographic image, write a very brief observation that could be "presented" to your instructor, the clinical sonographer, or the sonologist. Your observation will be based on Chapter 7 in the textbook, which describes how to write a technical observation. Please go back and review that chapter if needed.

For each image, your assessment should include: (1) a view of each major structure (axial or longitudinal; note: these are not the scanning planes) and (2) structures identified in the image with correct sonographic appearance description and measurements if shown (see Chapter 7 in the textbook for information on how to write a technical observation).

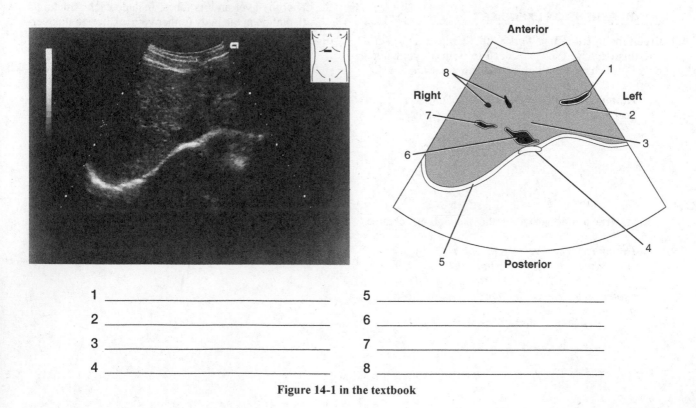

1 _____   5 _____

2 _____   6 _____

3 _____   7 _____

4 _____   8 _____

Figure 14-1 in the textbook

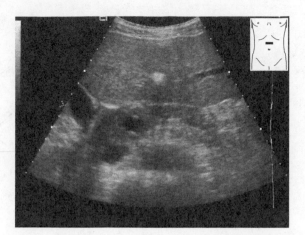

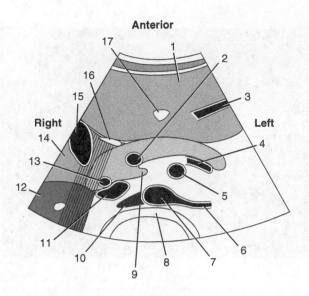

Anterior

17 1

16 2

15 3

Right **Left**

14 4

13

12 5

11 6

10 9 8 7

Posterior

1 _____	10 _____
2 _____	11 _____
3 _____	12 _____
4 _____	13 _____
5 _____	14 _____
6 _____	15 _____
7 _____	16 _____
8 _____	17 _____
9 _____	

Figure 14-5 in the textbook

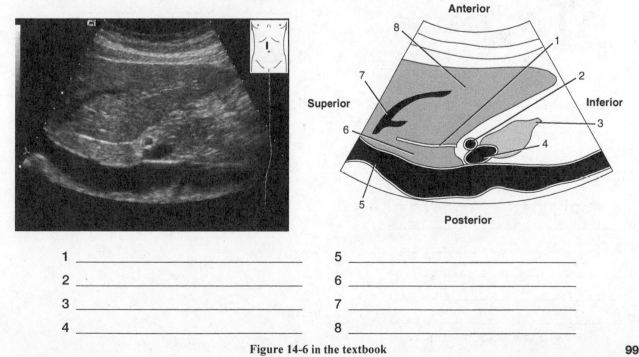

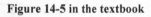

Anterior

8 1

7 2

Superior **Inferior**

6 3

5 4

Posterior

1 _____	5 _____
2 _____	6 _____
3 _____	7 _____
4 _____	8 _____

Figure 14-6 in the textbook

Chapter **14** **The Liver**

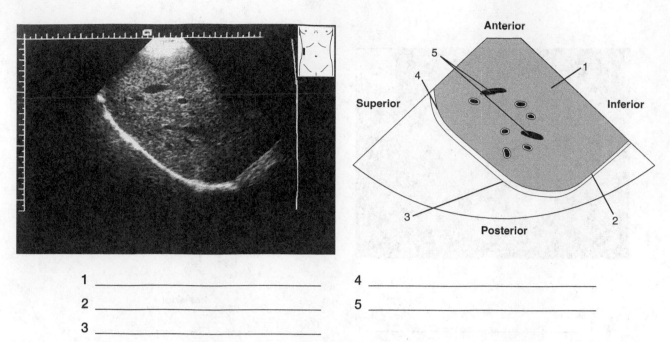

1 _____   4 _____

2 _____   5 _____

3 _____

Figure 14-7 in the textbook

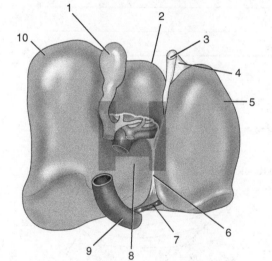

1 _____

2 _____

3 _____

4 _____

5 _____

6 _____

7 _____

8 _____

9 _____

10 _____

Figure 14-8, top, in the textbook

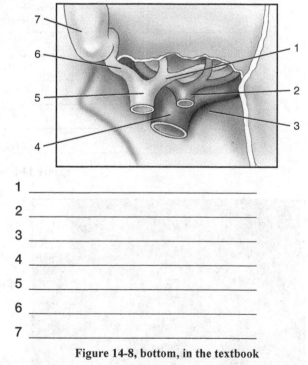

1 _____

2 _____

3 _____

4 _____

5 _____

6 _____

7 _____

Figure 14-8, bottom, in the textbook

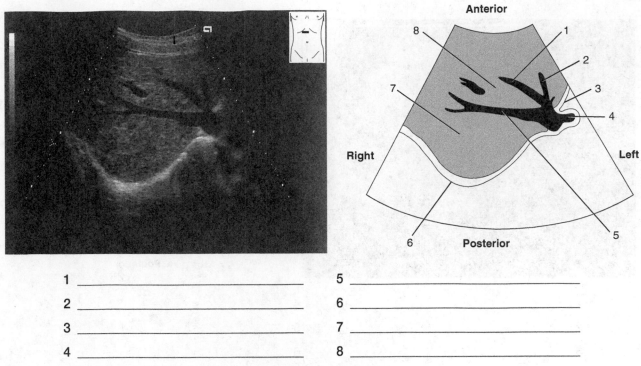

1 _____	5 _____
2 _____	6 _____
3 _____	7 _____
4 _____	8 _____

Figure 14-9 in the textbook

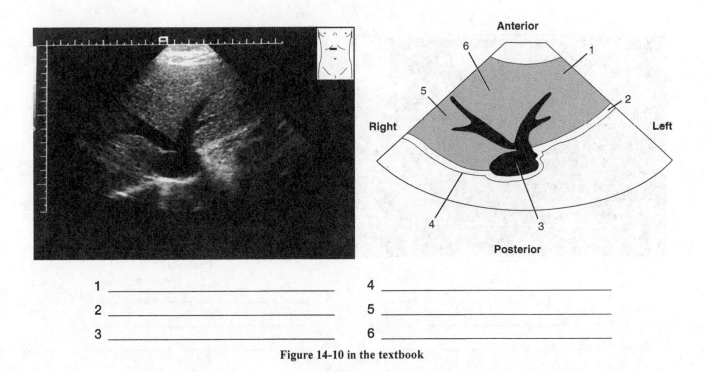

1 _____	4 _____
2 _____	5 _____
3 _____	6 _____

Figure 14-10 in the textbook

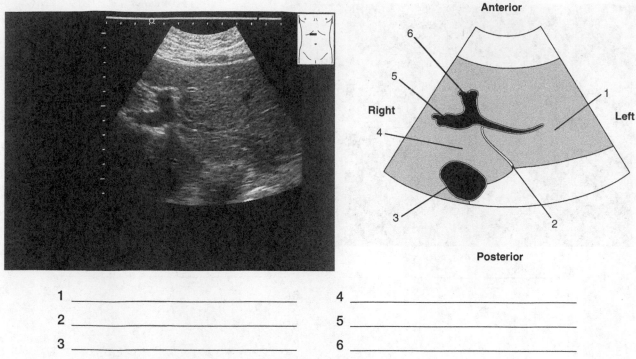

Figure 14-11 in the textbook

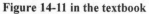

1 _____   4 _____

2 _____   5 _____

3 _____   6 _____

Figure 14-11 in the textbook

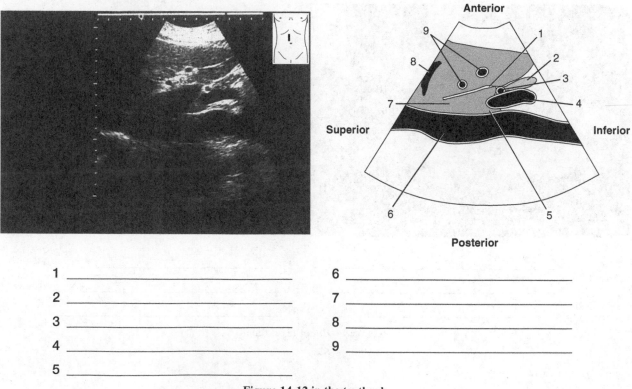

1 _____   6 _____

2 _____   7 _____

3 _____   8 _____

4 _____   9 _____

5 _____

Figure 14-12 in the textbook

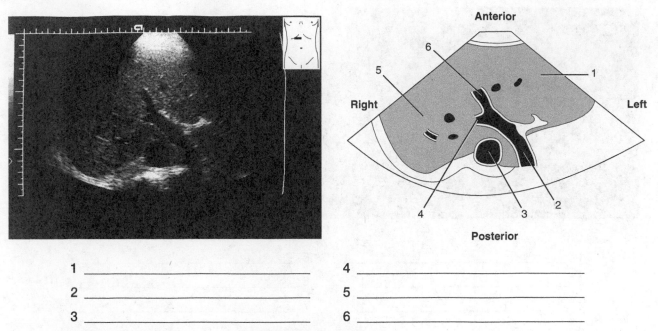

Figure 14-13 in the textbook

1 _____   4 _____
2 _____   5 _____
3 _____   6 _____

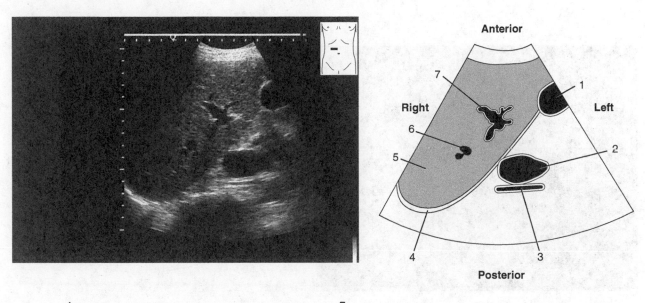

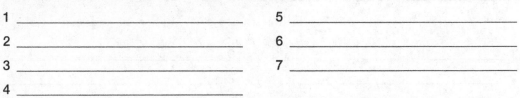

Figure 14-14 in the textbook

1 _____   5 _____
2 _____   6 _____
3 _____   7 _____
4 _____

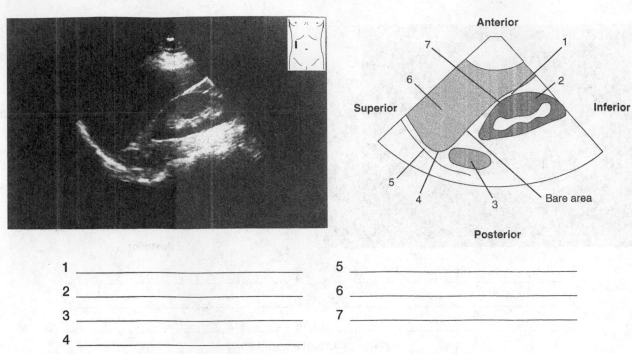

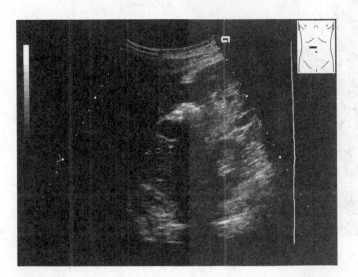

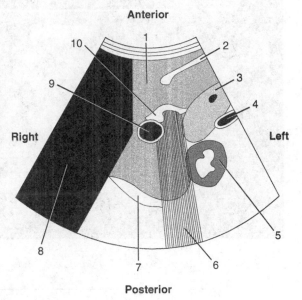

1 _____	5 _____
2 _____	6 _____
3 _____	7 _____
4 _____	

Figure 14-15 in the textbook

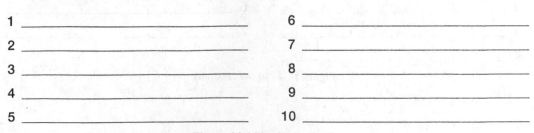

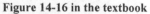

1 _____	6 _____
2 _____	7 _____
3 _____	8 _____
4 _____	9 _____
5 _____	10 _____

Figure 14-16 in the textbook

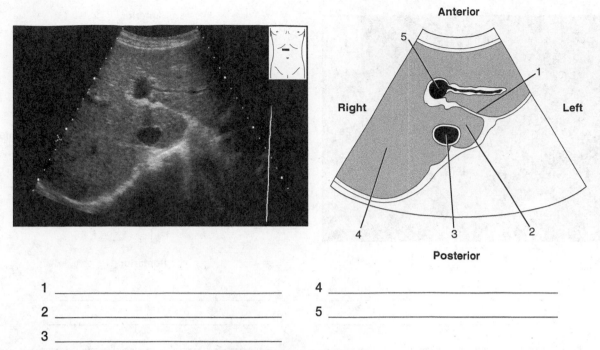

1	_____	4	_____
2	_____	5	_____
3	_____		

Figure 14-17 in the textbook

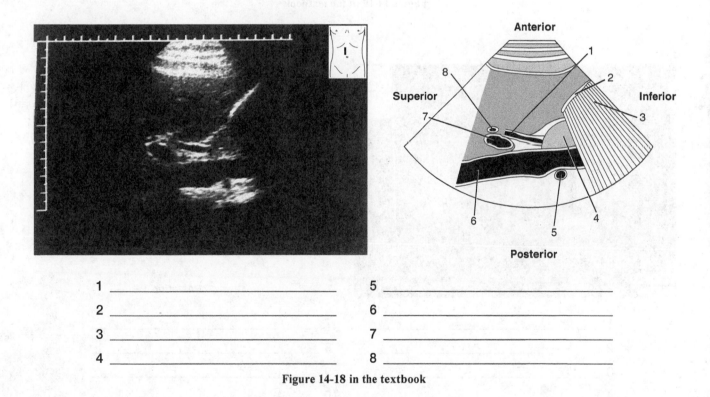

1	_____	5	_____
2	_____	6	_____
3	_____	7	_____
4	_____	8	_____

Figure 14-18 in the textbook

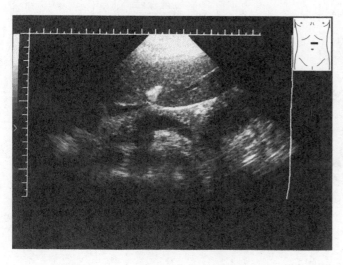

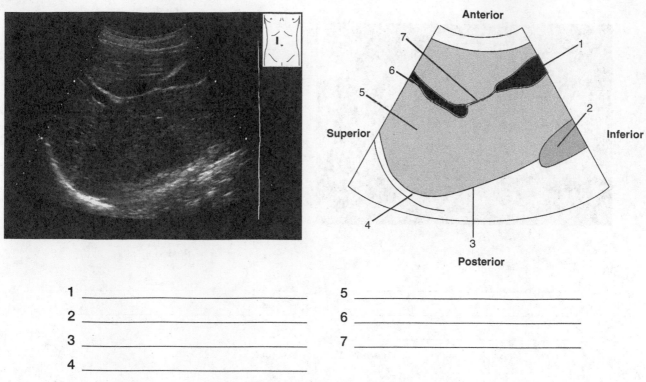

1 _____   5 _____
2 _____   6 _____
3 _____   7 _____
4 _____

Figure 14-19 in the textbook

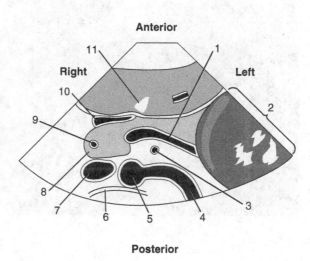

1 _____   7 _____
2 _____   8 _____
3 _____   9 _____
4 _____   10 _____
5 _____   11 _____
6 _____

Figure 14-20 in the textbook

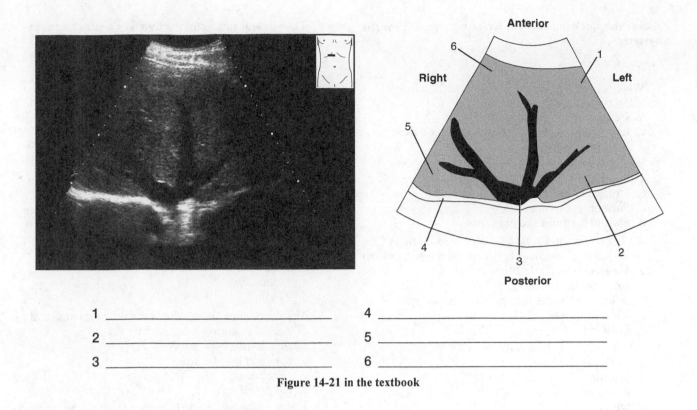

1 _____   4 _____

2 _____   5 _____

3 _____   6 _____

Figure 14-21 in the textbook

V. CHAPTER SUBHEADINGS EXERCISE

Directions to students

1. Convert each chapter subheading into a question; for example, change "Gross Anatomy" to "What is the gross anatomy of the liver?" Briefly write the answer to each question in a short paragraph in your notebook.

2. Exchange answers with your lab partner and check each other's work. Refer back to the textbook for further information and explanation.

3. What questions do you still have about the chapter? Write your questions in your notebook.

VI. CHAPTER EVALUATION EXERCISE

Directions to students: Use a fresh sheet of notebook paper. Based on your work with the chapter and its accompanying laboratory assignments, identify three concepts you believe are the most important. You may draw from any of the assignments you have already completed in the previous pages including learning objectives, anatomy and physiology, images, or chapter subheadings. Include a detailed rationale in your answers.

Answer the questions below. Refer to page 382 for the answers.

Multiple Choice

1. Which is NOT a principal function of the liver?
   a. Storage of nutrients
   b. Detoxification of the body
   c. Regulation of blood volume and blood flow
   d. Storage of bile

2. Which is NOT a metabolic function of the liver?
   a. Synthesis of blood plasma proteins
   b. Storage of minerals and vitamins
   c. Formation of vitamin A
   d. Steroid hormone metabolism

3. An intersegmental boundary observed on transverse plane scans of the liver between the medial and lateral segments of the left lobe is the
   a. coronary ligament.
   b. bifurcation of the common hepatic artery.
   c. left portal vein.
   d. main lobar fissure.

4. Which is NOT a component of bile?
   a. cholesterol
   b. lecithin
   c. bilirubin
   d. blood

5. Cholesterol, a major component of bile secreted by the liver, serves primarily to
   a. thicken sludge.
   b. color bile.
   c. solidify bile salts.
   d. emulsify fats.

6. The visceral surface of the liver is superior and anterior to each of the following EXCEPT
   a. the gallbladder.
   b. the right costal margin of the liver.
   c. the right hepatic flexure of colon.
   d. the pyloric canal.

7. Riedel's lobe is most accurately described as a liver extension found in the
   a. right lobe.
   b. quadrate lobe.
   c. caudate lobe.
   d. left lobe.

8. On longitudinal sections, the liver is said to measure _____ along the midclavicular line in its normal state.
   a. 20 cm
   b. 5 cm
   c. 13 cm
   d. 25 mm

9. The vasculature of the liver includes branches of all of the following vessels EXCEPT the
   a. right hypogastric artery.
   b. common hepatic artery.
   c. celiac artery.
   d. left portal vein.

10. Which structure forms the boundary of the bare area of the liver?
    a. left coronary ligament
    b. fissure for the ligamentum venosum
    c. falciform ligament
    d. right triangular ligament

15 The Biliary System

I. MEMORIZATION EXERCISE

Directions to students: Write the key words in your notebook or on note cards. Write the words on one side of the notepaper and then write the definitions on the opposite side of the page or on the back of the paper. If using note cards, write the key word on the front and the definition on the back. *This step should be completed before the lab session begins.*

Memorize the key word definitions silently for 5 minutes, then work with a lab partner and identify the words you still need help with. List the words here. Add additional rows if needed.

II. COMPREHENSION EXERCISE

Directions to students: Work with a lab partner to complete this exercise. You will need to write in your notebook. First, change each objective into a question.

> *Example: "Describe the basic function of the biliary system" becomes "What is the basic function of the biliary system?"*

Next, write a short answer to the question just created.

> *Example: "The biliary system conveys bile, manufactured in the liver, from the liver to the gallbladder for storage. The hormone cholecystokinin stimulates release of the bile from the gallbladder to the duodenum. Bile is transported to the duodenum via the common bile duct and enters the duodenum through the sphincter of Oddi. The purpose of bile is to help break down fats in the duodenum, aiding digestion."*

Highlight or circle any part of your answers about which you are unsure, and check the answers in your textbook. If you are still unsure of the answers, put a question mark next to the answer(s) for the review session of the lab.

III. APPLICATION OF ANATOMY AND PHYSIOLOGY EXERCISE

Directions to students: Work on the following with your lab partner.

1. In your notebook, draw as much of the biliary system as you can from memory.

2. Label the biliary system. Include each structure's orientation in the body (either vertical, horizontal, vertical oblique, or horizontal oblique). Ask your lab partner to critique your work. What did you miss? Check your drawing using the sketches in your textbook and complete any missing structures from your drawing.

3. Below your drawing, write two or three summary sentences of the physiology of the liver. Ask your lab partner to check your work. Now check your work against the physiology section in the textbook. What else can you add to your description?

IV. IMAGE ANALYSIS EXERCISE

Directions to students: Work on the following figures with your lab partner. It's your choice! You can label all the sketches at once, then go back and label each image with your lab partner, or label an image and its accompanying sketch at the same time. Either way, the goal is to correctly label all of the sketches and carefully compare the sketch with the sonographic image.

For each sonographic image, write a very brief observation that could be "presented" to your instructor, the clinical sonographer, or the sonologist. Your observation will be based on Chapter 7 in the textbook, which describes how to write a technical observation. Please go back and review that chapter if needed.

For each image, your assessment should include: (1) the view of each major structure (axial or longitudinal; note: these are not the scanning planes) and (2) structures identified in the image with correct sonographic appearance description and measurements if shown (see Chapter 7 in the textbook for information on how to write a technical observation).

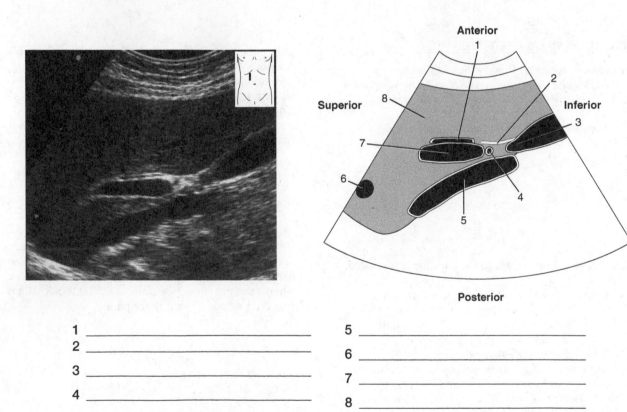

1 _____   5 _____
2 _____   6 _____
3 _____   7 _____
4 _____   8 _____

Figure 15-1 in the textbook

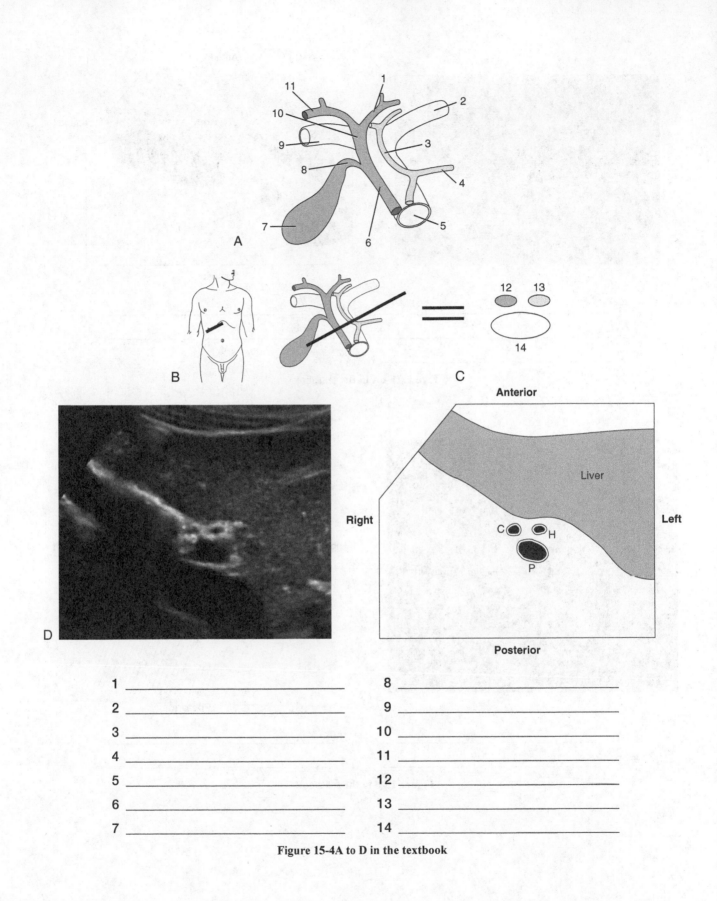

Figure 15-4A to D in the textbook

1 _____   8 _____

2 _____   9 _____

3 _____   10 _____

4 _____   11 _____

5 _____   12 _____

6 _____   13 _____

7 _____   14 _____

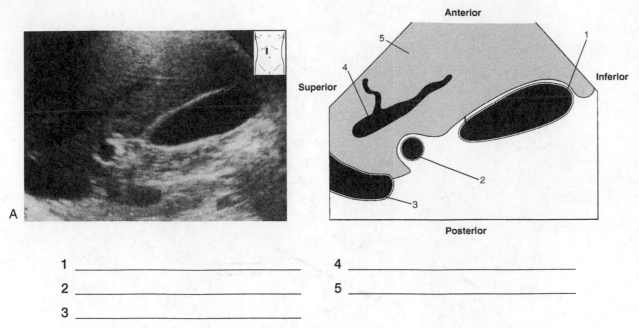

1	_____	4	_____
2	_____	5	_____
3	_____		

Figure 15-6A in the textbook

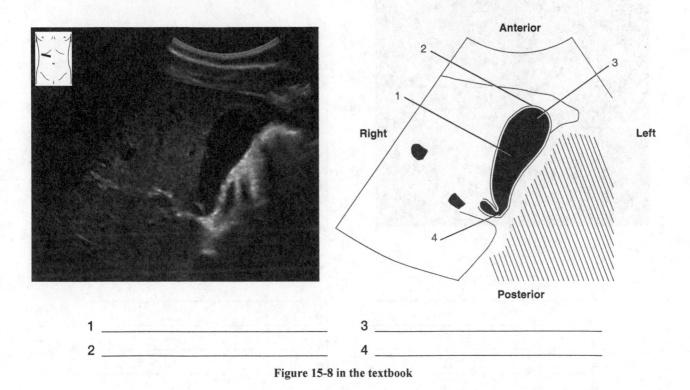

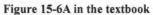

1	_____	3	_____
2	_____	4	_____

Figure 15-8 in the textbook

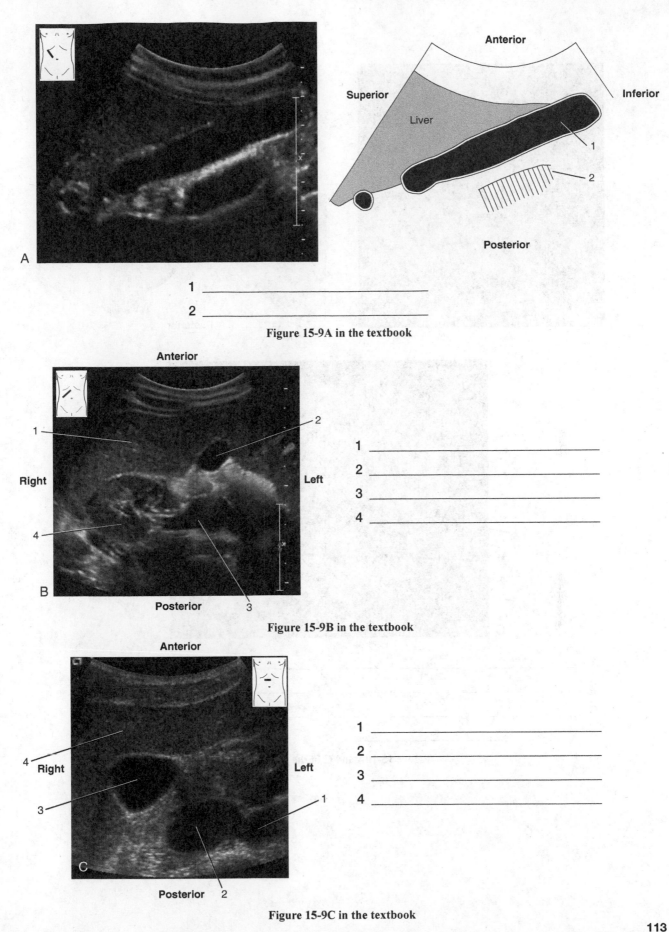

1 _____
2 _____

Figure 15-9A in the textbook

1 _____
2 _____
3 _____
4 _____

Figure 15-9B in the textbook

1 _____
2 _____
3 _____
4 _____

Figure 15-9C in the textbook

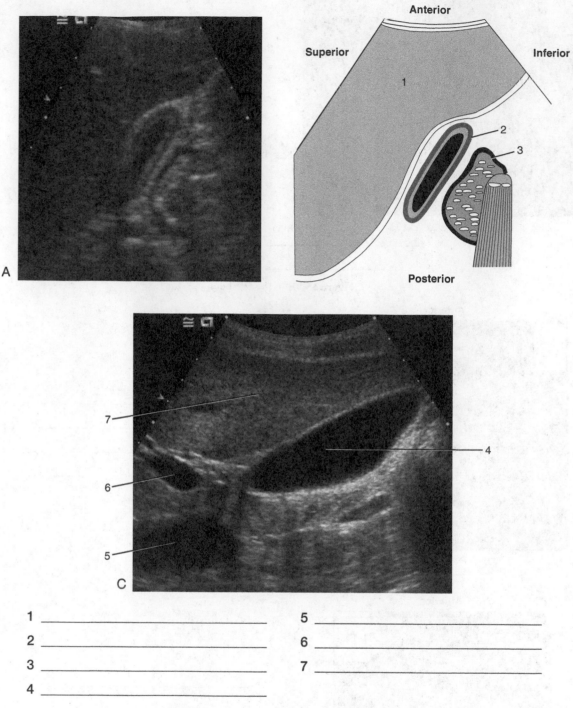

Label	
Anterior	
Superior	Inferior
1	
2	
3	
Posterior	

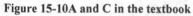

1 _____   5 _____

2 _____   6 _____

3 _____   7 _____

4 _____

Figure 15-10A and C in the textbook

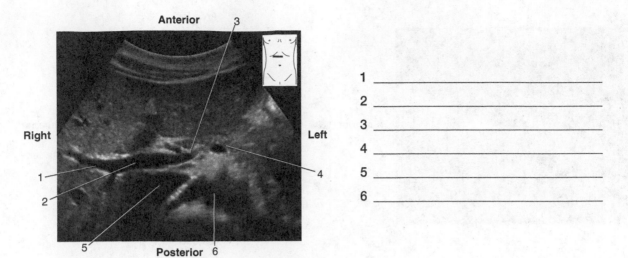

Anterior

Right   Left

1 _____
2 _____
3 _____

1 _____
2 _____
3 _____
4 _____
5 _____
6 _____

Posterior   6

Figure 15-12 in the textbook

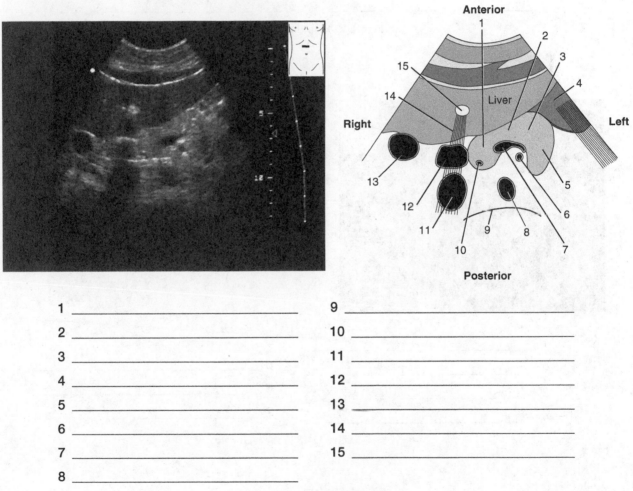

Anterior

Right   Liver   Left

Posterior

1 _____   9 _____
2 _____   10 _____
3 _____   11 _____
4 _____   12 _____
5 _____   13 _____
6 _____   14 _____
7 _____   15 _____
8 _____

Figure 15-13 in the textbook

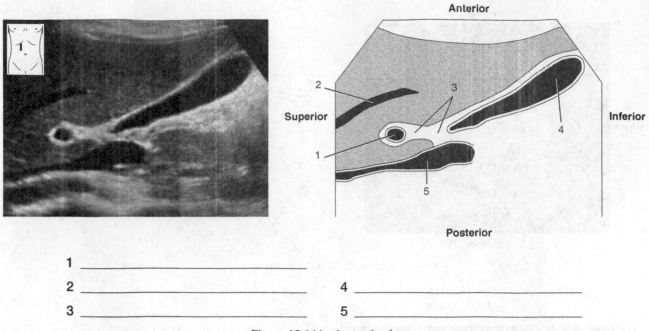

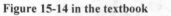

1 _____

2 _____   4 _____

3 _____   5 _____

Figure 15-14 in the textbook

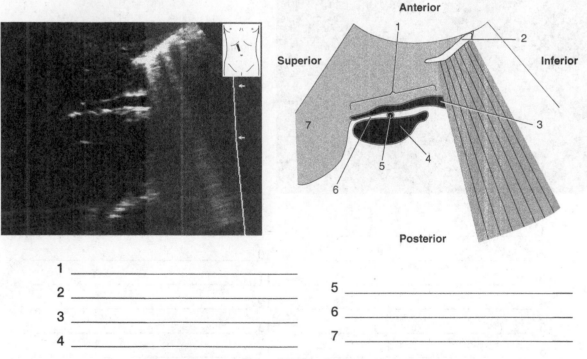

1 _____

2 _____

3 _____   5 _____

4 _____   6 _____

                                             7 _____

Figure 15-18 in the textbook

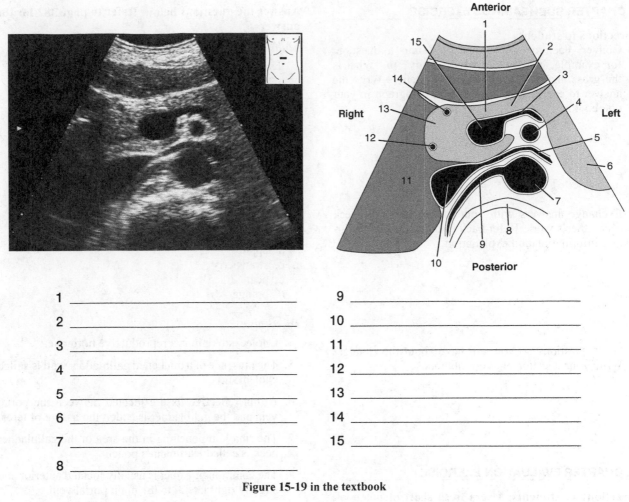

1	_____	9	_____
2	_____	10	_____
3	_____	11	_____
4	_____	12	_____
5	_____	13	_____
6	_____	14	_____
7	_____	15	_____
8	_____		

Figure 15-19 in the textbook

V. CHAPTER SUBHEADINGS EXERCISE

Directions to students

1. Convert each chapter subheading into a question; for example, change "Gross Anatomy" to "What is the gross anatomy of the biliary system?" Write the answer to each question in a short paragraph in your notebook.

2. Exchange answers with your lab partner and check each other's work. Refer back to the textbook for further information and explanation.

3. What questions do you still have about the chapter? Write your questions in your notebook.

VI. CHAPTER EVALUATION EXERCISE

Directions to students: Use a fresh sheet of notebook paper. Based on your work with the chapter and its accompanying laboratory assignments, identify three concepts you believe are the most important. You may draw from any of the assignments you have already completed in the previous pages including learning objectives, anatomy and physiology, images, or chapter subheadings. Include a detailed rationale in your answers.

Answer the questions below. Refer to page 382 for the answers.

Multiple Choice

1. The _____ supplies the gallbladder and liver.
   a. celiac artery
   b. proper hepatic artery
   c. splenic artery
   d. common hepatic artery

2. The latin word *porta* means _____.
   a. gallbladder
   b. liver
   c. duct
   d. gateway

3. The shape of the gallbladder resembles the shape of a(n) _____.
   a. apple
   b. strawberry
   c. pear
   d. orange

True/False

4. Cholecystokinin is a reproductive hormone.

5. The presence of a thickened gallbladder wall is called cholecystitis.

6. A thin reflective fissure located between the portal vein and the gallbladder is called the fissure of teres.

7. The small outpouching in the area of the gallbladder neck is called Hartmann's pouch.

8. The common bile duct is usually located anterior and slightly right lateral to the main portal vein.

9. The abbreviation LLD is known as left lateral deep.

10. The abbreviation LFT means liver function test.

16 The Pancreas

I. MEMORIZATION EXERCISE

Directions to students: Write the key words in your notebook or on note cards. Write the words on one side of the notepaper and then write the definitions on the opposite side of the page or on the back of the paper. If using note cards, write the key word on the front and the definition on the back. *This step should be completed before the lab session begins.*

Memorize the key word definitions silently for 5 minutes, then work with a lab partner and identify the words you still need help with. List the words here. Add additional rows if needed.

II. COMPREHENSION EXERCISE

Directions to students: Work with a lab partner to complete this exercise. You will need to write in your notebook. First, change each objective into a question.

> *Example: "Describe the basic function of the pancreas" becomes "What is the basic function of the pancreas?"*

Next, write a short answer to the question just created.

> *Example: "The pancreas is an endocrine and exocrine organ. Only 2% of the gland's weight is for its endocrine function. The endocrine function is to produce insulin, glucagon, and somatostatin to regulate blood glucose. The exocrine function is to produce pancreatic juice, a substance that helps digest fats, proteins, carbohydrates, and nucleic acids."*

Highlight or circle any part of your answers about which you are unsure, and check the answers in your textbook. If you are still unsure of the answers, put a question mark next to the answer(s) for the review session of the lab.

III. APPLICATION OF ANATOMY AND PHYSIOLOGY EXERCISE

Directions to students: Work on the following with your lab partner.
1. In your notebook, draw the pancreas and as much of the surrounding vasculature as you can from memory.

2. Label the pancreas and the surrounding vasculature. Include each structure's orientation in the body (either vertical, horizontal, vertical oblique, or horizontal oblique). Ask your lab partner to critique your work. What did you miss? Check your drawing using the sketches in your textbook and complete any missing structures from your drawing.

3. Below your drawing, write two or three summary sentences of the physiology of the pancreas. Ask your lab partner to check your work. Now check your work against the physiology section in the textbook. What else can you add to your description?

IV. IMAGE ANALYSIS EXERCISE

Directions to students: Work on the following figures with your lab partner. It's your choice! You can label all the sketches at once, then go back and label each image with your lab partner, or label an image and its accompanying sketch at the same time. Either way, the goal is to correctly label all of the sketches and carefully compare the sketch with the sonographic image.

For each sonographic image, write a very brief observation that could be "presented" to your instructor, the clinical sonographer, or the sonologist. Your observation will be based on Chapter 7 in the textbook, which describes how to write a technical observation. Please go back and review that chapter if needed.

For each image, your assessment should include: (1) the view of each major structure (axial or longitudinal; note: these are not the scanning planes) and (2) structures identified in the image with correct sonographic appearance description and measurements if shown (see Chapter 7 in the textbook for information on how to write a technical observation).

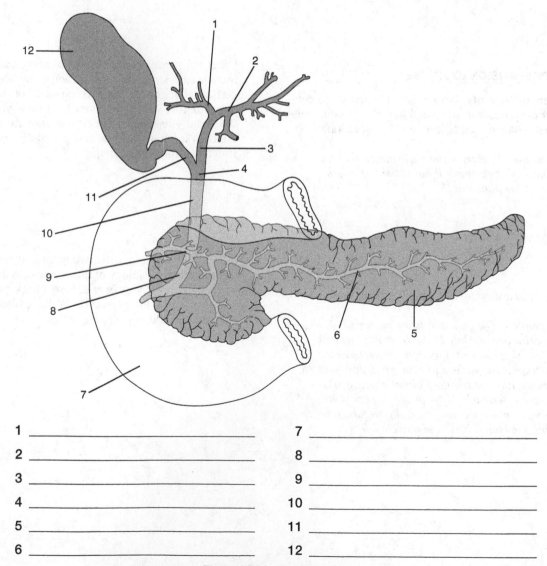

1 _____   7 _____

2 _____   8 _____

3 _____   9 _____

4 _____   10 _____

5 _____   11 _____

6 _____   12 _____

Figure 16-1 in the textbook

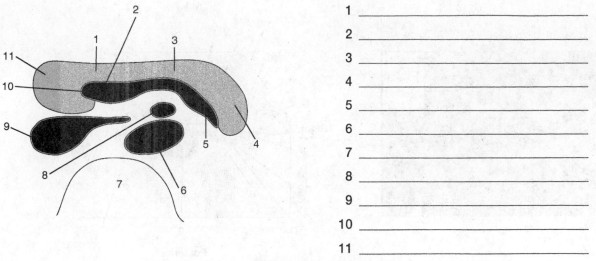

1	_____
2	_____
3	_____
4	_____
5	_____
6	_____
7	_____
8	_____
9	_____
10	_____
11	_____

Figure 16-2 in the textbook

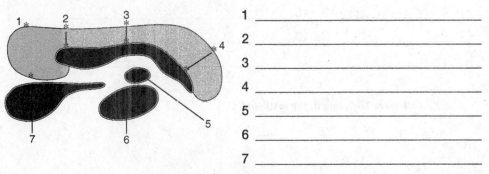

1	_____
2	_____
3	_____
4	_____
5	_____
6	_____
7	_____

Figure 16-3 in the textbook

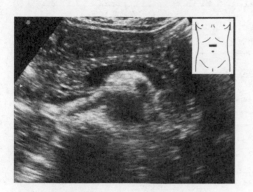

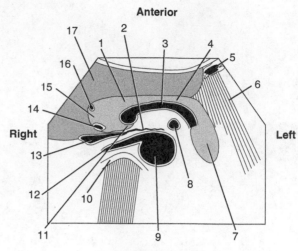

Anterior

17 2
16 1   3   4
15   5
14   6
Right   Left
13
12
11   10   9   8   7

Posterior

1 _____   10 _____
2 _____   11 _____
3 _____   12 _____
4 _____   13 _____
5 _____   14 _____
6 _____   15 _____
7 _____   16 _____
8 _____   17 _____
9 _____

Figure 16-7, top, in the textbook

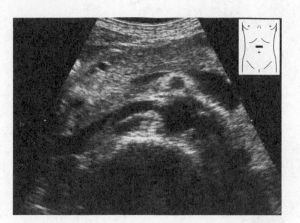

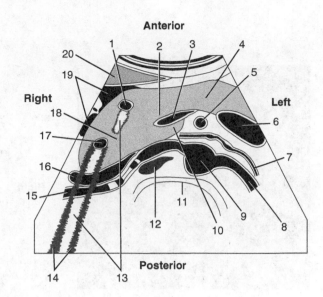

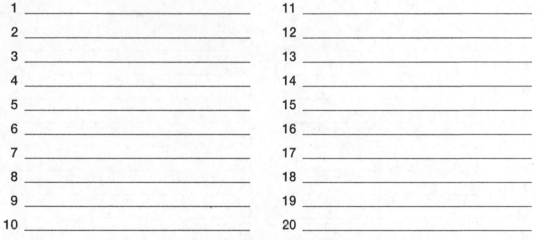

1 _____	11 _____
2 _____	12 _____
3 _____	13 _____
4 _____	14 _____
5 _____	15 _____
6 _____	16 _____
7 _____	17 _____
8 _____	18 _____
9 _____	19 _____
10 _____	20 _____

Figure 16-7, middle, in the textbook

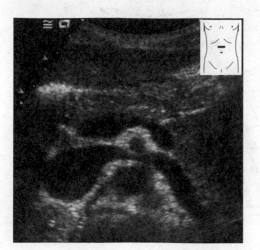

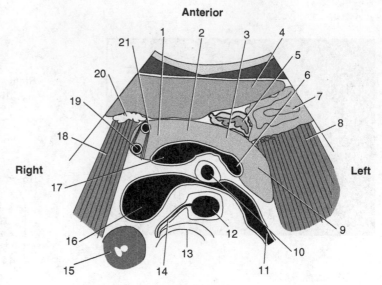

1 _____   12 _____

2 _____   13 _____

3 _____   14 _____

4 _____   15 _____

5 _____   16 _____

6 _____   17 _____

7 _____   18 _____

8 _____   19 _____

9 _____   20 _____

10 _____   21 _____

11 _____

Figure 16-7, bottom, in the textbook

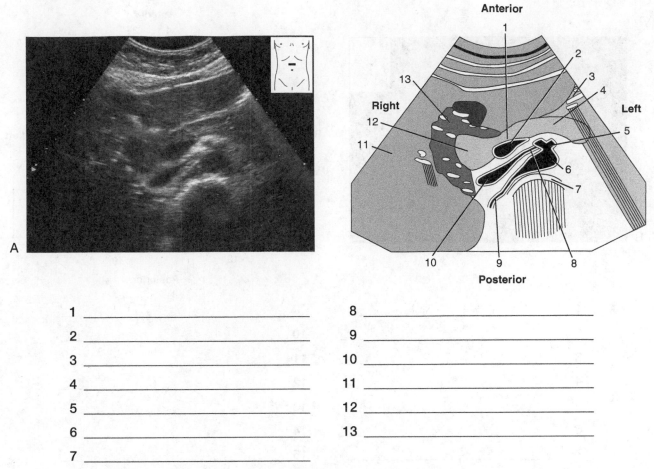

Figure 16-8A in the textbook

1 _____

2 _____

3 _____

4 _____

5 _____

6 _____

7 _____

8 _____

9 _____

10 _____

11 _____

12 _____

13 _____

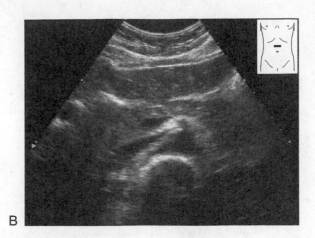

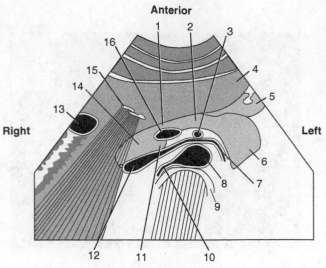

Anterior

Right

Left

Posterior

1 _____   9 _____
2 _____   10 _____
3 _____   11 _____
4 _____   12 _____
5 _____   13 _____
6 _____   14 _____
7 _____   15 _____
8 _____   16 _____

Figure 16-8B in the textbook

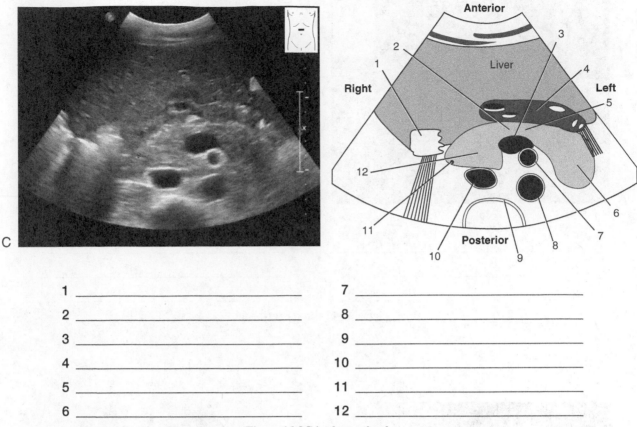

1	_____	7	_____
2	_____	8	_____
3	_____	9	_____
4	_____	10	_____
5	_____	11	_____
6	_____	12	_____

Figure 16-8C in the textbook

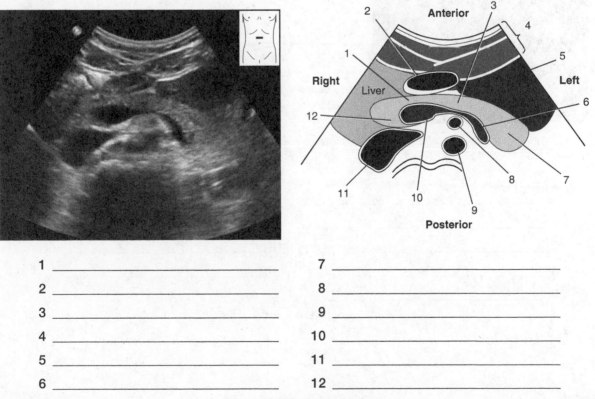

1	_____	7	_____
2	_____	8	_____
3	_____	9	_____
4	_____	10	_____
5	_____	11	_____
6	_____	12	_____

Figure 16-11 in the textbook

Chapter **16** **The Pancreas**

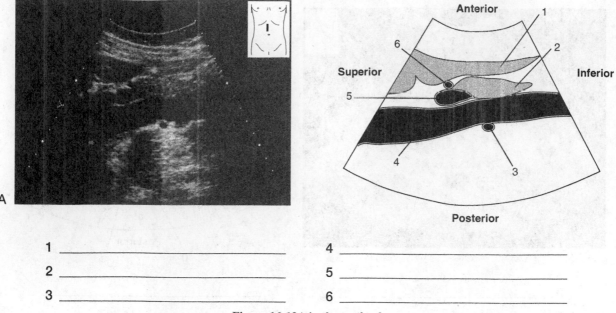

1	_____	4	_____
2	_____	5	_____
3	_____	6	_____

Figure 16-12A in the textbook

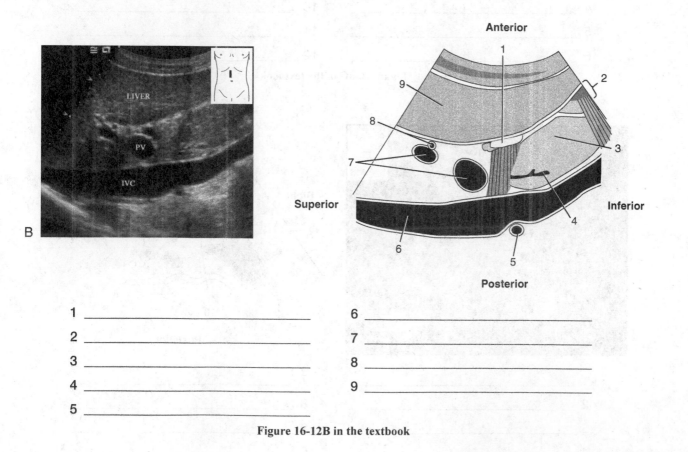

1	_____	6	_____
2	_____	7	_____
3	_____	8	_____
4	_____	9	_____
5	_____		

Figure 16-12B in the textbook

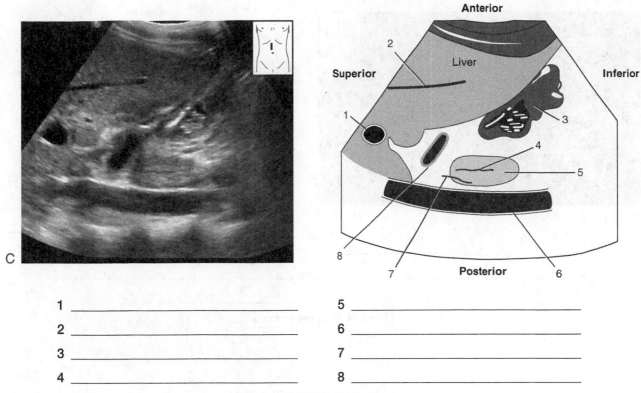

1 _____	5 _____
2 _____	6 _____
3 _____	7 _____
4 _____	8 _____

Figure 16-12C in the textbook

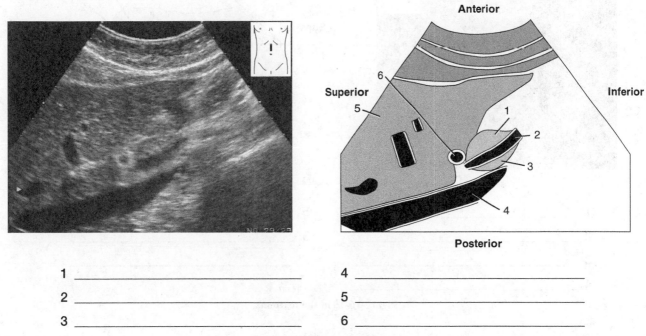

1 _____	4 _____
2 _____	5 _____
3 _____	6 _____

Figure 16-13 in the textbook

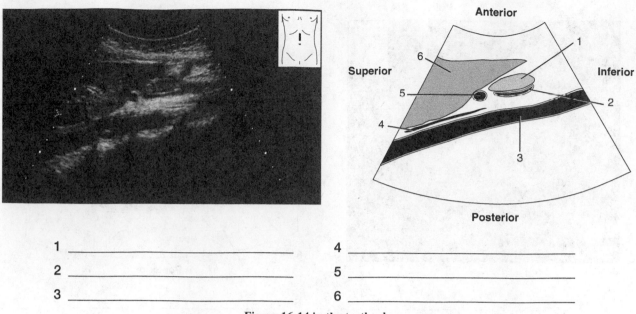

1 _____ 4 _____

2 _____ 5 _____

3 _____ 6 _____

Figure 16-14 in the textbook

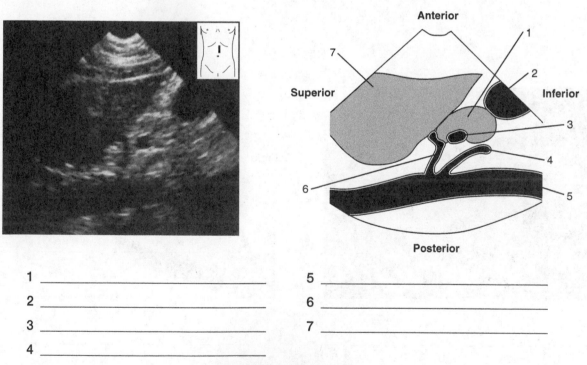

1 _____ 5 _____

2 _____ 6 _____

3 _____ 7 _____

4 _____

Figure 16-15 in the textbook

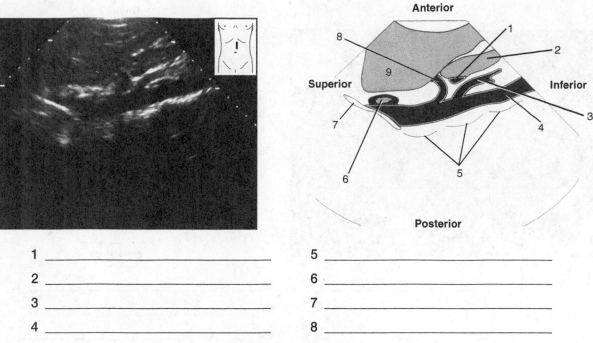

1	_____	5	_____
2	_____	6	_____
3	_____	7	_____
4	_____	8	_____

Figure 16-16 in the textbook

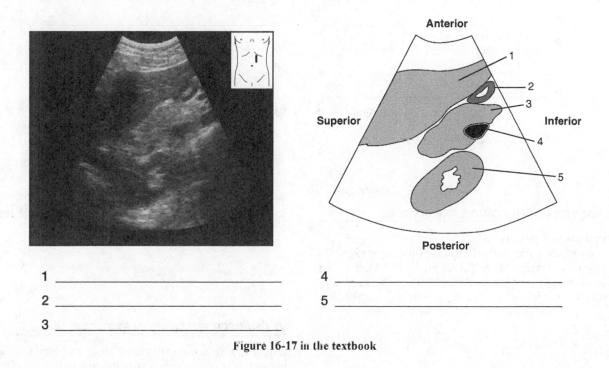

1	_____	4	_____
2	_____	5	_____
3	_____		

Figure 16-17 in the textbook

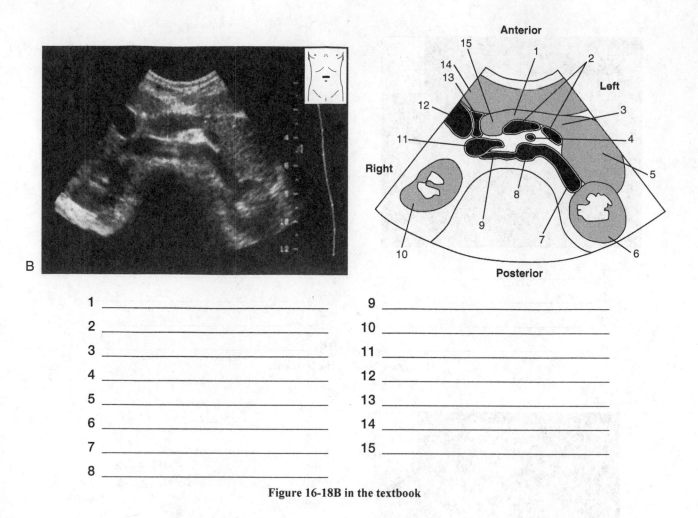

1 _____	9 _____	
2 _____	10 _____	
3 _____	11 _____	
4 _____	12 _____	
5 _____	13 _____	
6 _____	14 _____	
7 _____	15 _____	
8 _____		

Figure 16-18B in the textbook

V. CHAPTER SUBHEADINGS EXERCISE

Directions to students

1. Convert each chapter subheading into a question; for example, change "Gross Anatomy" to "What is the gross anatomy of the pancreas?" Write the answer to each question in a short paragraph in your notebook.

2. Exchange answers with your lab partner and check each other's work. Refer back to the textbook for further information and explanation.

3. What questions do you still have about the chapter? Write your questions in your notebook.

VI. CHAPTER EVALUATION EXERCISE

Directions to students: Use a fresh sheet of notebook paper. Based on your work with the chapter and its accompanying laboratory assignments, identify three concepts you believe are the most important. You may draw from any of the assignments you have already completed in the previous pages including learning objectives, anatomy and physiology, images, or chapter subheadings. Include a detailed rationale in your answers.

Answer the questions below. Refer to page 382 for the answers.

Multiple Choice

1. The pancreas is shaped like the upside down letter
   a. H.
   b. N.
   c. U.
   d. C.

2. Which structures are posterior to the pancreas?
   a. Inferior Vena Cava (IVC), stomach, transverse colon
   b. IVC, diaphragm, Aorta (AO)
   c. AO, stomach, duodenum
   d. Duodenum, connective prevertebral tissue, diaphragm

3. Which of the following structures enter the duodenum?
   a. Common bile duct, accessory pancreatic duct, duct of Wirsung
   b. Common bile duct, common hepatic duct, accessory pancreatic duct
   c. Common hepatic duct, cystic duct, main pancreatic duct
   d. Celiac duct, common hepatic duct, common bile duct

4. The body of the pancreas can best be described as lying anterior to
   a. Superior Mesenteric Artery (SMA), Splenic Vein (SV), AO.
   b. SMA, SV, IVC.
   c. IMA, Common Bile Duct (CBD), AO.
   d. Inferior Mesenteric Artery (IMA), SV, IVC.

5. The tail of the pancreas can best be described as is medial to the
   a. stomach.
   b. left kidney.
   c. splenic artery.
   d. splenic hilum.

Completion

Indicate the measurements of each of the following structures:

6. Anteroposterior measurement of pancreatic head _____

7. Anteroposterior measurement of pancreatic neck _____

8. Anteroposterior measurement of pancreatic body _____

9. Anteroposterior measurement of pancreatic tail _____

10. Total length of the pancreas _____

The Urinary and Adrenal Systems 17

I. MEMORIZATION EXERCISE

Directions to Students: Write the key words in your notebook or on note cards. Write the words on one side of the notepaper and then write the definitions on the opposite side of the page or on the back of the paper. If using note cards, write the key word on the front and the definition on the back. *This step should be completed before the lab session begins.*

Memorize the key word definitions silently for 5 minutes, then work with a lab partner and identify the words you still need help with. List the words here. Add additional rows if needed.

II. COMPREHENSION EXERCISE

Directions to Students: Work with a lab partner to complete this exercise. You will need to write in your notebook. First, change each objective into a question.

> *Example: "Explain the function of the nephron" becomes "What is the function of the nephron?"*

Next, write a short answer to the question just created.

> *Example: "The nephron moves products from areas of high to low concentration by osmosis and active transport. It consists of Bowman's capsule, glomerulus, afferent and efferent arterioles, proximal and distal convoluted tubules, and collecting duct."*

Highlight or circle any part of your answers about which you are unsure, and check the answers in your textbook. If you are still unsure of the answers, put a question mark next to the answer(s) for the review session of the lab.

III. APPLICATION OF ANATOMY AND PHYSIOLOGY EXERCISE

Directions to Students: Work on the following with your lab partner.

1. In your notebook, draw the kidney and as much vasculature as you can from memory.

2. Label the kidney and its vasculature. Include each structure's orientation in the body (either vertical, horizontal, vertical oblique, or horizontal oblique). Ask your lab partner to critique your work. What did you miss? Check your drawing using the sketches in your textbook and complete any missing structures from your drawing.

3. Below your drawing, write two or three summary sentences of the physiology of the urinary and adrenal systems. Ask your lab partner to check your work. Now check your work against the physiology section in the textbook. What else can you add to your description?

IV. IMAGE ANALYSIS EXERCISE

Directions to Students: Work on the following figures with your lab partner. It's your choice! You can label all the sketches at once, then go back and label each image with your lab partner, or label an image and its accompanying sketch at the same time. Either way, the goal is to correctly label all of the sketches and carefully compare the sketch with the sonographic image.

For each image, your assessment should include: (1) the view of each major structure (axial or longitudinal; note: these are not the scanning planes) and (2) structures identified in the image with the correct sonographic appearance, description, and measurements if shown (see Chapter 7 in the textbook for information on how to write a technical observation).

For each sonographic image, write a very brief observation that could be "presented" to your instructor, the clinical sonographer, or the sonologist. Your observation will be based on Chapter 7 in the textbook, which describes how to write a technical observation. Please go back and review that chapter if needed.

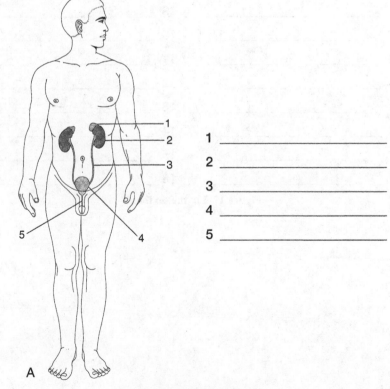

1 _____

2 _____

3 _____

4 _____

5 _____

Figure 17-1A in the textbook

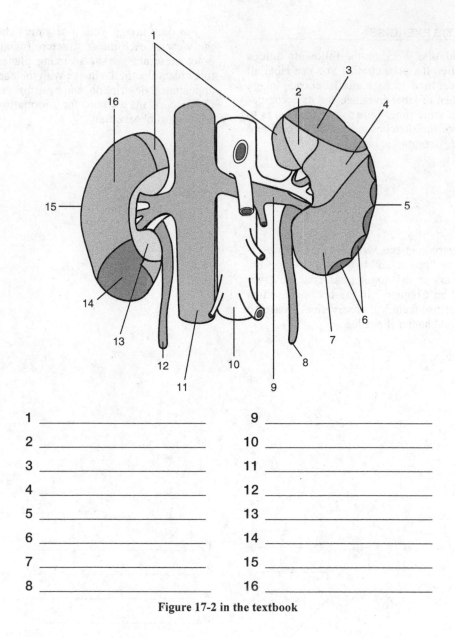

Figure 17-2 in the textbook

1 _____   9 _____

2 _____   10 _____

3 _____   11 _____

4 _____   12 _____

5 _____   13 _____

6 _____   14 _____

7 _____   15 _____

8 _____   16 _____

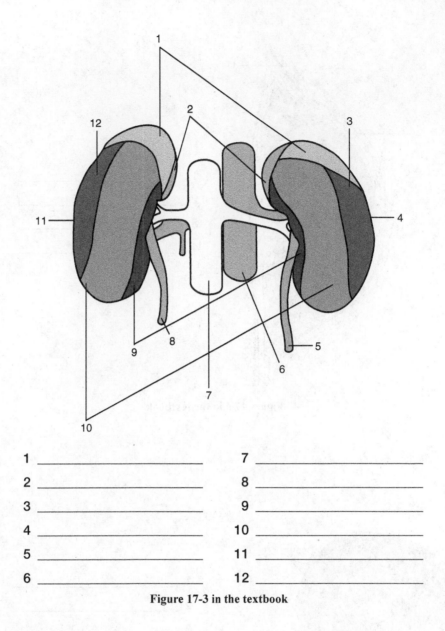

Figure 17-3 in the textbook

1	_____	7	_____
2	_____	8	_____
3	_____	9	_____
4	_____	10	_____
5	_____	11	_____
6	_____	12	_____

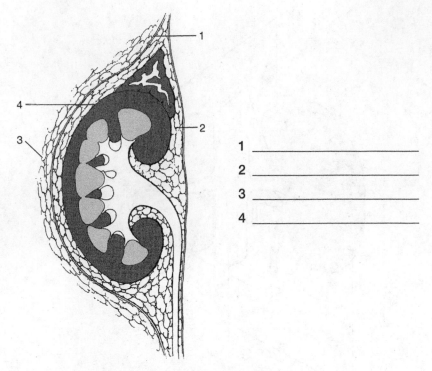

1 _____
2 _____
3 _____
4 _____

Figure 17-6 in the textbook

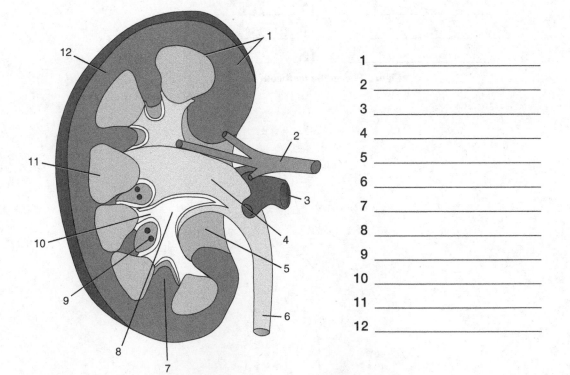

1 _____
2 _____
3 _____
4 _____
5 _____
6 _____
7 _____
8 _____
9 _____
10 _____
11 _____
12 _____

Figure 17-7 in the textbook

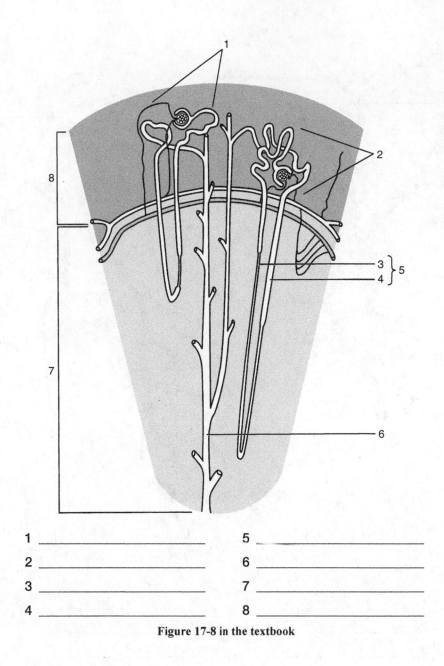

Figure 17-8 in the textbook

1 _____   5 _____

2 _____   6 _____

3 _____   7 _____

4 _____   8 _____

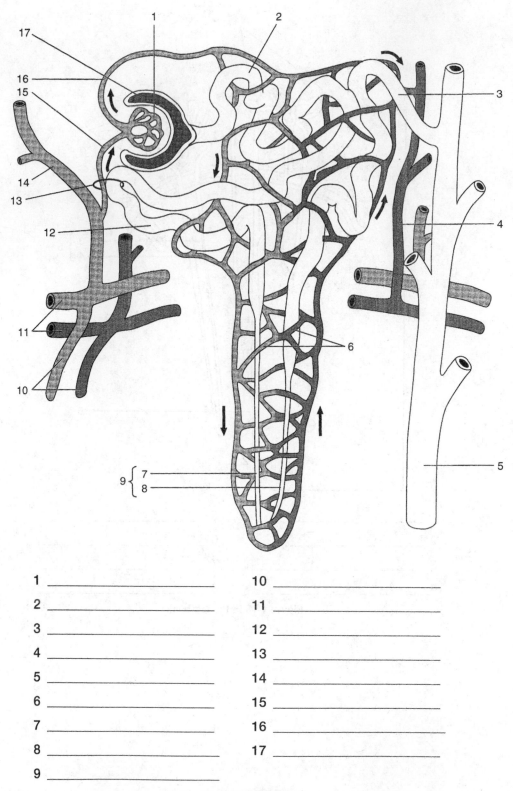

Figure 17-12 in the textbook

1 _____   10 _____

2 _____   11 _____

3 _____   12 _____

4 _____   13 _____

5 _____   14 _____

6 _____   15 _____

7 _____   16 _____

8 _____   17 _____

9 _____

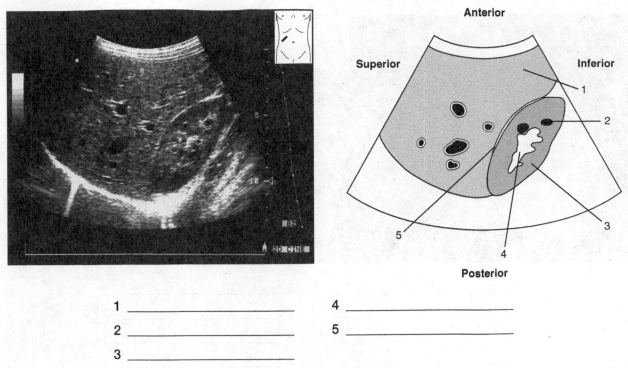

1	_____	4	_____
2	_____	5	_____
3	_____		

Figure 17-15 in the textbook

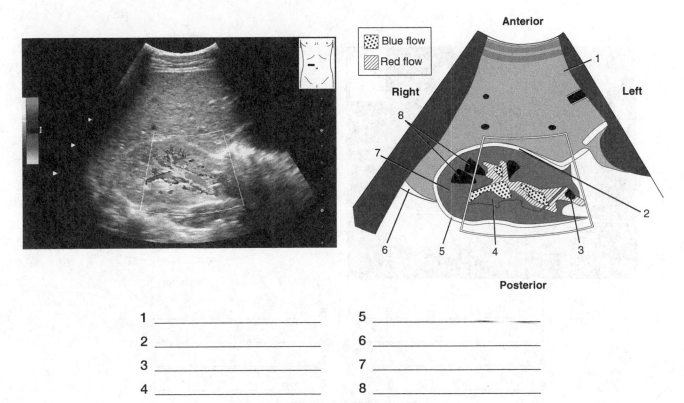

1	_____	5	_____
2	_____	6	_____
3	_____	7	_____
4	_____	8	_____

Figure 17-16 in the textbook

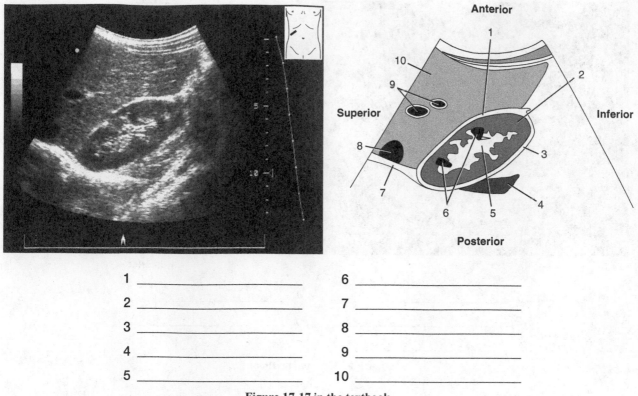

1	_____	6	_____
2	_____	7	_____
3	_____	8	_____
4	_____	9	_____
5	_____	10	_____

Figure 17-17 in the textbook

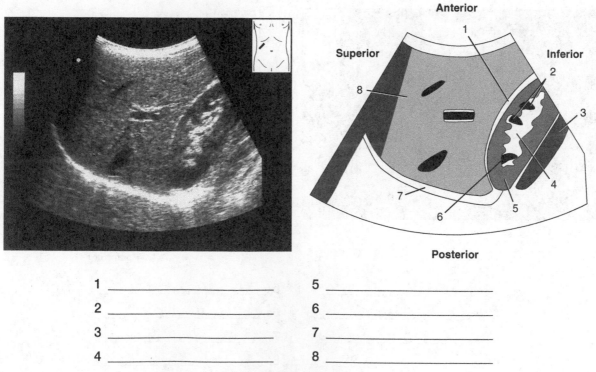

1	_____	5	_____
2	_____	6	_____
3	_____	7	_____
4	_____	8	_____

Figure 17-18 in the textbook

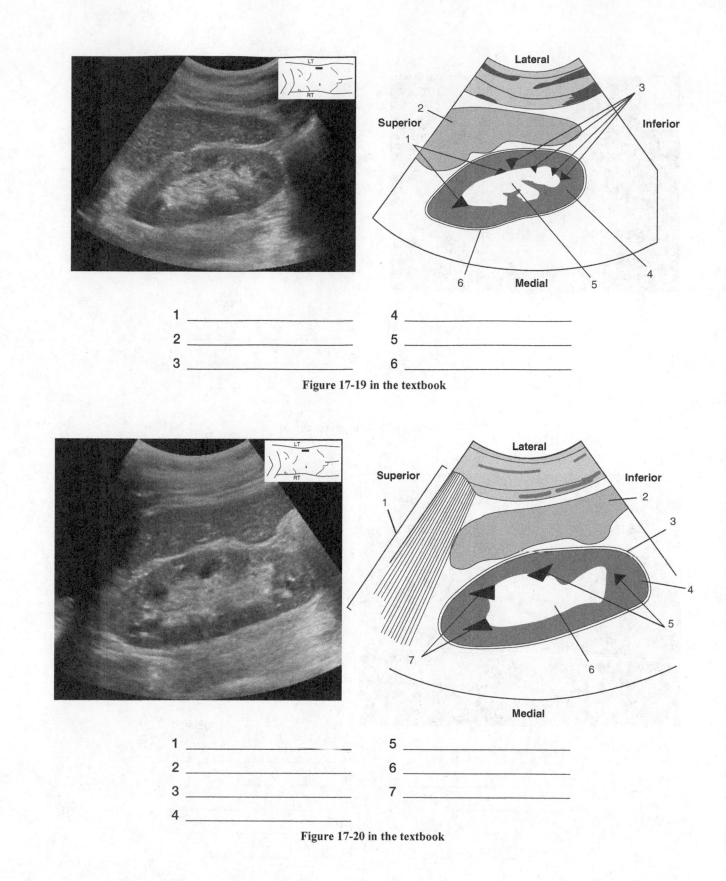

1	_____	4	_____
2	_____	5	_____
3	_____	6	_____

Figure 17-19 in the textbook

1	_____	5	_____
2	_____	6	_____
3	_____	7	_____
4	_____		

Figure 17-20 in the textbook

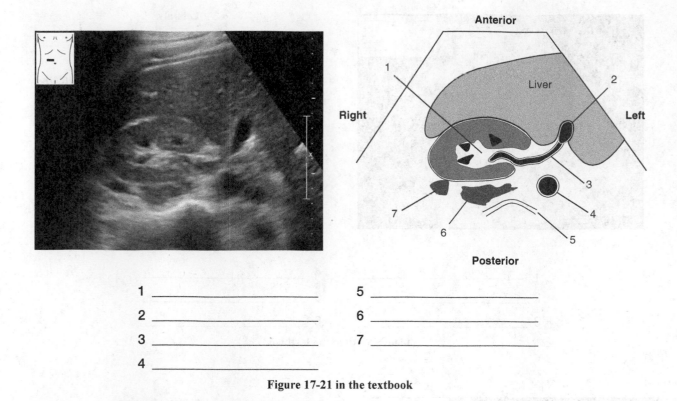

Anterior

Right

Liver

Left

1

2

3

4

5

7

6

Posterior

1 _____   5 _____

2 _____   6 _____

3 _____   7 _____

4 _____

Figure 17-21 in the textbook

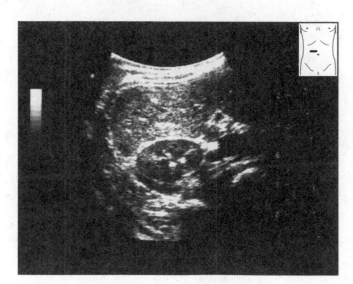

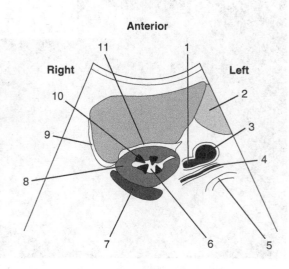

Anterior

11   1

Right   Left

10   2

9   3

8   4

7   6   5

Posterior

1 _____   7 _____

2 _____   8 _____

3 _____   9 _____

4 _____   10 _____

5 _____   11 _____

6 _____

Figure 17-22 in the textbook

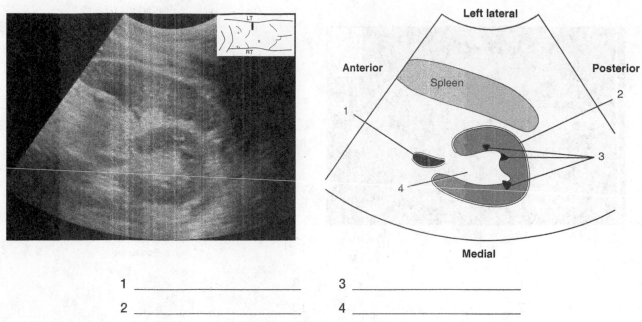

1 _____   3 _____

2 _____   4 _____

Figure 17-23 in the textbook

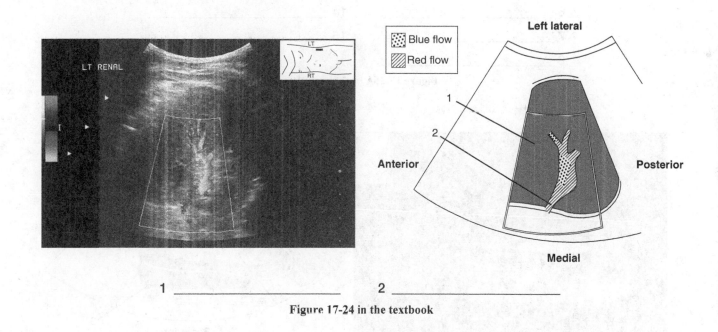

1 _____   2 _____

Figure 17-24 in the textbook

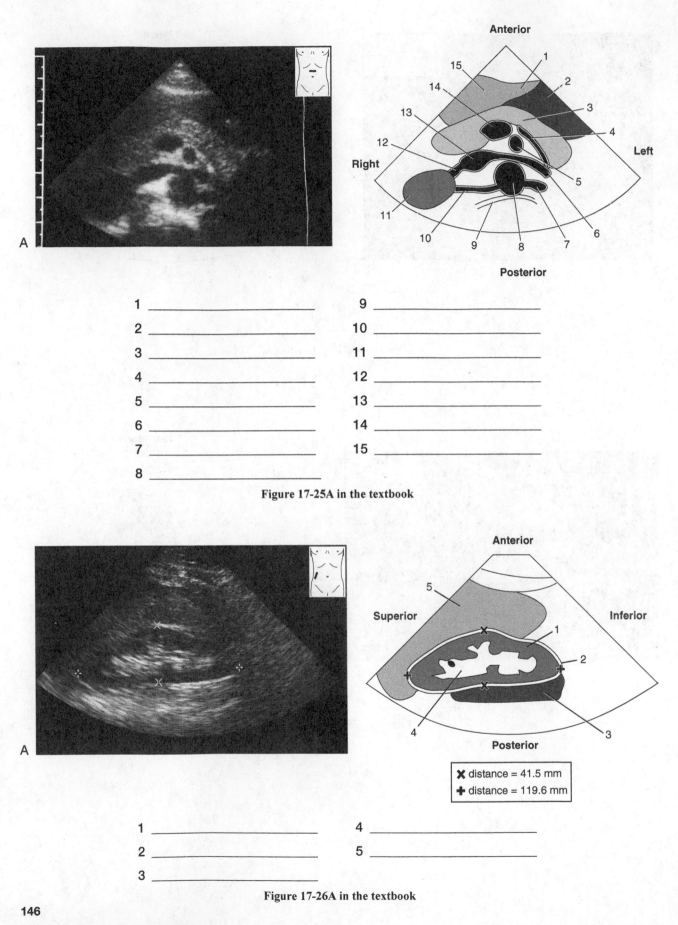

Figure 17-25A in the textbook

1	_____	9	_____
2	_____	10	_____
3	_____	11	_____
4	_____	12	_____
5	_____	13	_____
6	_____	14	_____
7	_____	15	_____
8	_____		

✖ distance = 41.5 mm
✚ distance = 119.6 mm

1	_____	4	_____
2	_____	5	_____
3	_____		

Figure 17-26A in the textbook

Chapter **17** **The Urinary and Adrenal Systems**

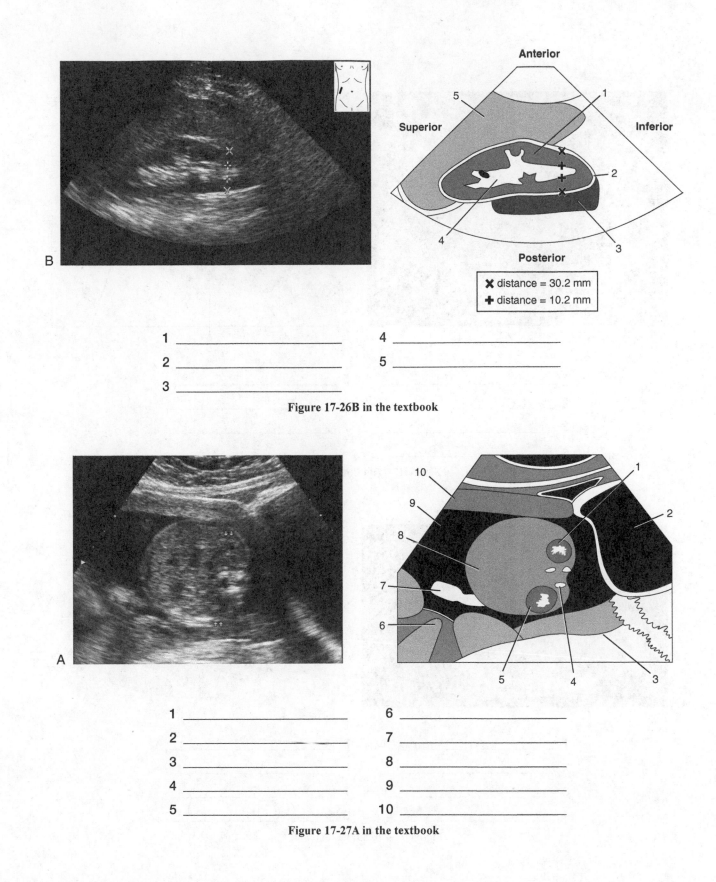

Figure 17-26B in the textbook

1 _____   4 _____

2 _____   5 _____

3 _____

distance = 30.2 mm
distance = 10.2 mm

1 _____   6 _____

2 _____   7 _____

3 _____   8 _____

4 _____   9 _____

5 _____   10 _____

Figure 17-27A in the textbook

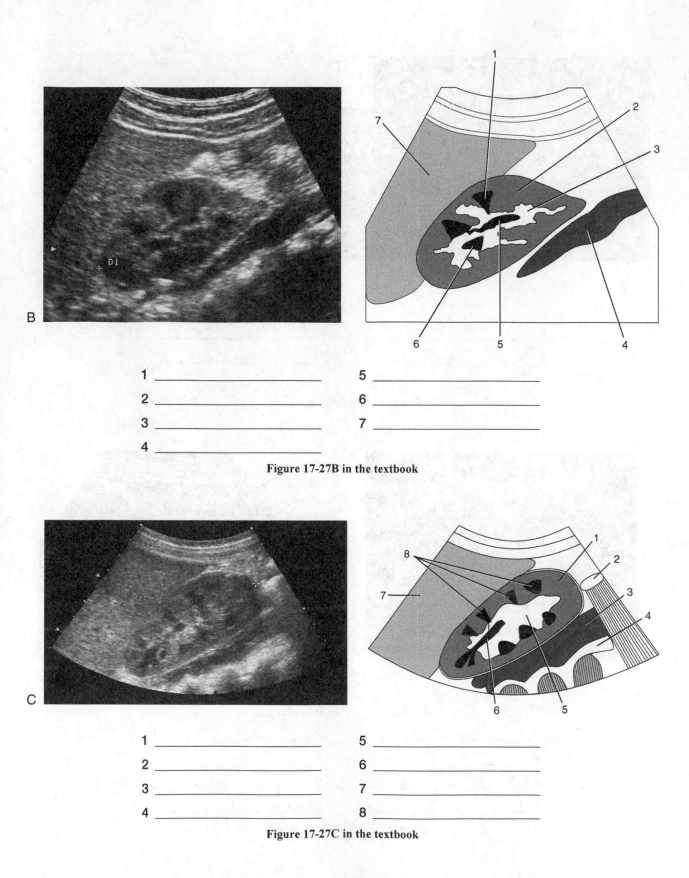

B

1	_____	5	_____
2	_____	6	_____
3	_____	7	_____
4	_____		

Figure 17-27B in the textbook

C

1	_____	5	_____
2	_____	6	_____
3	_____	7	_____
4	_____	8	_____

Figure 17-27C in the textbook

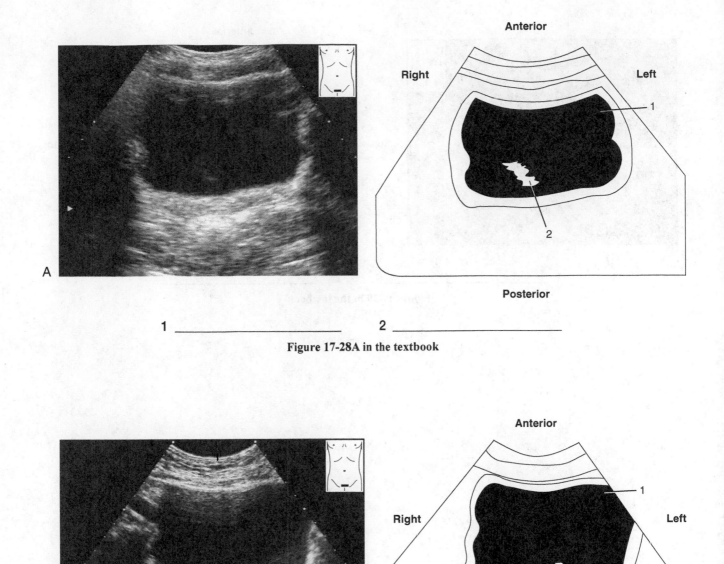

1 _____   2 _____

Figure 17-28A in the textbook

1 _____   2 _____

Figure 17-28B in the textbook

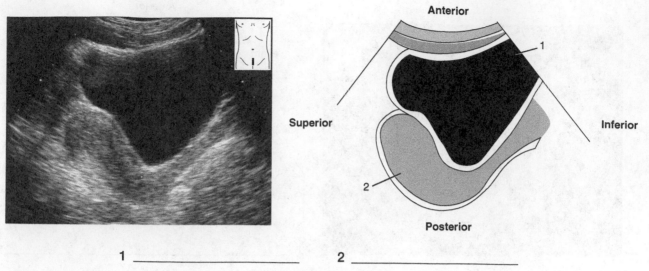

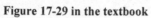

1 _____ 2 _____

Figure 17-29 in the textbook

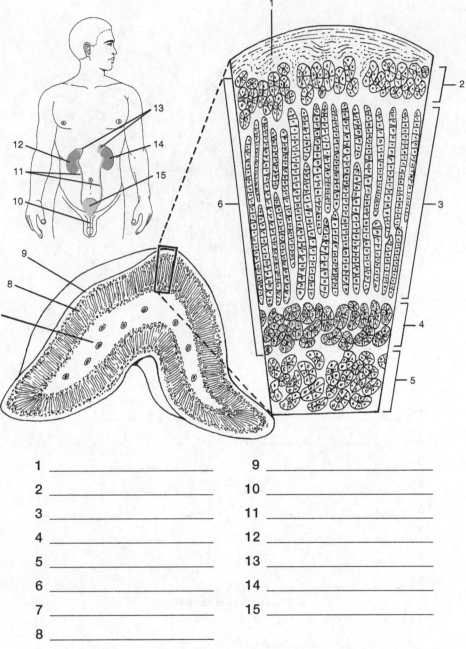

1	_____	9	_____
2	_____	10	_____
3	_____	11	_____
4	_____	12	_____
5	_____	13	_____
6	_____	14	_____
7	_____	15	_____
8	_____		

Figure 17-30 in the textbook

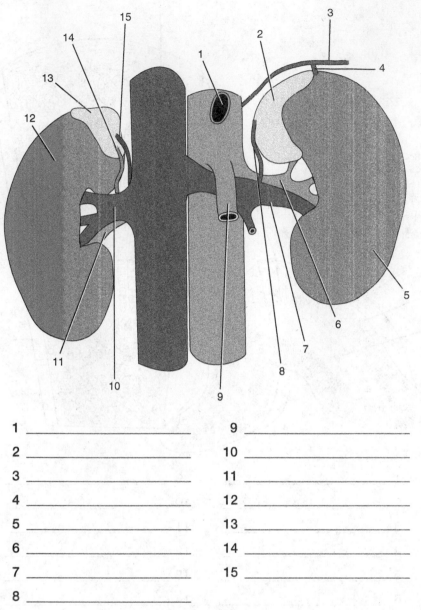

1	_____	9	_____
2	_____	10	_____
3	_____	11	_____
4	_____	12	_____
5	_____	13	_____
6	_____	14	_____
7	_____	15	_____
8	_____		

Figure 17-31 in the textbook

V. CHAPTER SUBHEADINGS EXERCISE

Directions to Students:

1. Convert each chapter subheading into a question; for example, change "Gross Anatomy" to "What is the gross anatomy of the kidney?" Write the answer to each question in a short paragraph in your notebook.

2. Exchange answers with your lab partner and check each other's work. Refer back to the textbook for further information and explanation.

3. What questions do you still have about the chapter? Write your questions in your notebook.

VI. CHAPTER EVALUATION EXERCISE

Directions to Students: Use a fresh sheet of notebook paper. Based on your work with the chapter and its accompanying laboratory assignments, identify three concepts you believe are the most important. You may draw from any of the assignments you have already completed in the previous pages including learning objectives, anatomy and physiology, images, or chapter subheadings. Include a detailed rationale in your answers.

Answer the questions below. Refer to page 382 for the answers.

Matching

1. ____ Location where the renal artery enters.
2. ____ Central area of the kidney that houses the renal vessels, nerves, and lymphatics.
3. ____ Contains the renal corpuscle and proximal and distal convoluted tubules of the nephron.
4. ____ Area where filtration and reabsorption occur.
5. ____ Composed of major and minor calyces.
6. ____ Upper expanded end of the ureter.

A. Renal cortex
B. Renal sinus
C. Renal medulla
D. Renal hilum
E. Infundibulum
F. Renal pelvis

True/False

7. The female urethra is longer than the male urethra.
8. The adrenal gland is easily visualized sonographically in neonates.
9. The kidneys are intraperitoneal in location.
10. At birth, the adrenal glands are one-half the size of the kidneys but then rapidly shrink.

The Spleen 18

I. MEMORIZATION EXERCISE

Directions to Students: Write the key words in your notebook or on note cards. Write the words on one side of the notepaper and then write the definitions on the opposite side of the page or on the back of the paper. If using note cards, write the key word on the front and the definition on the back. *This step should be completed before the lab session begins.*

Memorize the key word definitions silently for 5 minutes, then work with a lab partner and identify the words you still need help with. List the words here. Add additional rows if needed.

II. COMPREHENSION EXERCISE

Directions to Students: Work with a lab partner to complete this exercise. You will need to write in your notebook. First, change each objective into a question.

> *Example: "Describe the location of the spleen" becomes "What is the location of the spleen?"*

Next, write a short answer to the question just created.

> *Example: "The spleen is in the left hypochondrium. It lies posterior and lateral to the stomach fundus and body, tail of the pancreas, and left colic flexure."*

Highlight or circle any part of your answers about which you are unsure, and check the answers in your textbook. If you are still unsure of the answers, put a question mark next to the answer(s) for the review session of the lab.

III. APPLICATION OF ANATOMY AND PHYSIOLOGY EXERCISE

Directions to Students: Work on the following with your lab partner.

1. In your notebook, draw the spleen and as much surrounding vasculature as you can from memory.

2. Label the spleen and its vasculature. Include each structure's orientation in the body (either vertical, horizontal, vertical oblique, or horizontal oblique). Ask your lab partner to critique your work. What did you miss? Check your drawing using the sketches in your textbook, and complete any missing structures from your drawing.

3. Below your drawing, write two or three summary sentences of the physiology of the spleen. Ask your lab partner to check your work. Now check your work against the physiology section in the textbook. What else can you add to your description?

IV. IMAGE ANALYSIS EXERCISE

Directions to Students: Work on the following figures with your lab partner. It's your choice! You can label all the sketches at once, then go back and label each image with your lab partner, or label an image and its accompanying sketch at the same time. Either way, the goal is to label all of the sketches correctly and carefully compare the sketch with the sonographic image.

For each sonographic image, write a very brief observation that could be presented to your instructor, the clinical sonographer, or the sonologist. Your observation will be based on Chapter 7 in the textbook, which describes how to write a technical observation. Please go back and review that chapter if needed.

For each image, your assessment should include (1) the view of each major structure (axial or longitudinal; note: these are not the scanning planes) and (2) structures identified in the image with the correct sonographic appearance, description, and measurements if shown (see Chapter 7 in the textbook for information on how to write a technical observation).

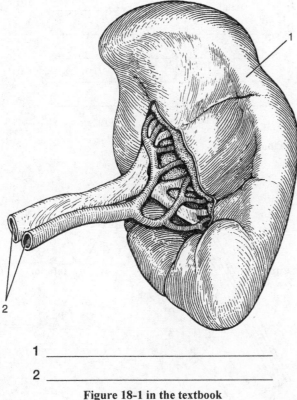

1 _____

2 _____

Figure 18-1 in the textbook

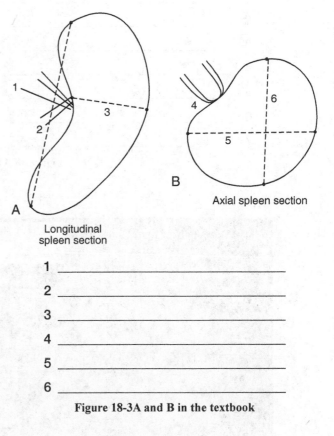

1 _____

2 _____

3 _____

4 _____

5 _____

6 _____

Figure 18-3A and B in the textbook

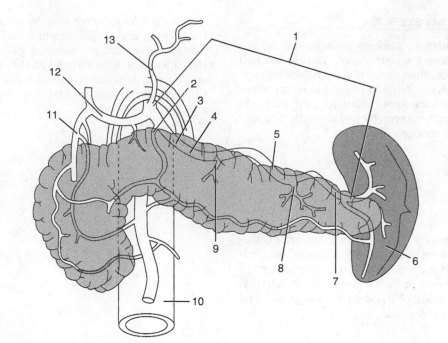

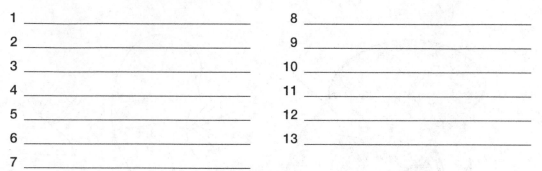

1 _____	8 _____
2 _____	9 _____
3 _____	10 _____
4 _____	11 _____
5 _____	12 _____
6 _____	13 _____
7 _____	

Figure 18-4 in the textbook

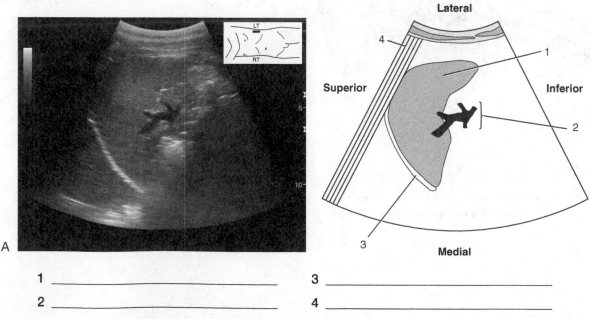

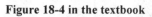

1 _____	3 _____
2 _____	4 _____

Figure 18-5A in the textbook

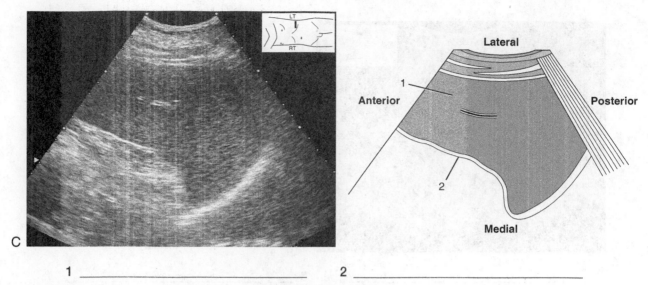

1 _____ 2 _____

Figure 18-5C in the textbook

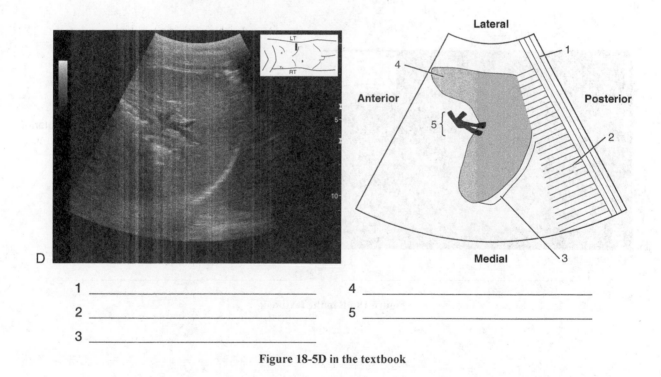

1 _____ 4 _____

2 _____ 5 _____

3 _____

Figure 18-5D in the textbook

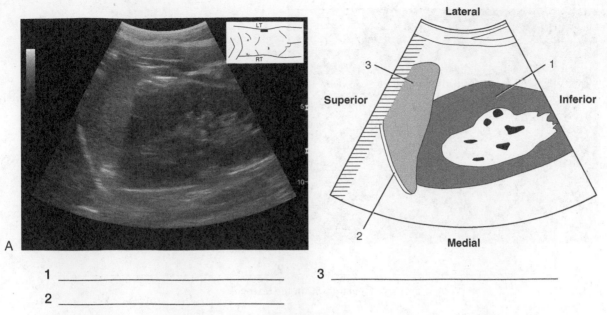

1 _____   3 _____

2 _____

Figure 18-6A in the textbook

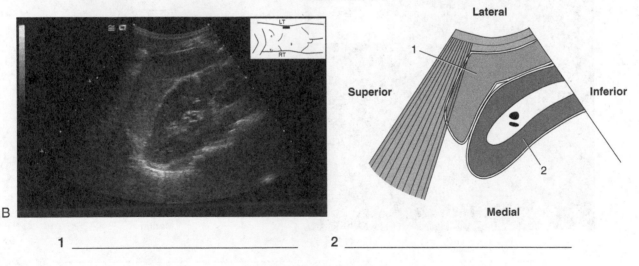

1 _____   2 _____

Figure 18-6B in the textbook

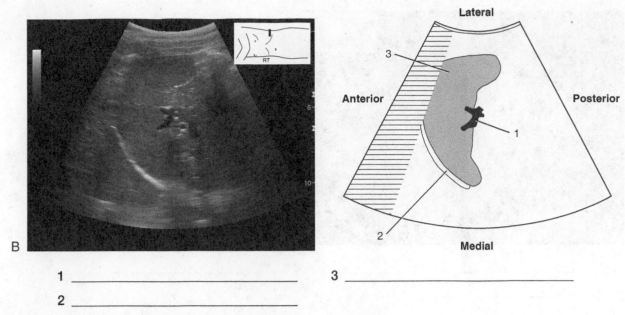

1 _____   3 _____

2 _____

Figure 18-7B in the textbook

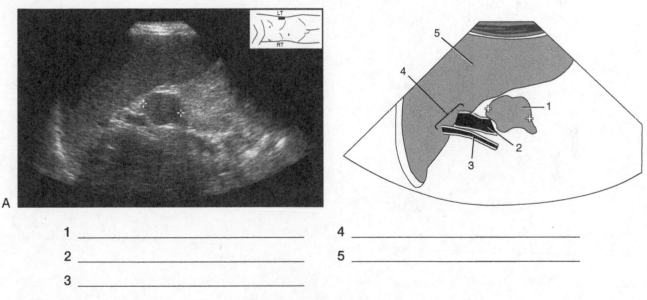

1 _____   4 _____

2 _____   5 _____

3 _____

Figure 18-8A in the textbook

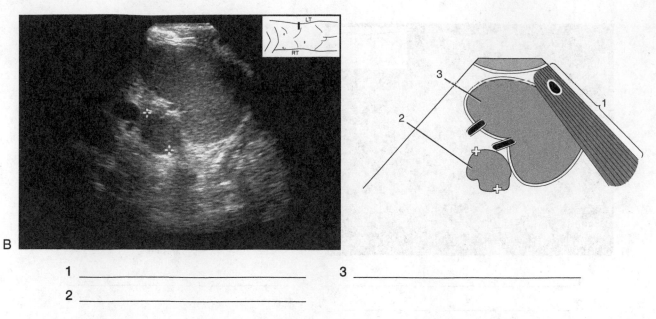

B

1 _____   3 _____

2 _____

Figure 18-8B in the textbook

V. CHAPTER SUBHEADINGS EXERCISE

Directions to Students:

1. Convert each chapter subheading into a question; for example, change "Gross Anatomy" to "What is the gross anatomy of the spleen?" Write the answer to each question in a short paragraph in your notebook.

2. Exchange answers with your lab partner and check each other's work. Refer back to the textbook for further information and explanations.

3. What questions do you still have about the chapter? Write your questions in your notebook.

VI. CHAPTER EVALUATION EXERCISE

Directions to Students: Use a fresh sheet of notebook paper. Based on your work with the chapter and its accompanying laboratory assignments, identify three concepts you believe are the most important. You may draw from any of the assignments you've already completed in the previous pages including learning objectives, anatomy and physiology, images, or chapter subheadings. Include a detailed rationale in your answers.

Answer the questions below. Refer to page 383 for the answers.

Multiple Choice

1. The splenic vein conveys venous blood from the spleen and courses along the gastrolienal ligament to its confluence with the
   a. Superior mesenteric artery
   b. Splenic artery
   c. Superior mesenteric vein
   d. Main portal vein

2. All of the following are functions of the spleen except:
   a. Defense
   b. Hematopoiesis
   c. Serves as a blood reservoir
   d. Stores bile

Matching

____ 3. The process of removing abnormal red blood cells by the spleen.

____ 4. Oxygen-carrying and iron-containing pigment of red blood cells.

____ 5. The process that produces erythrocytes and white blood cells in the developing fetus.

____ 6. The term for a red blood cell.

____ 7. The process of removing nuclei from old red blood cells.

____ 8. Responsible for phagocytosis of damaged or old cells.

____ 9. Found in the spleen, consists of lymphatic tissue, and is where immune functions take place.

____ 10. The process of removing worn-out and abnormal red blood cells and platelets from the bloodstream by phagocyte cells in the spleen.

A. Erythrocyte
B. Phagocytosis
C. Hematopoiesis
D. White pulp
E. Culling
F. Hemoglobin
G. Reticuloendothelial system
H. Pitting

The Gastrointestinal System 19

I. MEMORIZATION EXERCISE

Directions to Students: Write the key words in your notebook or on note cards. Write the words on one side of the notepaper and then write the definitions on the opposite side of the page or on the back of the paper. If using note cards, write the key word on the front and the definition on the back. *This step should be completed before the lab session begins.*

Memorize the key word definitions silently for 5 minutes, then work with a lab partner and identify the words you still need help with. List the words here. Add additional rows if needed.

II. COMPREHENSION EXERCISE

Directions to Students: Work with a lab partner to complete this exercise. You will need to write in your notebook. First, change each objective into a question.

> *Example: "Identify the five principal layers of bowel, known as the gut signature" becomes "What are the five principal layers of bowel, known as the gut signature?"*

Next, write a short answer to the question just created.

> *Example: "The five layers of bowel, from the inside out, are the innermost layer, the mucosa, which is in contact with the intestinal contents; next is the submucosa; the muscular layer, muscularis; serosa; and the outermost layer, mesothelium, which covers the bowel loops."*

Highlight or circle any part of your answers about which you are unsure and check the answers in your textbook. If you are still unsure of the answers, put a question mark next to the answer(s) for the review session of the lab.

III. APPLICATION OF ANATOMY AND PHYSIOLOGY EXERCISE

Directions to Students: Work on the following with your lab partner.

1. In your notebook, draw as much of the gastrointestinal (GI) tract as you can from memory.

2. Label the parts of the GI tract. Include each structure's orientation in the body (either vertical, horizontal, vertical oblique, or horizontal oblique). Ask your lab partner to critique your work. What did you miss? Check your drawing using the sketches in your textbook, and complete any missing structures from your drawing.

3. Below your drawing, write two or three summary sentences on the physiology of the GI tract. Ask your lab partner to check your work. Now check your work against the physiology section in the textbook. What else can you add to your description?

IV. IMAGE ANALYSIS EXERCISE

Directions to Students: Work on the following figures with your lab partner. It's your choice! You can label all the sketches at once, then go back and label each image with your lab partner, or label an image and its accompanying sketch at the same time. Either way, the goal is to label all of the sketches correctly and carefully compare the sketch with the sonographic image.

For each sonographic image, write a very brief observation that could be presented to your instructor, a clinical sonographer, or a sonologist. Your observation will be based on Chapter 7 in the textbook, which describes how to write a technical observation. Please go back and review that chapter if needed.

For each image, your assessment should include (1) the view of each major structure (axial or longitudinal; note: these are not the scanning planes) and (2) structures identified in the image with the correct sonographic appearance, description, and measurements if shown (see Chapter 7 in the textbook for information on how to write a technical observation).

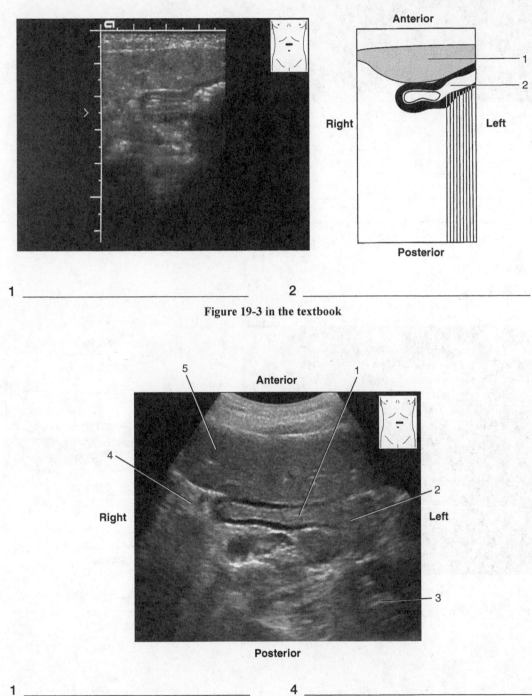

1 _____ 2 _____

Figure 19-3 in the textbook

1 _____ 4 _____

2 _____ 5 _____

3 _____

Figure 19-4 in the textbook

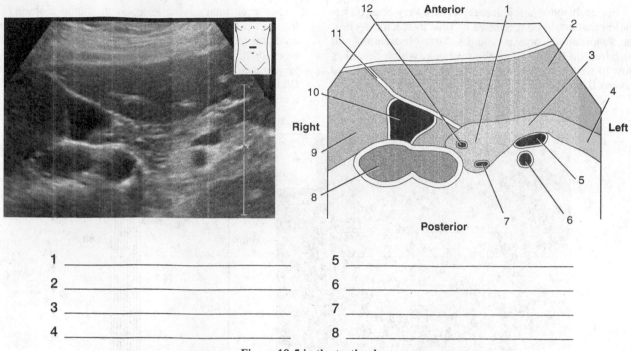

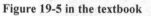

1	_____	5	_____
2	_____	6	_____
3	_____	7	_____
4	_____	8	_____

Figure 19-5 in the textbook

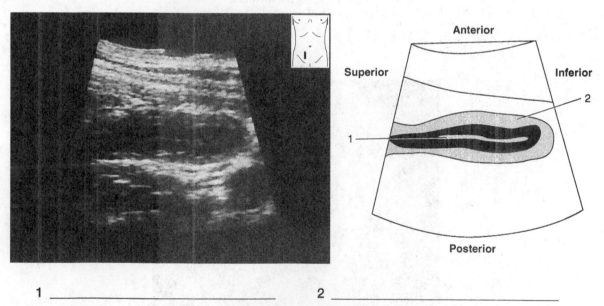

| 1 | _____ | 2 | _____ |

Figure 19-6 in the textbook

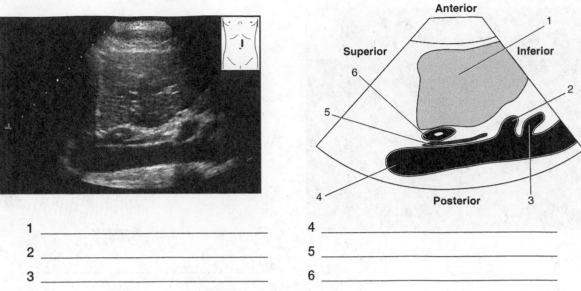

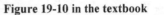

1 _____   4 _____

2 _____   5 _____

3 _____   6 _____

Figure 19-10 in the textbook

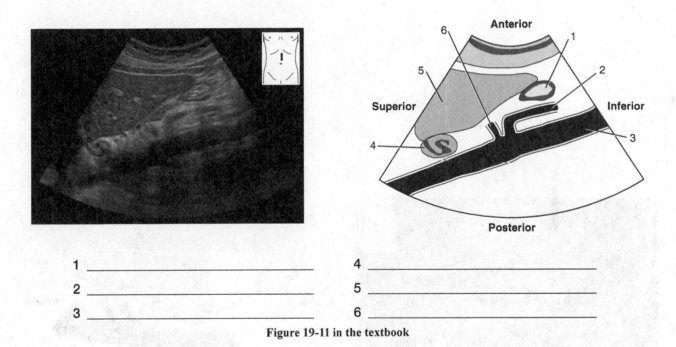

1 _____   4 _____

2 _____   5 _____

3 _____   6 _____

Figure 19-11 in the textbook

Chapter **19** **The Gastrointestinal System**

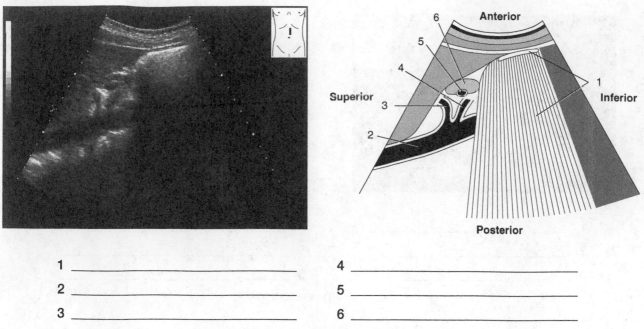

1 _____   4 _____
2 _____   5 _____
3 _____   6 _____

Figure 19-13 in the textbook

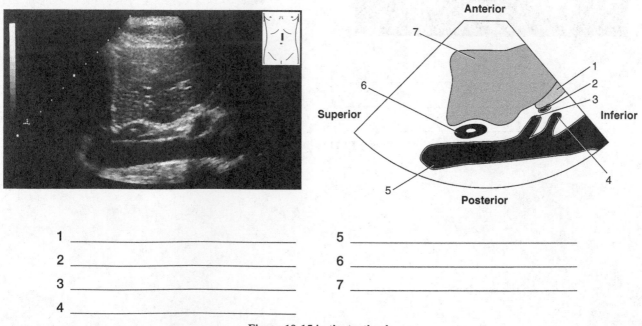

1 _____   5 _____
2 _____   6 _____
3 _____   7 _____
4 _____

Figure 19-15 in the textbook

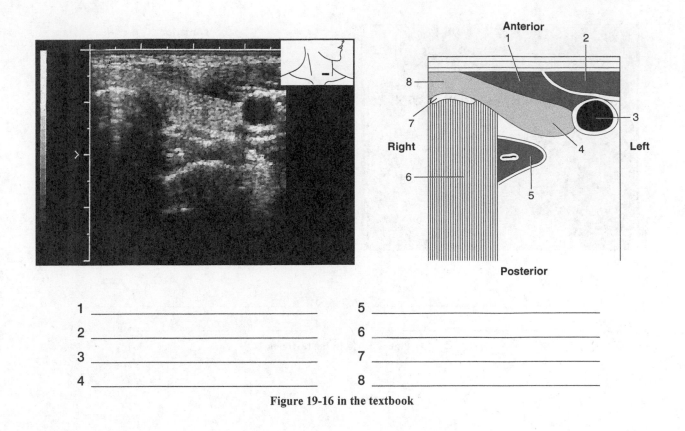

1 _____   5 _____

2 _____   6 _____

3 _____   7 _____

4 _____   8 _____

Figure 19-16 in the textbook

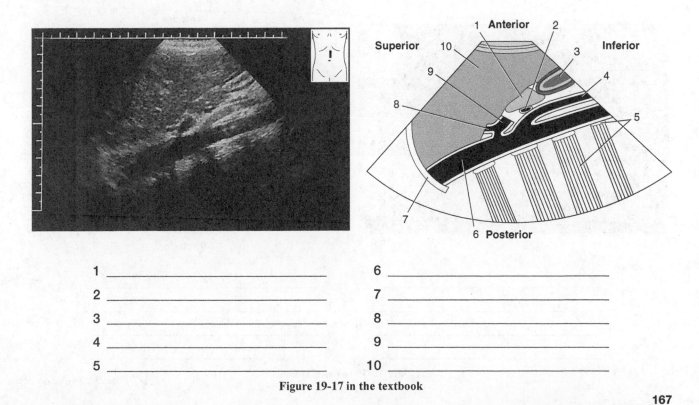

1 _____   6 _____

2 _____   7 _____

3 _____   8 _____

4 _____   9 _____

5 _____   10 _____

Figure 19-17 in the textbook

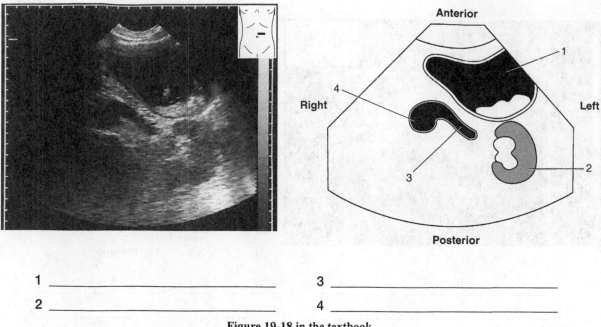

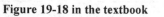

1 _____ 3 _____

2 _____ 4 _____

Figure 19-18 in the textbook

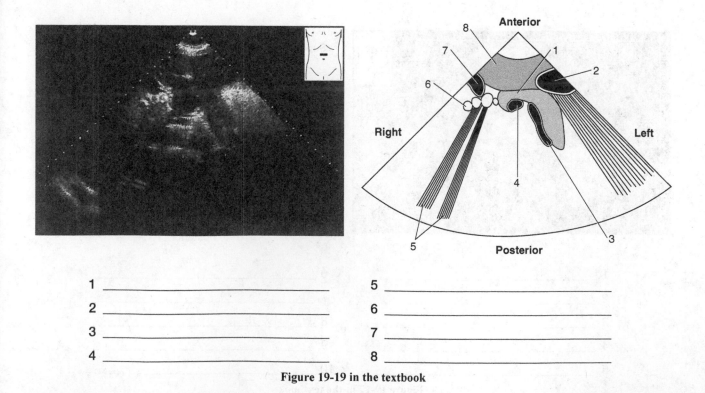

1 _____ 5 _____

2 _____ 6 _____

3 _____ 7 _____

4 _____ 8 _____

Figure 19-19 in the textbook

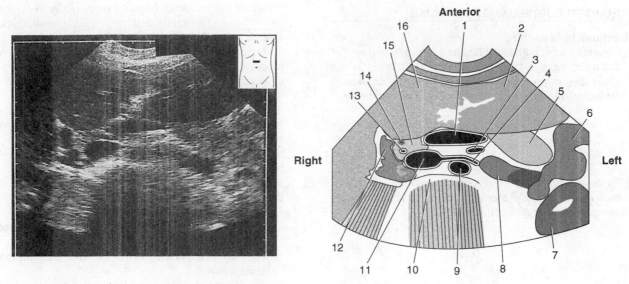

Anterior

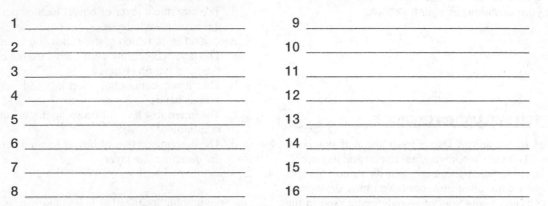

1 _____	9 _____
2 _____	10 _____
3 _____	11 _____
4 _____	12 _____
5 _____	13 _____
6 _____	14 _____
7 _____	15 _____
8 _____	16 _____

Figure 19-20 in the textbook

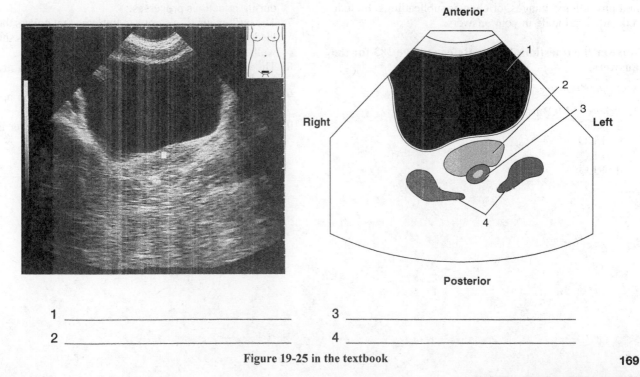

Anterior

1 _____	3 _____
2 _____	4 _____

Figure 19-25 in the textbook

Chapter **19 The Gastrointestinal System**

V. CHAPTER SUBHEADINGS EXERCISE

Directions to Students:

1. Convert each chapter subheading into a question; for example, change "Gross Anatomy" to "What is the gross anatomy of the GI tract?" Write the answer to each question in a short paragraph in your notebook.

2. Exchange answers with your lab partner and check each other's work. Refer back to the textbook for further information and explanations.

3. What questions do you still have about the chapter? Write your questions in your notebook.

VI. CHAPTER EVALUATION EXERCISE

Directions to Students: Use a fresh sheet of notebook paper. Based on your work with the chapter and its accompanying laboratory assignments, identify three concepts you believe are the most important. You may draw from any of the assignments you've already completed in the previous pages including learning objectives, anatomy and physiology, images, or chapter subheadings. Include a detailed rationale in your answers.

Answer the questions below. Refer to page 383 for the answers.

Multiple Choice

1. Where is McBurney's point located?
   a. RUQ
   b. LUQ
   c. LLQ
   d. RLQ

2. Diseased inflammatory bowel is more likely to exhibit _____ peristalsis and _____ wall thickness or hyperemia.
   a. increased; decreased
   b. decreased; increased
   c. decreased; decreased
   d. increased; increased

3. The _____ and _____ segments of the large bowel are located on the right and left sides of the body, medial to the paracolic gutters.
   a. transverse; ascending
   b. ascending; descending
   c. transverse; descending
   d. descending; sigmoid

4. Mucosa refers to which of the following layers?
   a. The layer containing blood vessels and lymph channels
   b. The layer containing circular and longitudinal fibrous bands
   c. The innermost layer of bowel in direct contact with intraluminal contents
   d. The outermost layer of bowel located peripheral to the outer muscle layer

5. Serosa refers to which of the following layers?
   a. The layer containing connective tissue, blood vessels, and lymph channels
   b. The layer containing circular and longitudinal fibrous bands
   c. The innermost layer of bowel in direct contact with intraluminal contents
   d. The outermost layer of bowel located peripheral to the outer muscle layer

True/False

6. Sonographic localization is less likely to occur when the peritoneal coverings of the bowel stick together during infectious processes.

7. The peritoneum is a serous membrane that covers the visceral organs of the peritoneal cavity and lines the walls of the abdomen and pelvis.

8. The ascending and descending colon segments are considered retroperitoneal in location.

9. The stomach and the first part of the duodenum are retroperitoneal structures.

10. The source of the major blood supply to the liver is from veins draining the digestive tract.

20 The Male Pelvis: Prostate Gland and Seminal Vesicles Sonography

I. MEMORIZATION EXERCISE

Directions to Students: Write the key words in your notebook or on note cards. Write the words on one side of the notepaper and then write the definitions on the opposite side of the page or on the back of the paper. If using note cards, write the key word on the front and the definition on the back. *This step should be completed before the lab session begins.*

Memorize the key word definitions silently for 5 minutes, then work with a lab partner and identify the words you still need help with. List the words here. Add additional rows if needed.

II. COMPREHENSION EXERCISE

Directions to Students: Work with a lab partner to complete this exercise. You will need to write in your notebook. First, change each objective into a question.

> *Example: "Describe the location of the prostate gland and seminal vesicles" becomes "Where are the prostate gland and seminal vesicles located?"*

Next, write a short answer to the question just created.

> *Example: "The prostate gland is a doughnut-like gland that lies inferior to the urinary bladder surrounding the proximal urethra. The seminal vesicles are paired glands that lie posterior to the urinary bladder just superior to the prostate."*

Highlight or circle any part of your answers about which you are unsure, and check the answers in your textbook. If you are still unsure of the answers, put a question mark next to the answer(s) for the review session of the lab.

III. APPLICATION OF ANATOMY AND PHYSIOLOGY EXERCISE

Directions to Students: Work on the following with your lab partner.
1. In your notebook, draw the prostate and seminal vesicles from memory.

2. Label the prostate gland and seminal vesicles. Include each structure's orientation in the body (either vertical, horizontal, vertical oblique, or horizontal oblique). Ask your lab partner to critique your work. What did you miss? Check your drawing using the sketches in your textbook, and complete any missing structures from your drawing.

3. Below your drawing, write two or three summary sentences on the physiology of the prostate gland and seminal vesicles. Ask your lab partner to check your work. Now check your work against the physiology section in the textbook. What else can you add to your description?

IV. IMAGE ANALYSIS EXERCISE

Directions to Students: Work on the following figures with your lab partner. It's your choice! You can label all the sketches at once, then go back and label each image with your lab partner, or label an image and its accompanying sketch at the same time. Either way, the goal is to label all of the sketches correctly and carefully compare the sketch with the sonographic image.

For each sonographic image, write a very brief observation that could be presented to your instructor, the clinical sonographer, or the sonologist. Your observation will be based on Chapter 7 in the textbook, which describes how to write a technical observation. Please go back and review that chapter if needed.

For each image, your assessment should include (1) the view of each major structure (axial or longitudinal; note: these are not the scanning planes) and (2) structures identified in the image with the correct sonographic appearance, description, and measurements if shown (see Chapter 7 in the textbook for information on how to write a technical observation).

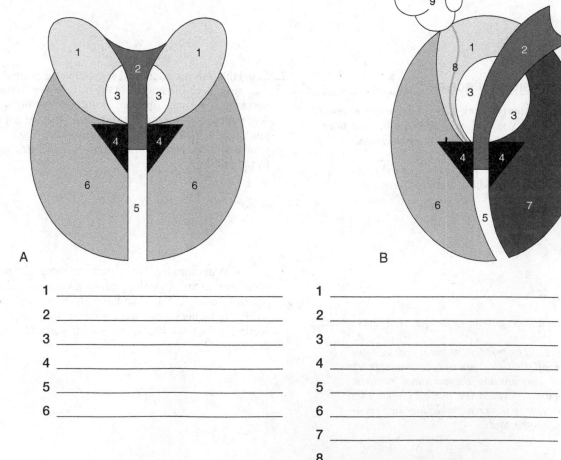

A

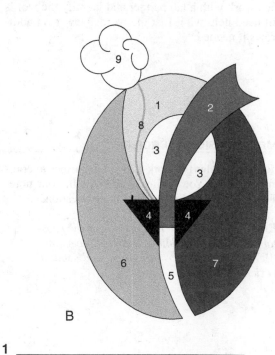

B

1 _____

2 _____

3 _____

4 _____

5 _____

6 _____

1 _____

2 _____

3 _____

4 _____

5 _____

6 _____

7 _____

8 _____

9 _____

Figure 20-2A and B in the textbook

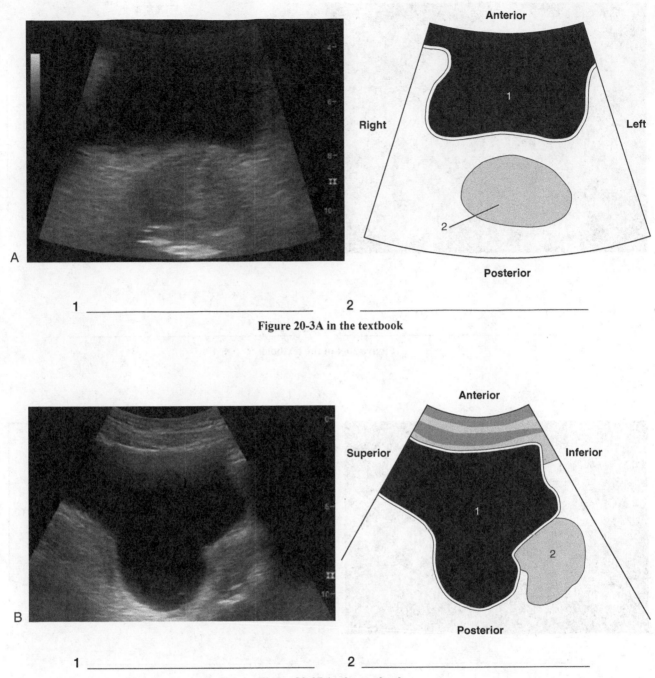

1 _____   2 _____

Figure 20-3A in the textbook

1 _____   2 _____

Figure 20-3B in the textbook

Chapter **20   The Male Pelvis: Prostate Gland and Seminal Vesicles Sonography**

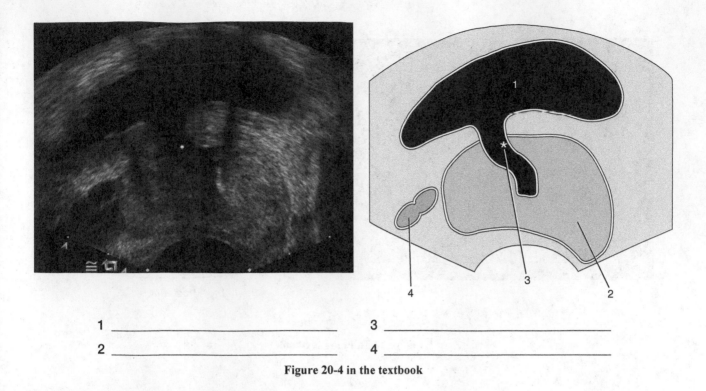

1 _____   3 _____

2 _____   4 _____

Figure 20-4 in the textbook

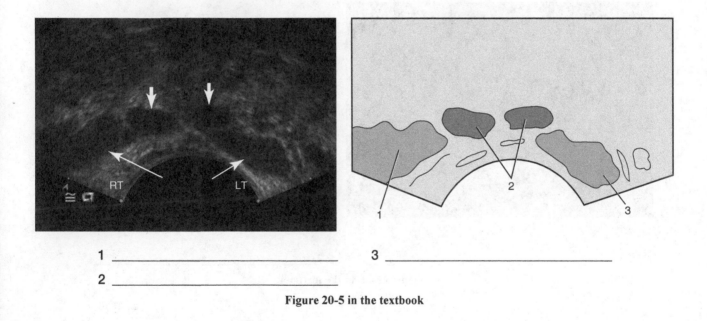

1 _____   3 _____

2 _____

Figure 20-5 in the textbook

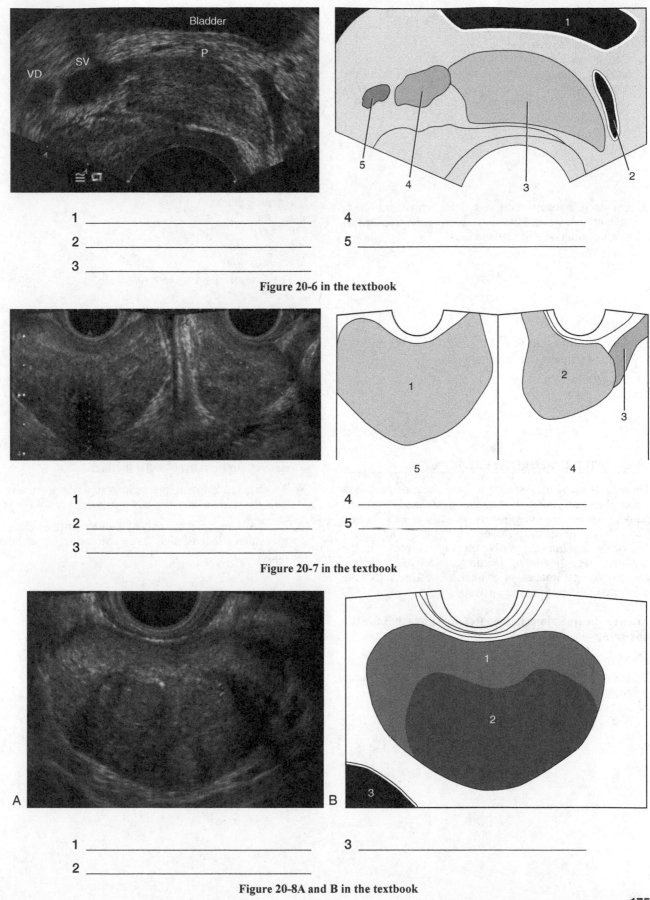

1 _____   4 _____

2 _____   5 _____

3 _____

Figure 20-6 in the textbook

1 _____   4 _____

2 _____   5 _____

3 _____

Figure 20-7 in the textbook

1 _____   3 _____

2 _____

Figure 20-8A and B in the textbook

Chapter **20**   **The Male Pelvis: Prostate Gland and Seminal Vesicles Sonography**

V. CHAPTER SUBHEADINGS EXERCISE

Directions to Students:

1. Convert each chapter subheading into a question; for example, change "Gross Anatomy" to "What is the gross anatomy of the prostate?" Write the answer to each question in a short paragraph in your notebook.

2. Exchange answers with your lab partner and check each other's work. Refer back to the textbook for further information and explanations.

3. What questions do you still have about the chapter? Write your questions in your notebook.

VI. CHAPTER EVALUATION EXERCISE

Directions to Students: Use a fresh sheet of notebook paper. Based on your work with the chapter and its accompanying laboratory assignments, identify three concepts you believe are the most important. You may draw from any of the assignments you've already completed in the previous pages including learning objectives, anatomy and physiology, images, or chapter subheadings. Include a detailed rationale in your answers.

Answer the questions below. Refer to page 383 for the answers.

Multiple Choice

1. The length of each seminal vesicle measures approximately
   a. 1 cm
   b. 5 cm
   c. 1 mm
   d. 5 mm

2. With age, the prostate sometimes
   a. Flattens
   b. Calcifies
   c. Enlarges
   d. Atrophies

3. Of the glandular prostate, the transition zone accounts for about
   a. 5%
   b. 10%
   c. 13%
   d. 33%

4. Seminal vesicles in the long axis are seen using which scanning plane?
   a. Long
   b. Axial
   c. Transverse
   d. Tangential

5. The prostate gland is sonographically
   a. Asymmetric
   b. Hyperechoic
   c. Homogeneous
   d. Heterogeneous

True/False

6. The prostate gland and seminal vesicles contribute to sperm viability by secreting alkaline fluids.

7. The fluid secreted by the seminal vesicles constitutes about 33% of semen volume.

8. The seminal vesicles empty into the distal ductus deferens to form the ejaculatory ducts.

9. The transabdominal approach is superior for scanning the seminal vesicles and prostate.

10. The prostate gland consists of a small anterior verumontanum and a much larger posterior glandular region.

21 The Female Pelvis

I. MEMORIZATION EXERCISE

Directions to Students: Write the key words in your notebook or on note cards. Write the words on one side of the notepaper and then write the definitions on the opposite side of the page or on the back of the paper. If using note cards, write the key word on the front and the definition on the back. *This step should be completed before the lab session begins.*

Memorize the key word definitions silently for 5 minutes, then work with a lab partner and identify the words you still need help with. List the words here. Add additional rows if needed.

II. COMPREHENSION EXERCISE

Directions to Students: Work with a lab partner to complete this exercise. You will need to write in your notebook. First, change each objective into a question.

> *Example: "Describe the location of the female pelvic anatomy with relation to the immediate adjacent structures" becomes "Where is the female pelvic anatomy located in relation to adjacent structures?"*

Next, write a short answer to the question just created.

> *Example: "The female pelvis lies in three regions: the right and left iliac, and the hypogastric areas. It is the inferior part of the peritoneal cavity that is bordered by the iliac crests superiorly and the pelvic diaphragm inferiorly."*

Highlight or circle any part of your answers about which you are unsure, and check the answers in your textbook. If you are still unsure of the answers, put a question mark next to the answer(s) for the review session of the lab.

III. APPLICATION OF ANATOMY AND PHYSIOLOGY EXERCISE

Directions to Students: Work on the following with your lab partner.
1. In your notebook, draw as many structures of the female pelvis as you can from memory.

2. Label the structures in the female pelvis. Include each structure's orientation in the body (either vertical, horizontal, vertical oblique, or horizontal oblique). Ask your lab partner to critique your work. What did you miss? Check your drawing using the sketches in your textbook, and complete any missing structures from your drawing.

3. Below your drawing, write two or three summary sentences on the physiology of the female pelvis. Ask your lab partner to check your work. Now check your work against the physiology section in the textbook. What else can you add to your description?

IV. IMAGE ANALYSIS EXERCISE

Directions to Students: Work on the following figures with your lab partner. It's your choice! You can label all the sketches at once, then go back and label each image with your lab partner, or label an image and its accompanying sketch at the same time. Either way, the goal is to label all of the sketches correctly and carefully compare the sketch with the sonographic image.

For each sonographic image, write a very brief observation that could be presented to your instructor, the clinical sonographer, or the sonologist. Your observation will be based on Chapter 7 in the textbook, which describes how to write a technical observation. Please go back and review that chapter if needed.

For each image, your assessment should include (1) the view of each major structure (axial or longitudinal; note: these are not the scanning planes) and (2) structures identified in the image with the correct sonographic appearance, description, and measurements if shown (see Chapter 7 in the textbook for information on how to write a technical observation).

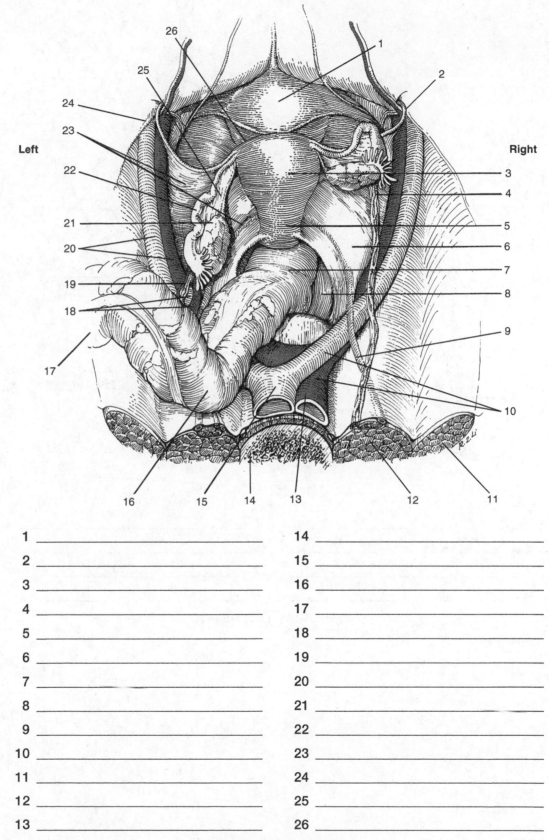

Left

Right

1	_____	14	_____
2	_____	15	_____
3	_____	16	_____
4	_____	17	_____
5	_____	18	_____
6	_____	19	_____
7	_____	20	_____
8	_____	21	_____
9	_____	22	_____
10	_____	23	_____
11	_____	24	_____
12	_____	25	_____
13	_____	26	_____

Figure 21-9 in the textbook

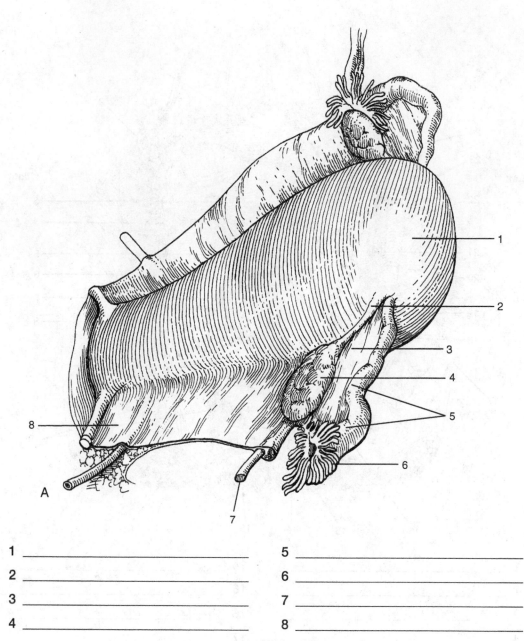

1 _____   5 _____
2 _____   6 _____
3 _____   7 _____
4 _____   8 _____

Figure 21-10A in the textbook

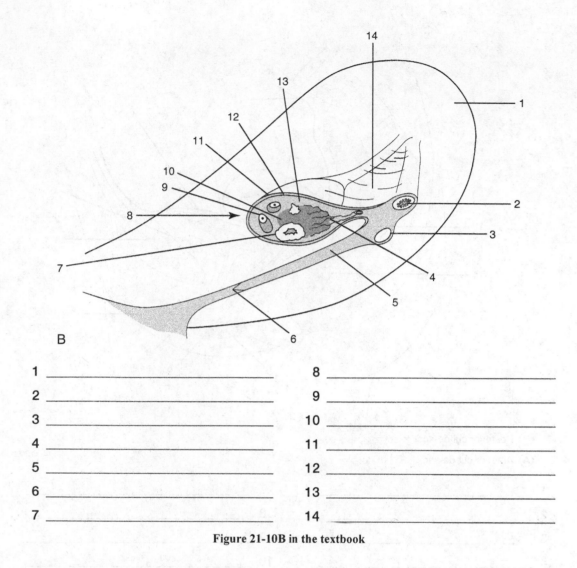

B

1	_____	8	_____
2	_____	9	_____
3	_____	10	_____
4	_____	11	_____
5	_____	12	_____
6	_____	13	_____
7	_____	14	_____

Figure 21-10B in the textbook

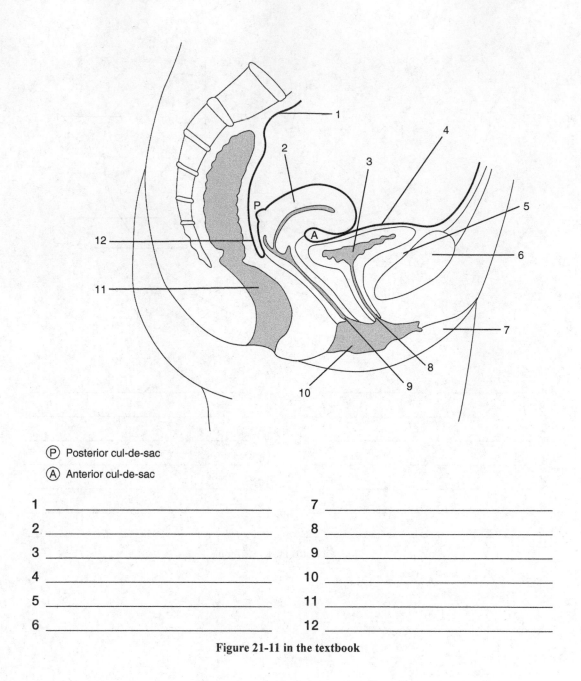

P   Posterior cul-de-sac

A   Anterior cul-de-sac

1 _____   7 _____
2 _____   8 _____
3 _____   9 _____
4 _____   10 _____
5 _____   11 _____
6 _____   12 _____

Figure 21-11 in the textbook

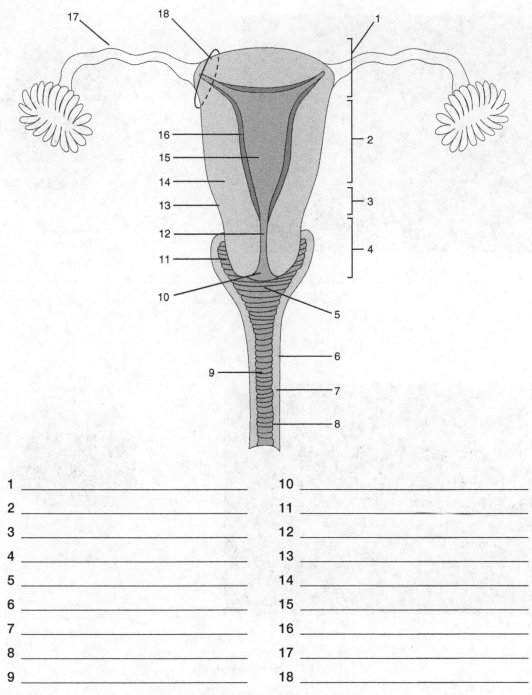

Figure 21-15 in the textbook

1 _____   10 _____

2 _____   11 _____

3 _____   12 _____

4 _____   13 _____

5 _____   14 _____

6 _____   15 _____

7 _____   16 _____

8 _____   17 _____

9 _____   18 _____

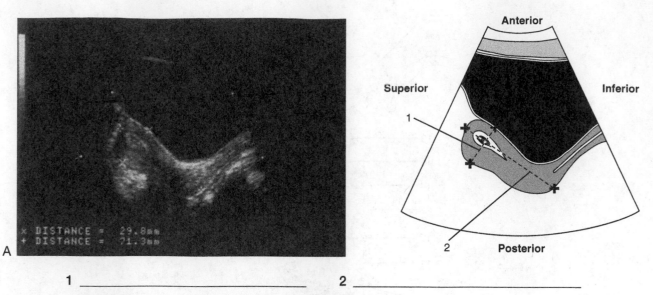

Figure 21-16A in the textbook

1 _____   2 _____

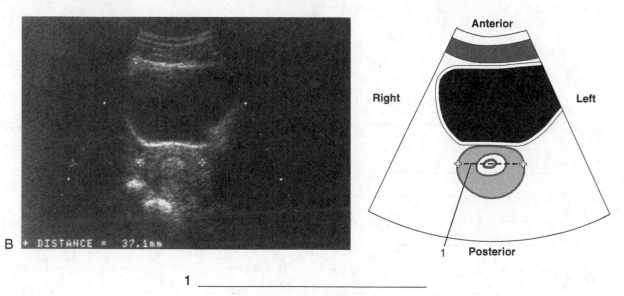

1 _____

Figure 21-16B in the textbook

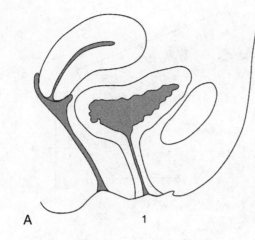

A   1

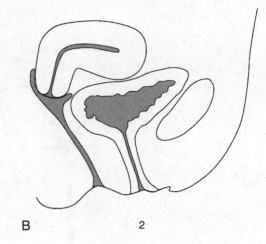

B   2

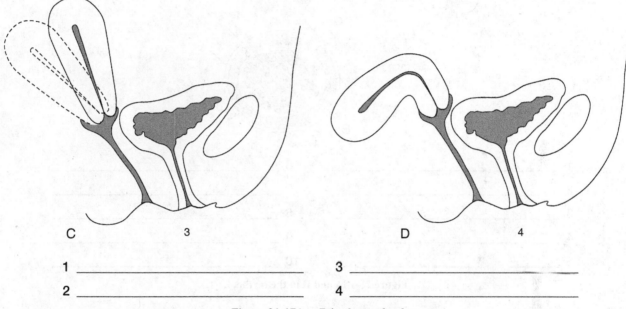

C   3   D   4

1 _____   3 _____

2 _____   4 _____

Figure 21-17A to D in the textbook

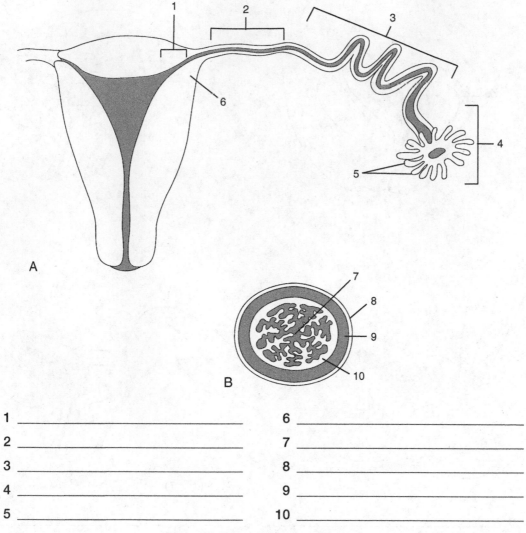

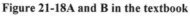

B

1	_____	6	_____
2	_____	7	_____
3	_____	8	_____
4	_____	9	_____
5	_____	10	_____

Figure 21-18A and B in the textbook

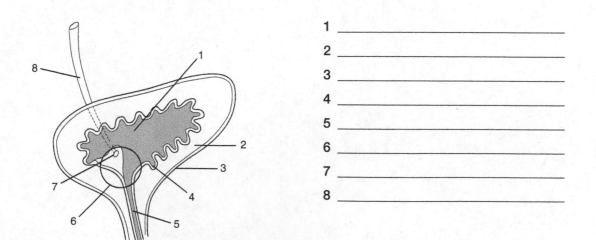

1	_____
2	_____
3	_____
4	_____
5	_____
6	_____
7	_____
8	_____

Figure 21-19 in the textbook

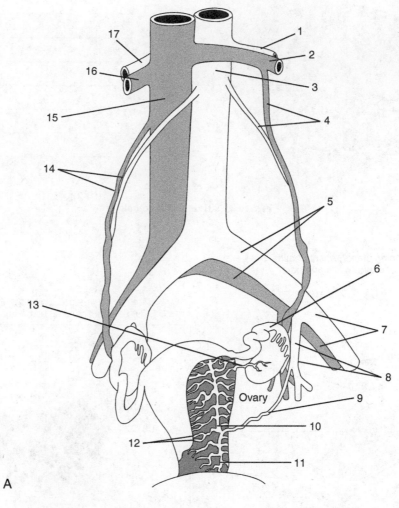

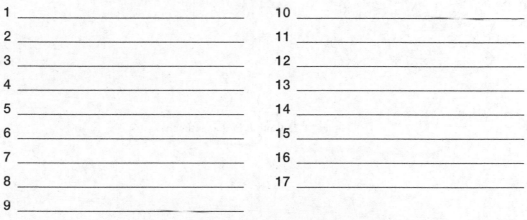

A

1	_____	10	_____
2	_____	11	_____
3	_____	12	_____
4	_____	13	_____
5	_____	14	_____
6	_____	15	_____
7	_____	16	_____
8	_____	17	_____
9	_____		

Figure 21-20A in the textbook

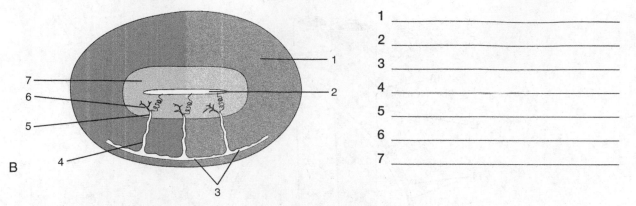

1 _____

2 _____

3 _____

4 _____

5 _____

6 _____

7 _____

Figure 21-20B in the textbook

Sagittal scanning plane/transabdominal (TA)
anterior sound wave approach

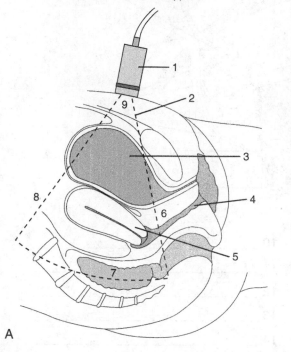

Image display monitor
TA sagittal scanning plane image orientation

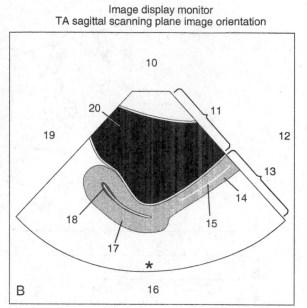

Figure 21-23A and B in the textbook

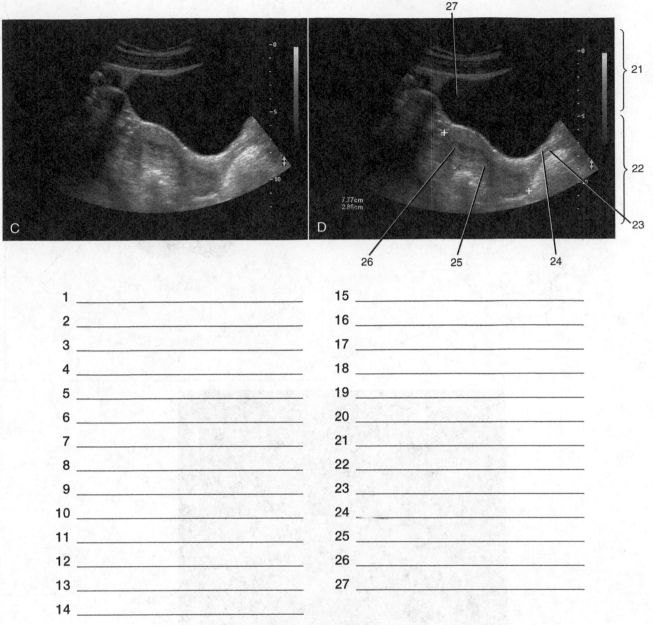

Figure 21-23C and D in the textbook

1 _____   15 _____
2 _____   16 _____
3 _____   17 _____
4 _____   18 _____
5 _____   19 _____
6 _____   20 _____
7 _____   21 _____
8 _____   22 _____
9 _____   23 _____
10 _____   24 _____
11 _____   25 _____
12 _____   26 _____
13 _____   27 _____
14 _____

Transverse scanning plane/transabdominal (TA) anterior sound wave approach

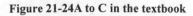

A

Image display monitor
TA transverse scanning plane image orientation

B

C

Figure 21-24A to C in the textbook

1 _____	10 _____
2 _____	11 _____
3 _____	12 _____
4 _____	13 _____
5 _____	14 _____
6 _____	15 _____
7 _____	16 _____
8 _____	17 _____
9 _____	18 _____

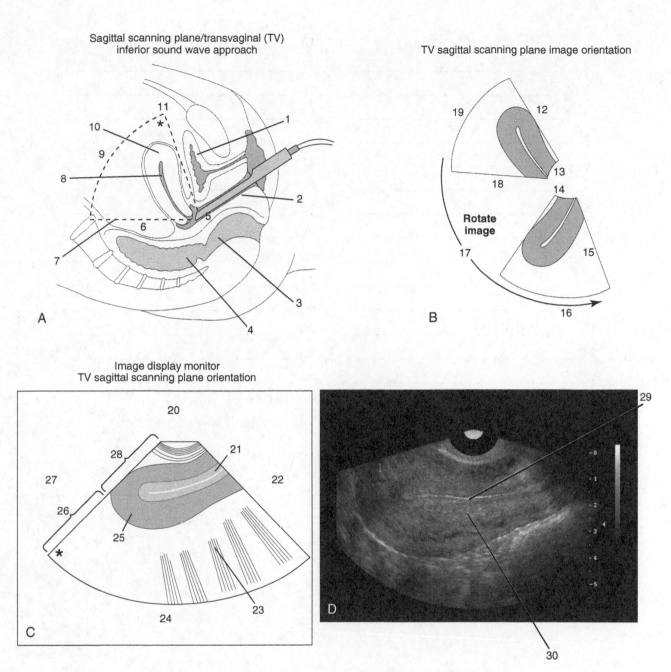

Sagittal scanning plane/transvaginal (TV)
inferior sound wave approach

11
10
9
8
1
2
5
6
7
3
4

A

TV sagittal scanning plane image orientation

19
12
18
13
14
15
Rotate image
17
16

B

Image display monitor
TV sagittal scanning plane orientation

20
28
21
27
22
26
25
23
*
24

C

29
30

D

Figure 21-25A to D in the textbook Answer blanks are on following page.

1 _____

2 _____

3 _____

4 _____

5 _____

6 _____

7 _____

8 _____

9 _____

10 _____

11 _____

12 _____

13 _____

14 _____

15 _____

16 _____

17 _____

18 _____

19 _____

20 _____

21 _____

22 _____

23 _____

24 _____

25 _____

26 _____

27 _____

28 _____

29 _____

30 _____

Figure 21-25A to D in the textbook

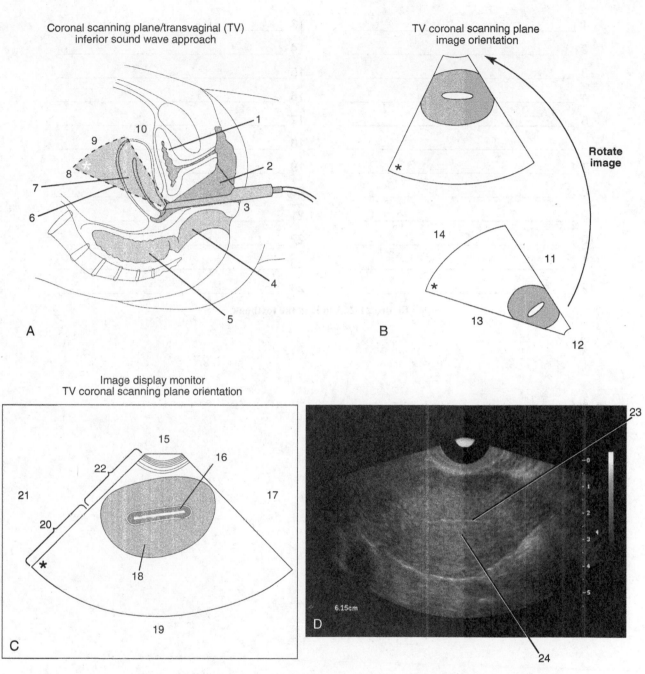

Coronal scanning plane/transvaginal (TV) inferior sound wave approach

A

TV coronal scanning plane image orientation

Rotate image

B

Image display monitor TV coronal scanning plane orientation

C

6.15cm

D

Figure 21-26A to D in the textbook Answer blanks are on following page.

1 _____

2 _____

3 _____

4 _____

5 _____

6 _____

7 _____

8 _____

9 _____

10 _____

11 _____

12 _____

13 _____

14 _____

15 _____

16 _____

17 _____

18 _____

19 _____

20 _____

21 _____

22 _____

23 _____

24 _____

Figure 21-26A to D in the textbook

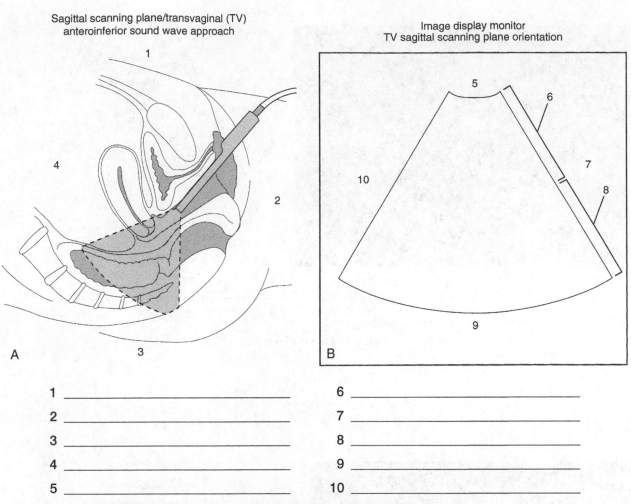

Sagittal scanning plane/transvaginal (TV)
anteroinferior sound wave approach

Image display monitor
TV sagittal scanning plane orientation

1

4

2

3

A

5

6

10

7

8

9

B

1 _____
2 _____
3 _____
4 _____
5 _____

6 _____
7 _____
8 _____
9 _____
10 _____

Figure 21-27A and B in the textbook

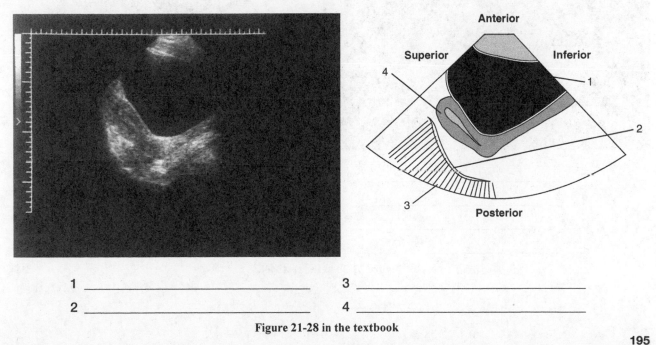

Anterior

Superior

Inferior

4

1

2

3

Posterior

1 _____
2 _____

3 _____
4 _____

Figure 21-28 in the textbook

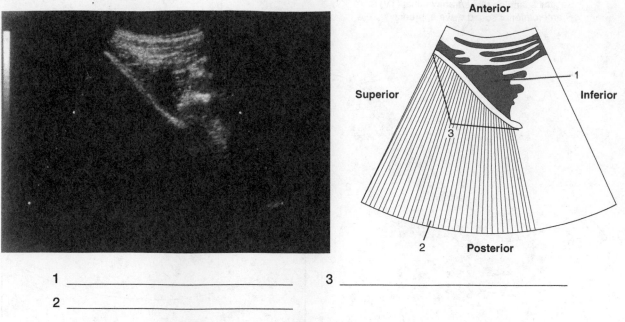

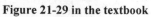

1 _____   3 _____

2 _____

Figure 21-29 in the textbook

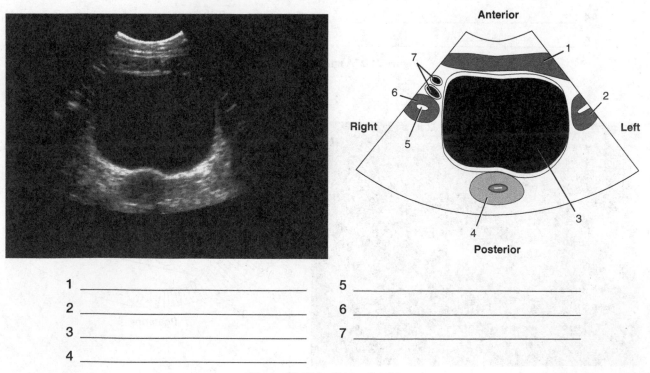

1 _____   5 _____

2 _____   6 _____

3 _____   7 _____

4 _____

Figure 21-30 in the textbook

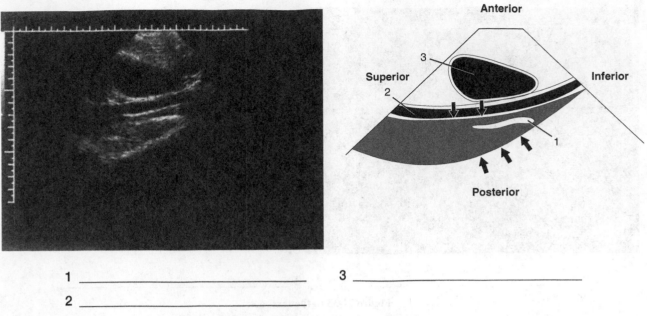

1 _____   3 _____
2 _____

Figure 21-31 in the textbook

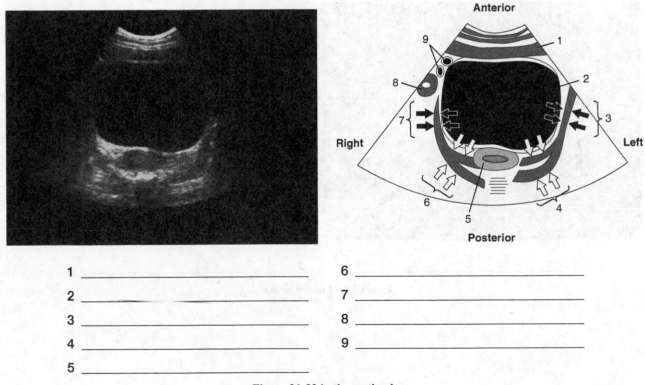

1 _____   6 _____
2 _____   7 _____
3 _____   8 _____
4 _____   9 _____
5 _____

Figure 21-32 in the textbook

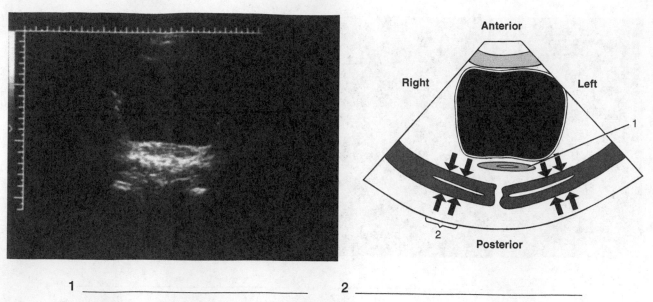

1 _____ 2 _____

Figure 21-33 in the textbook

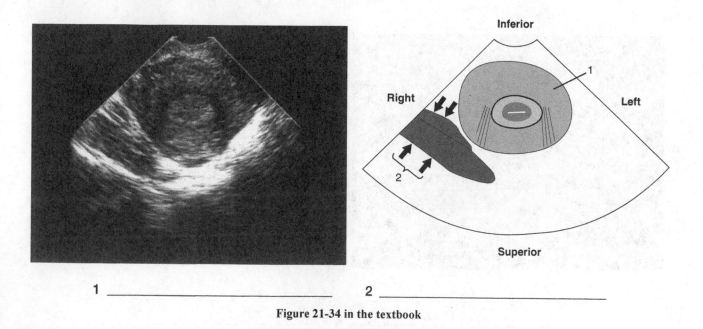

1 _____ 2 _____

Figure 21-34 in the textbook

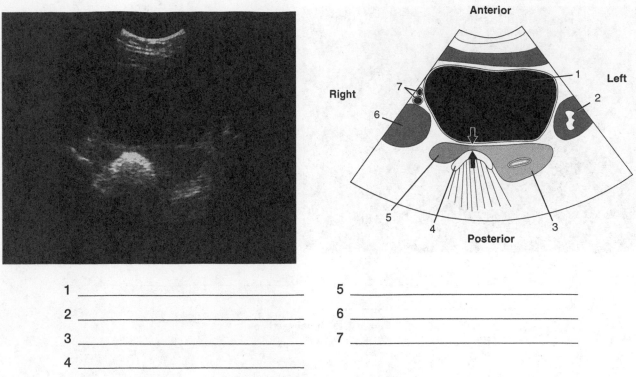

1	_____	5	_____
2	_____	6	_____
3	_____	7	_____
4	_____		

Figure 21-35 in the textbook

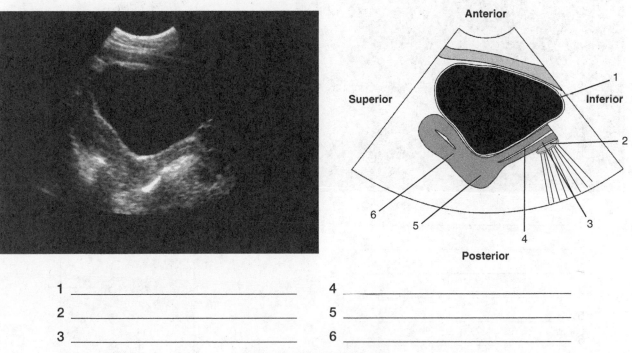

1	_____	4	_____
2	_____	5	_____
3	_____	6	_____

Figure 21-36 in the textbook

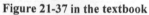

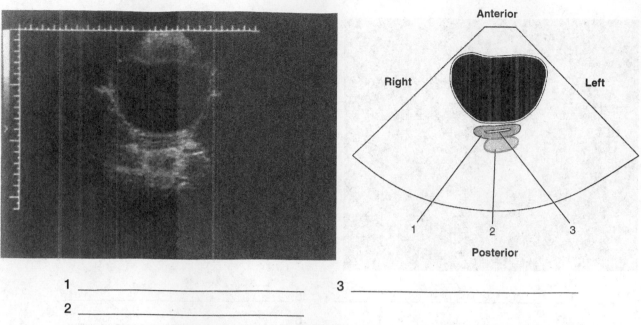

1 _____	3 _____
2 _____	

Figure 21-37 in the textbook

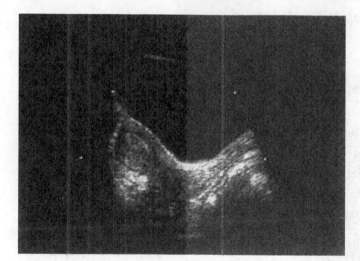

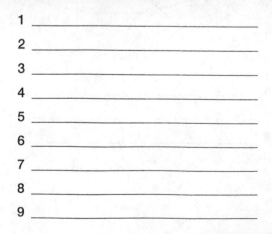

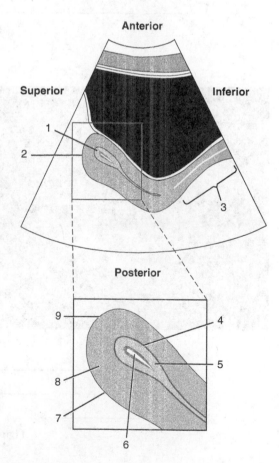

1 _____

2 _____

3 _____

4 _____

5 _____

6 _____

7 _____

8 _____

9 _____

Figure 21-38 in the textbook

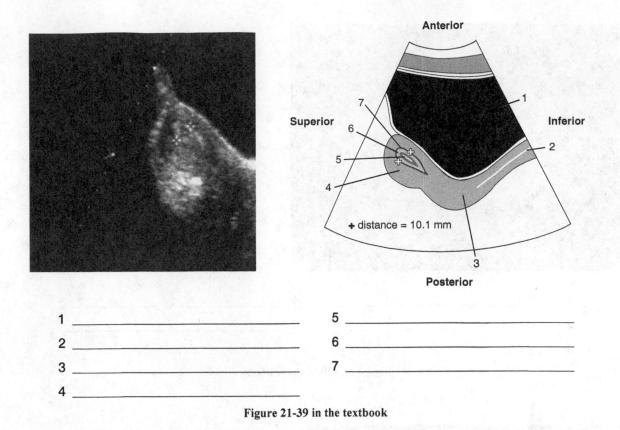

1 _____   5 _____

2 _____   6 _____

3 _____   7 _____

4 _____

Figure 21-39 in the textbook

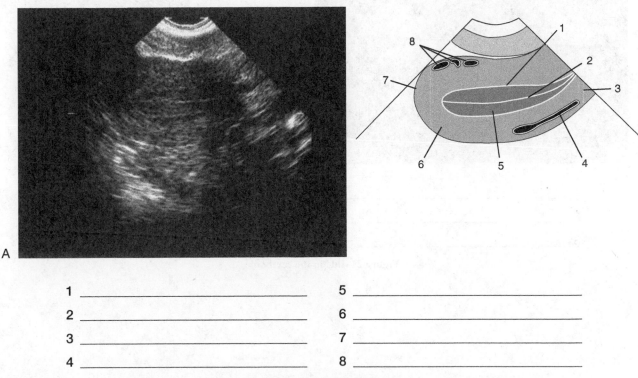

1 _____   5 _____

2 _____   6 _____

3 _____   7 _____

4 _____   8 _____

Figure 21-40A in the textbook

Chapter **21**   **The Female Pelvis**

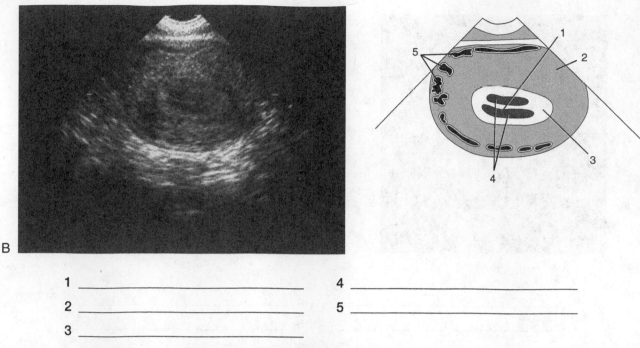

Figure 21-40B in the textbook

1 _____   4 _____

2 _____   5 _____

3 _____

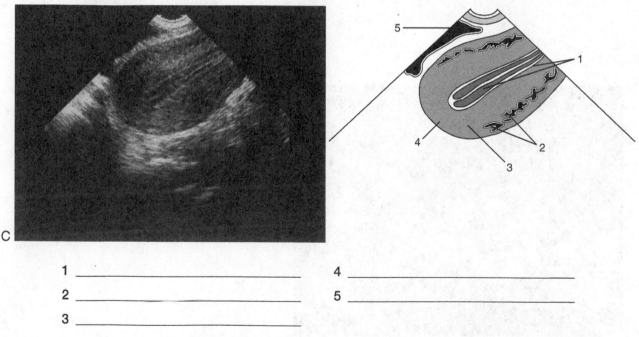

Figure 21-40C in the textbook

1 _____   4 _____

2 _____   5 _____

3 _____

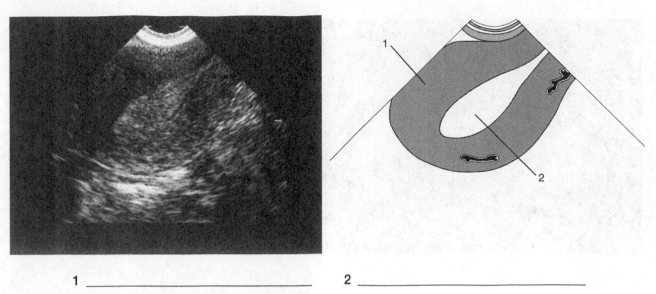

1 _____   2 _____

Figure 21-41 in the textbook

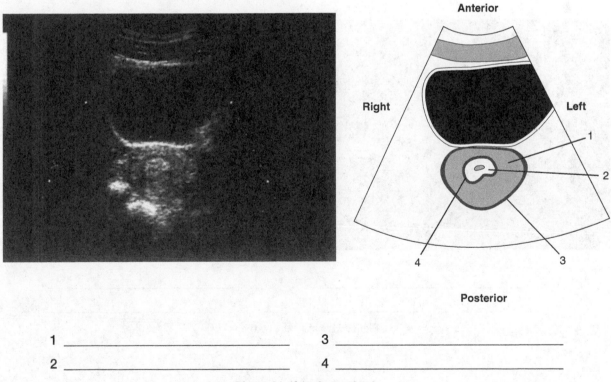

1 _____   3 _____
2 _____   4 _____

Figure 21-42 in the textbook

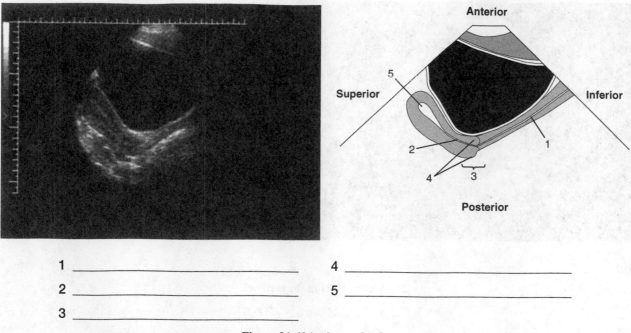

1 _____   4 _____

2 _____   5 _____

3 _____

Figure 21-43 in the textbook

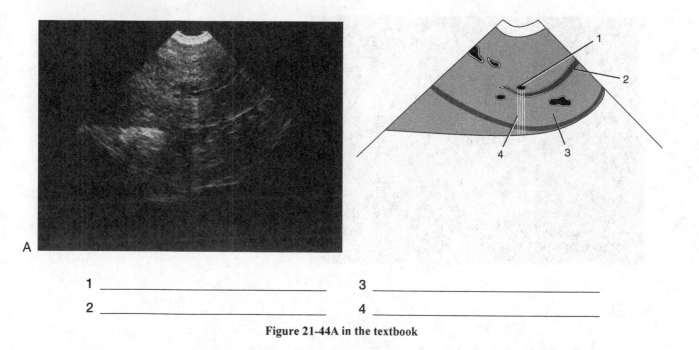

1 _____   3 _____

2 _____   4 _____

Figure 21-44A in the textbook

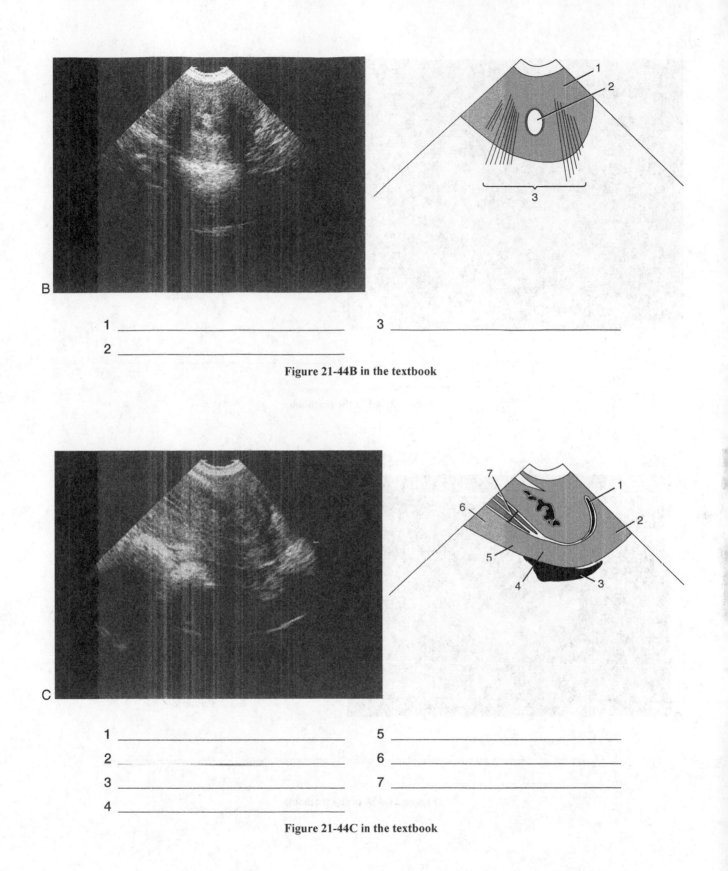

B

1 _____   3 _____

2 _____

Figure 21-44B in the textbook

C

1 _____   5 _____

2 _____   6 _____

3 _____   7 _____

4 _____

Figure 21-44C in the textbook

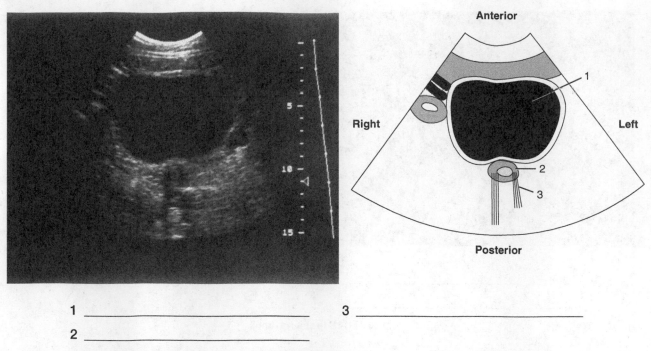

1 _____ 3 _____

2 _____

Figure 21-45 in the textbook

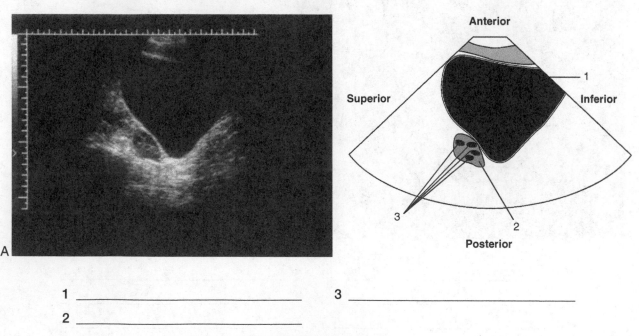

1 _____ 3 _____

2 _____

Figure 21-46A in the textbook

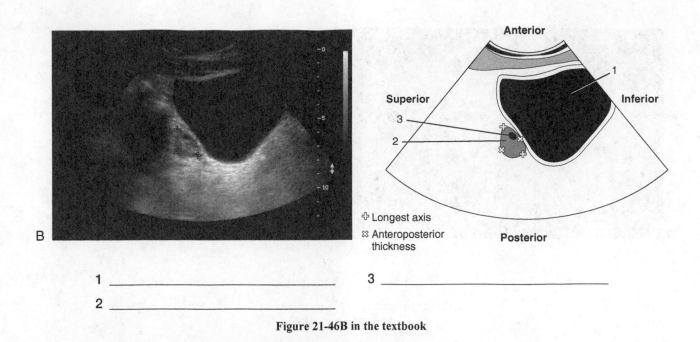

1 _____   3 _____
2 _____

Figure 21-46B in the textbook

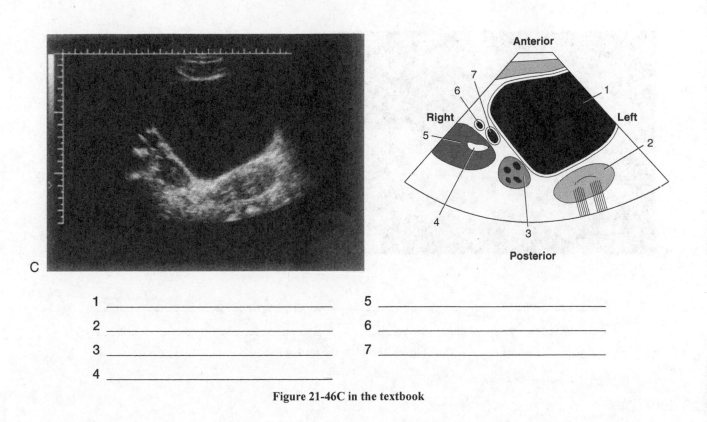

1 _____   5 _____
2 _____   6 _____
3 _____   7 _____
4 _____

Figure 21-46C in the textbook

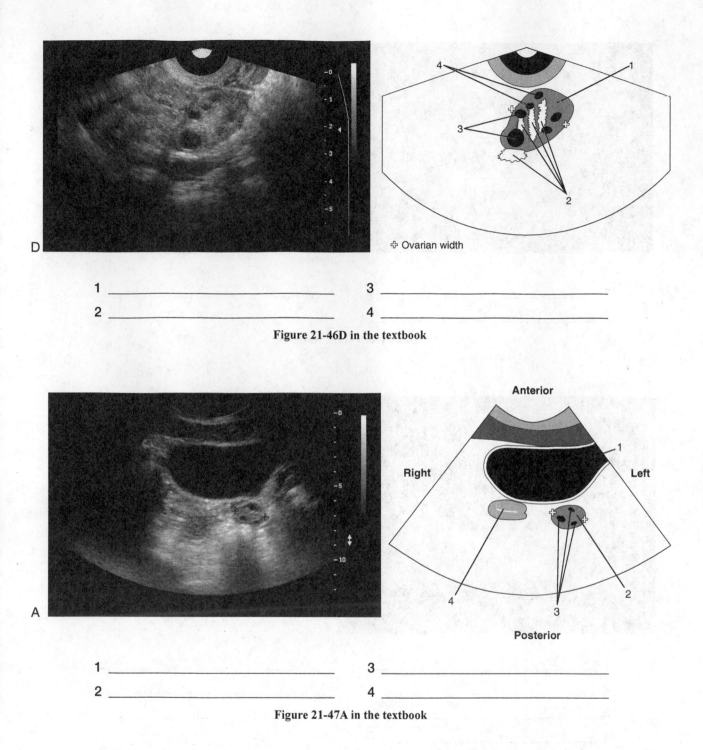

D

⊕ Ovarian width

1 _____ 3 _____

2 _____ 4 _____

Figure 21-46D in the textbook

Anterior

Right

Left

Posterior

A

1 _____ 3 _____

2 _____ 4 _____

Figure 21-47A in the textbook

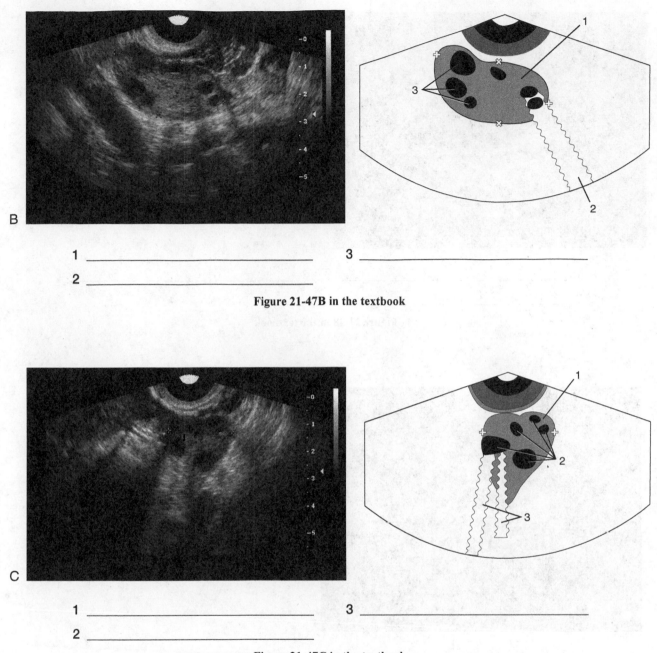

B

1 _____   3 _____

2 _____

Figure 21-47B in the textbook

C

1 _____   3 _____

2 _____

Figure 21-47C in the textbook

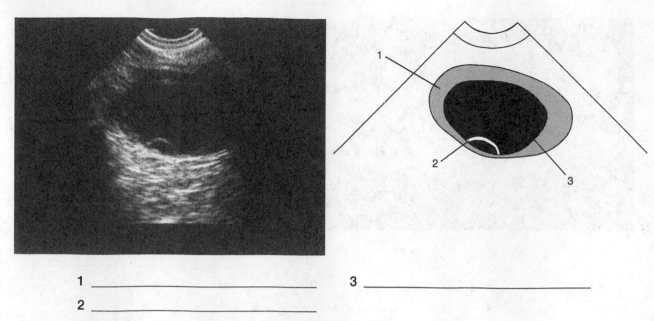

1 _____   3 _____

2 _____

Figure 21-48 in the textbook

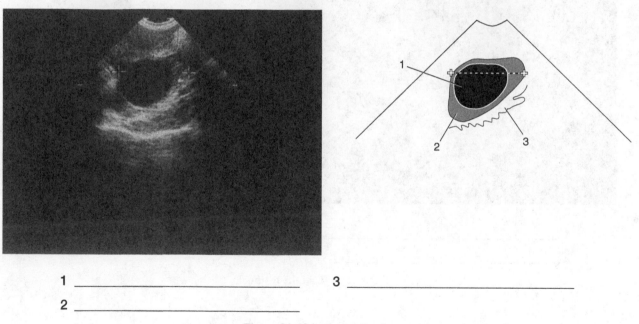

1 _____   3 _____

2 _____

Figure 21-49 in the textbook

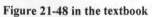

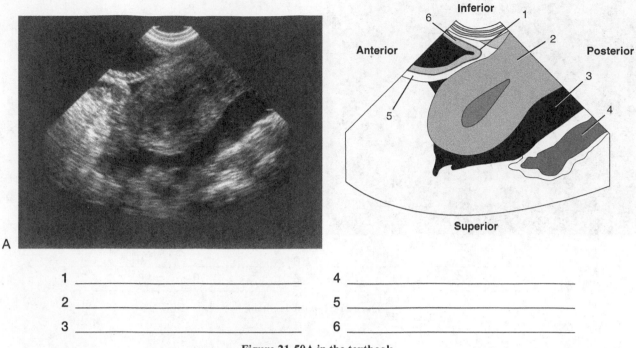

A

1	_____	4	_____
2	_____	5	_____
3	_____	6	_____

Figure 21-50A in the textbook

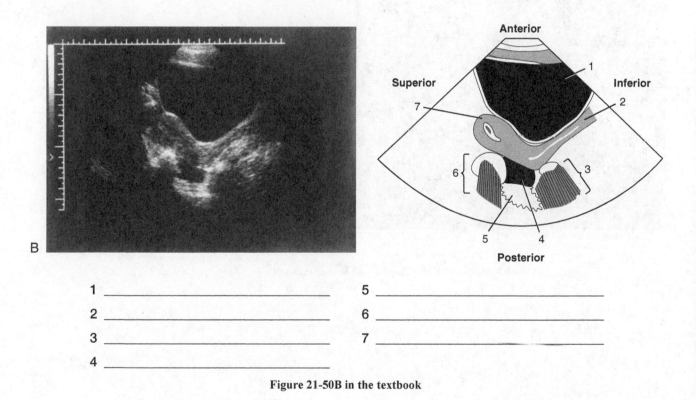

B

1	_____	5	_____
2	_____	6	_____
3	_____	7	_____
4	_____		

Figure 21-50B in the textbook

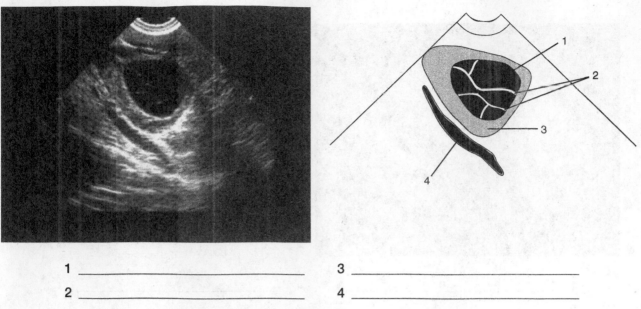

1 _____   3 _____

2 _____   4 _____

Figure 21-51 in the textbook

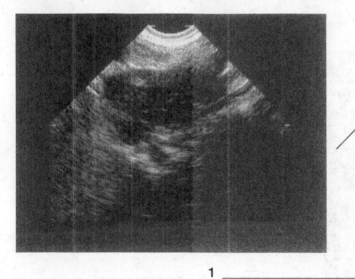
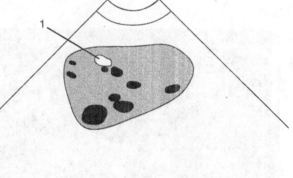

1 _____

Figure 21-52 in the textbook

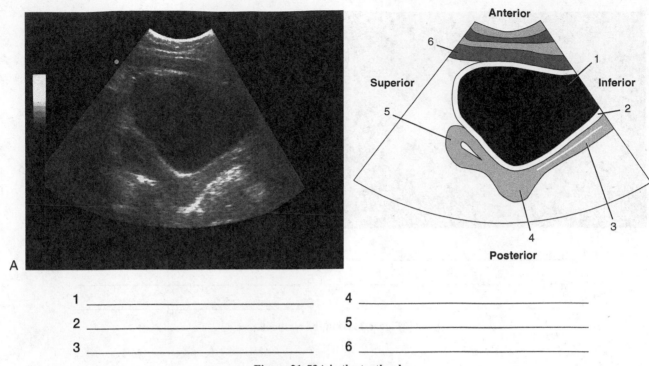

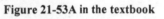

1 _____ 4 _____

2 _____ 5 _____

3 _____ 6 _____

Figure 21-53A in the textbook

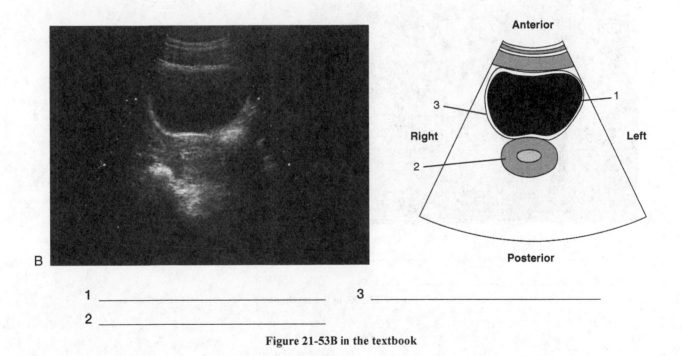

1 _____ 3 _____

2 _____

Figure 21-53B in the textbook

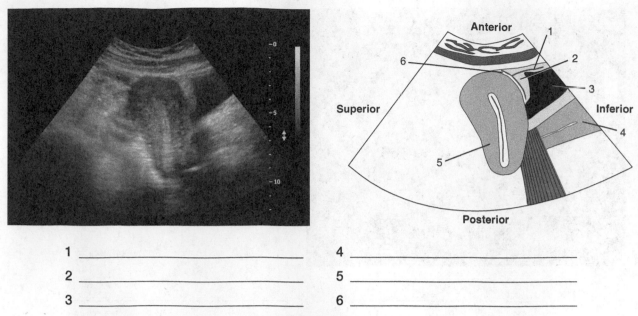

1 _____   4 _____

2 _____   5 _____

3 _____   6 _____

Figure 21-54 in the textbook

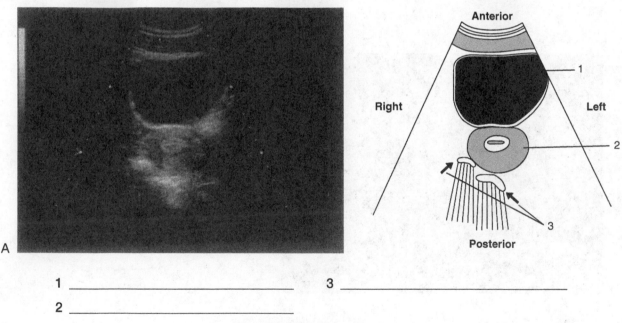

1 _____   3 _____

2 _____

Figure 21-55A in the textbook

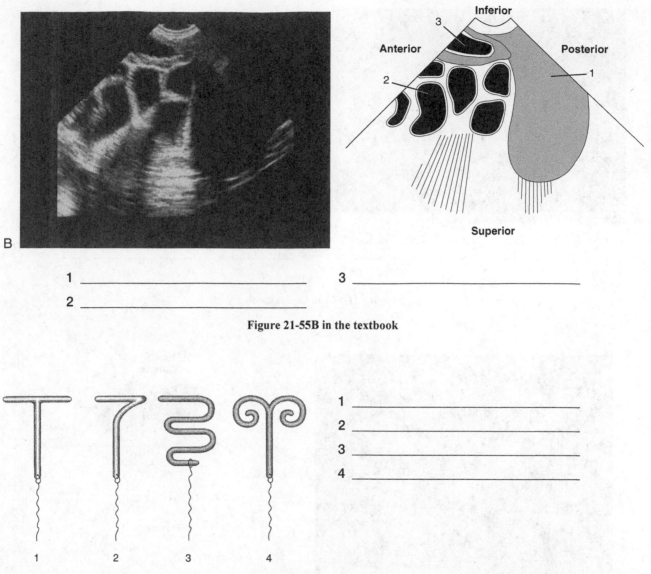

B

1 _____   3 _____

2 _____

Figure 21-55B in the textbook

1 _____

2 _____

3 _____

4 _____

Figure 21-56 in the textbook

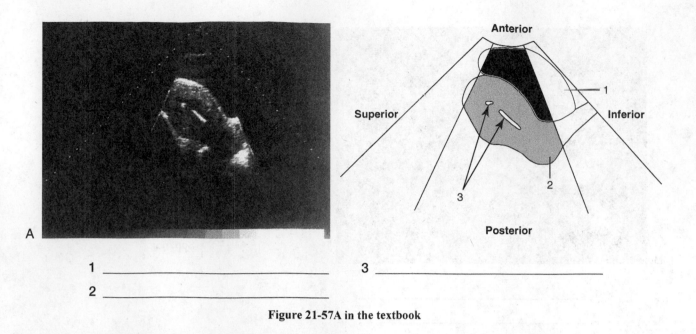

1 _____

2 _____

3 _____

Figure 21-57A in the textbook

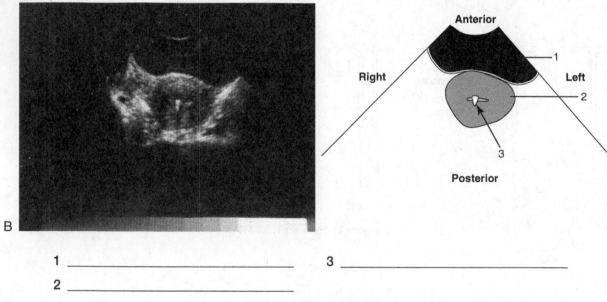

1 _____

2 _____

3 _____

Figure 21-57B in the textbook

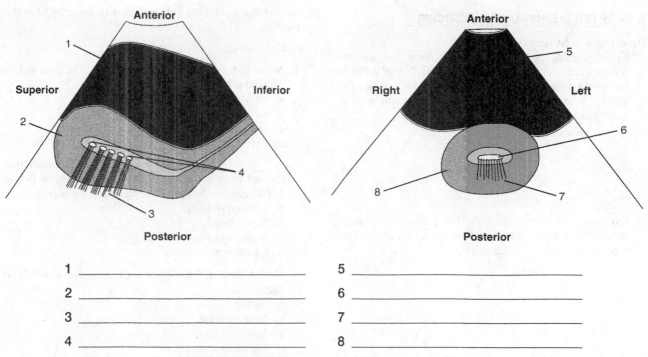

1 _____   5 _____

2 _____   6 _____

3 _____   7 _____

4 _____   8 _____

Figure 21-58 in the textbook

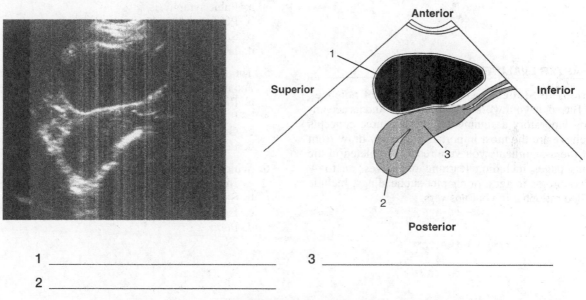

1 _____   3 _____

2 _____

Figure 21-60 in the textbook

V. CHAPTER SUBHEADINGS EXERCISE

Directions to Students:
1. Convert each chapter subheading into a question; for example, change "Gross Anatomy" to "What is the gross anatomy of the female pelvis?" Write the answer to each question in a short paragraph in your notebook.

2. Exchange answers with your lab partner and check each other's work. Refer back to the textbook for further information and explanations.

3. What questions do you still have about the chapter? Write your questions in your notebook.

VI. CHAPTER EVALUATION EXERCISE

Directions to Students: Use a fresh sheet of notebook paper. Based on your work with the chapter and its accompanying laboratory assignments, identify three concepts you believe are the most important. You may draw from any of the assignments you've already completed in the previous pages including learning objectives, anatomy and physiology, images, or chapter subheadings. Include a detailed rationale in your answers.

Answer the questions below. Refer to page 383 for the answers.

Multiple Choice

1. What is the name of the regions of the true pelvis located posterior to the broad ligaments?
   a. Pelvic cavity
   b. Pelvis major
   c. Adnexa
   d. Pelvic diaphragm

2. _____ are double folds of peritoneum that extend from the uterine cornua to the lateral pelvic walls and provide minor support for the uterus.
   a. Linea terminalis
   b. Spiral bands
   c. Broad ligaments
   d. Circular muscularis

3. Which layer of the uterine wall comprises the bulk of the uterus?
   a. Serosal
   b. Endometrium
   c. Myometrium
   d. Parametrium

4. The palpable external landmark that aids in evaluating the pelvis and is formed from an anterior fusion of bones is known as the
   a. Pubic symphysis
   b. Pelvic inlet
   c. Space of Retzius
   d. Ischium

5. The innominate bones encircle and form the lateral and anterior margins of the
   a. Iliac crest
   b. Pelvic diaphragm
   c. Greater sac
   d. Pelvic cavity

6. Which is not part of the innominate bones?
   a. Ilium
   b. Sacrum
   c. Ischium
   d. Pubis

7. Which false pelvic muscles appear closest to the anterior abdominal wall on transverse sonographic images?
   a. Piriformis
   b. Obturator internus
   c. Iliopsoas
   d. Levator ani

8. Which muscle pairs may be visualized outside the pelvic diaphragm?
   a. Obturator internus
   b. Pubococcygeus
   c. Levator ani
   d. Iliococcygeus

9. Sonographic landmarks of the ovaries include all except
   a. Spiral uterine arteries
   b. External iliac veins
   c. Internal iliac arteries
   d. Iliopsoas muscles

10. Which of the following sonographic findings are most likely to be visualized when viewing a graafian follicle?
    a. Irregular, thickened walls
    b. Fluid–fluid level
    c. Cellular layers
    d. 20 mm diameter

First Trimester Obstetrics 22

I. MEMORIZATION EXERCISE

Directions to Students: Write the key words in your notebook or on note cards. Write the words on one side of the notepaper and then write the definitions on the opposite side of the page or on the back of the paper. If using note cards, write the key word on the front and the definition on the back. *This step should be completed before the lab session begins.*

Memorize the key word definitions silently for 5 minutes, then work with a lab partner and identify the words you still need help with. List the words here. Add additional rows if needed.

II. COMPREHENSION EXERCISE

Directions to Students: Work with a lab partner to complete this exercise. You will need to write in your notebook. First, change each objective into a question.

> *Example: "Describe the sonographic appearance of the gestational sac and early embryo" becomes "What is the sonographic appearance of the gestational sac and early embryo?"*

Next, write a short answer to the question just created.

> *Example: "The gestational sac appears on ultrasound as an oval or round, anechoic, fluid-filled sac in the fundus or midportion of the endometrium. A collection of echoes against the wall of the gestational sac represents the early embryo. The gestational sac can be seen as early as 3 weeks' gestational age with transvaginal imaging. The early embryo can be seen at 5 to 6 weeks' gestational age with transvaginal imaging."*

Highlight or circle any part of your answers about which you are unsure, and check the answers in your textbook. If you are still unsure of the answers, put a question mark next to the answer(s) for the review session of the lab.

III. APPLICATION OF ANATOMY AND PHYSIOLOGY EXERCISE

Directions to Students: Work on the following with your lab partner.

1. In your notebook, draw the gestational sac at three different stages: implantation of the blastocyst, 5 weeks' gestational age, and 7 to 8 weeks' gestational age.

2. Label as many structures as you can in each of the drawings. Ask your lab partner to critique your work. What did you miss? Check your drawing using the sketches in your textbook, and complete any missing structures from your drawing.

3. Below your drawing, write two or three summary sentences on the physiology of the formation of the early gestational sac and embryo. Ask your lab partner to check your work. Now check your work against the physiology section in the textbook. What else can you add to your description?

IV. IMAGE ANALYSIS EXERCISE

Directions to Students: Work on the following figures with your lab partner. It's your choice! You can label all the sketches at once, then go back and label each image with your lab partner, or label an image and its accompanying sketch at the same time. Either way, the goal is to label all of the sketches correctly and carefully compare the sketch with the sonographic image.

For each sonographic image, write a very brief observation that could be presented to your instructor, the clinical sonographer, or the sonologist. Your observation will be based on Chapter 7 in the textbook, which describes how to write a technical observation. Please go back and review that chapter if needed.

For each image, your assessment should include (1) the view of each major structure (axial or longitudinal; note: these are not the scanning planes) and (2) structures identified in the image with the correct sonographic appearance, description, and measurements if shown (see Chapter 7 in the textbook for information on how to write a technical observation).

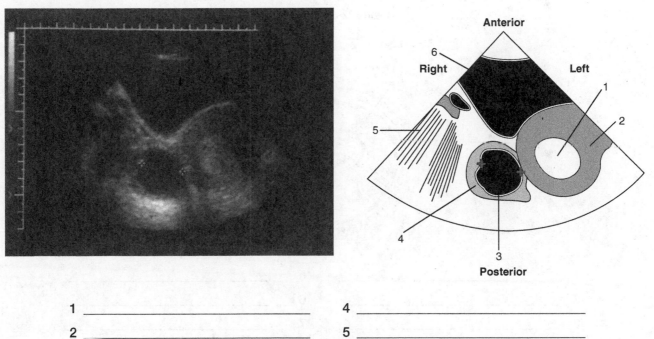

1 _____ 4 _____

2 _____ 5 _____

3 _____ 6 _____

Figure 22-2 in the textbook

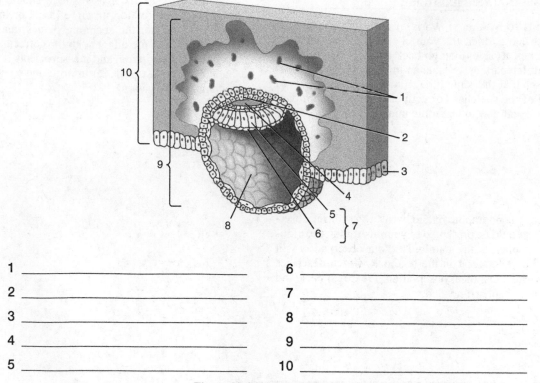

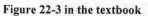

1 _____   6 _____
2 _____   7 _____
3 _____   8 _____
4 _____   9 _____
5 _____   10 _____

Figure 22-3 in the textbook

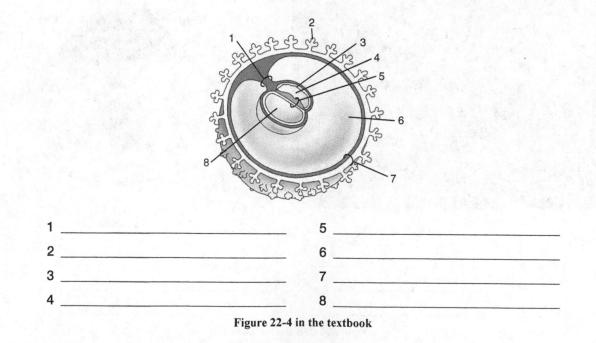

1 _____   5 _____
2 _____   6 _____
3 _____   7 _____
4 _____   8 _____

Figure 22-4 in the textbook

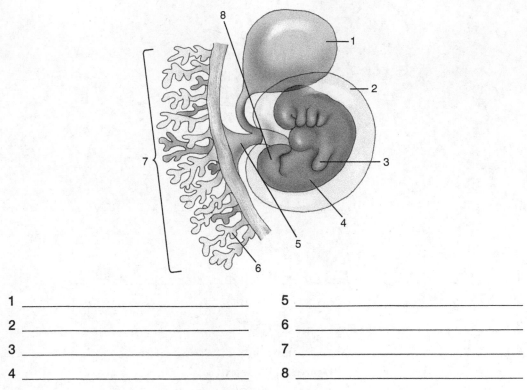

1 _____	5 _____
2 _____	6 _____
3 _____	7 _____
4 _____	8 _____

Figure 22-5 in the textbook

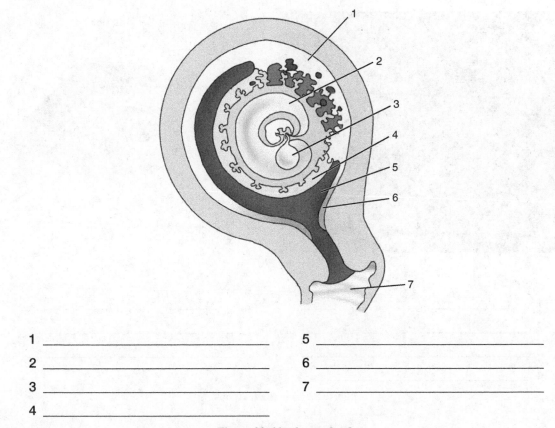

1 _____	5 _____
2 _____	6 _____
3 _____	7 _____
4 _____	

Figure 22-6 in the textbook

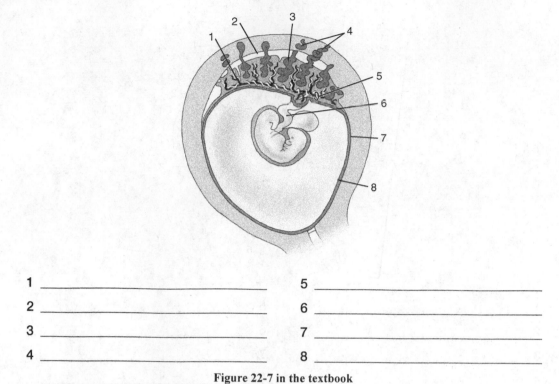

1 _____   5 _____
2 _____   6 _____
3 _____   7 _____
4 _____   8 _____

Figure 22-7 in the textbook

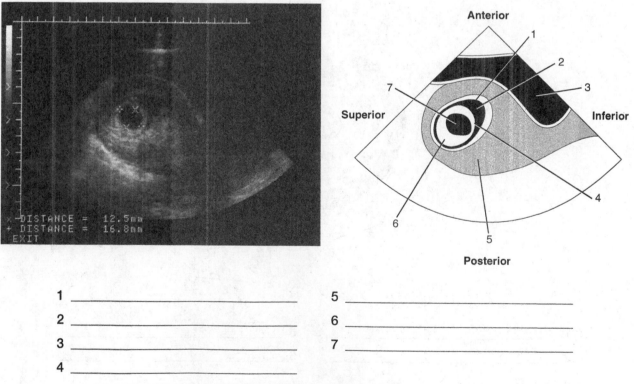

1 _____   5 _____
2 _____   6 _____
3 _____   7 _____
4 _____

Figure 22-10 in the textbook

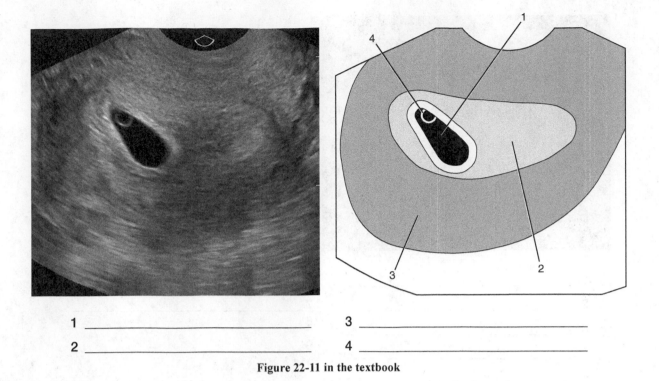

| 1 _____ | 3 _____ |
| 2 _____ | 4 _____ |

Figure 22-11 in the textbook

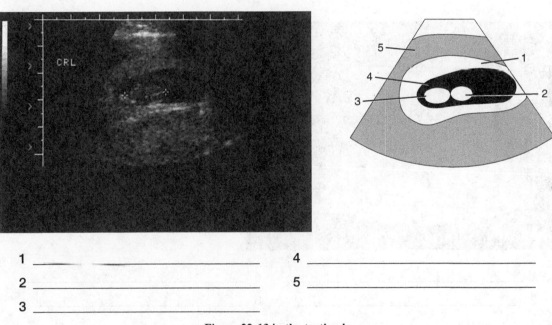

1 _____	4 _____
2 _____	5 _____
3 _____	

Figure 22-13 in the textbook

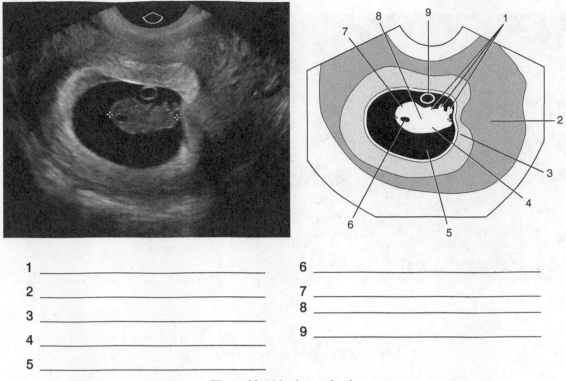

1	_____	6	_____
2	_____	7	_____
3	_____	8	_____
4	_____	9	_____
5	_____		

Figure 22-14 in the textbook

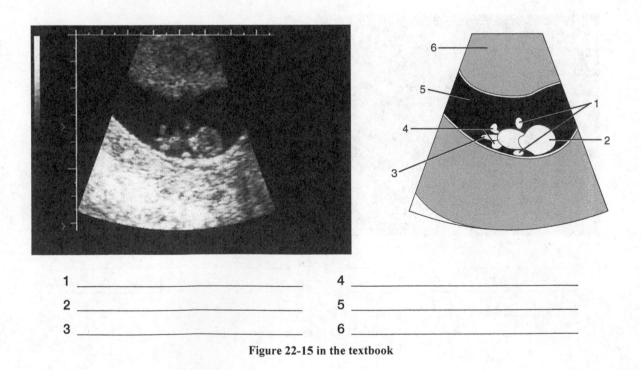

1	_____	4	_____
2	_____	5	_____
3	_____	6	_____

Figure 22-15 in the textbook

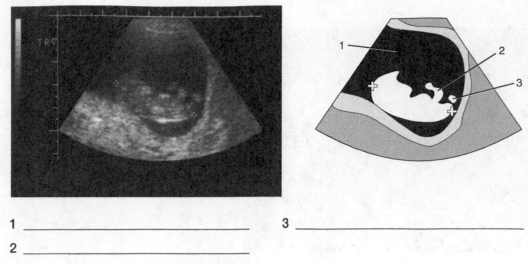

1 _____   3 _____

2 _____

Figure 22-16 in the textbook

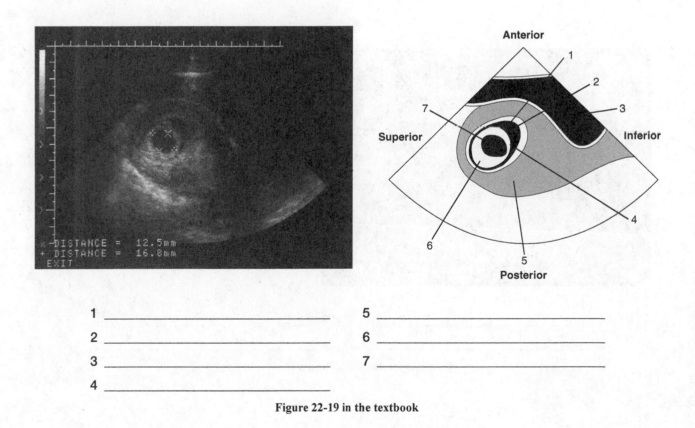

1 _____   5 _____

2 _____   6 _____

3 _____   7 _____

4 _____

Figure 22-19 in the textbook

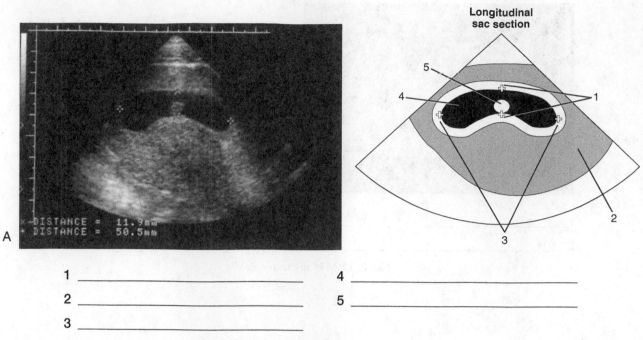

A

1 _____   4 _____

2 _____   5 _____

3 _____

Figure 22-22A in the textbook

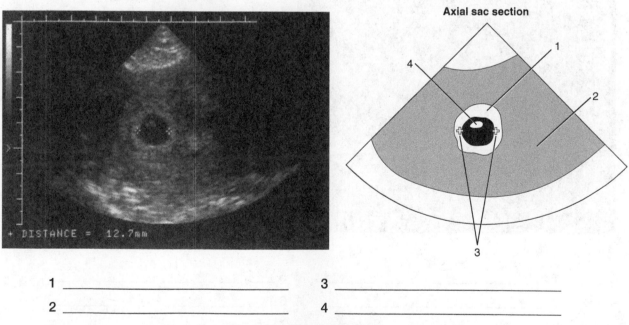

B

1 _____   3 _____

2 _____   4 _____

Figure 22-22B in the textbook

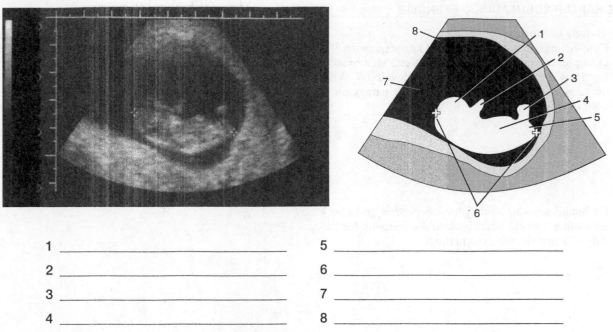

1	_____	5	_____
2	_____	6	_____
3	_____	7	_____
4	_____	8	_____

Figure 22-23 in the textbook

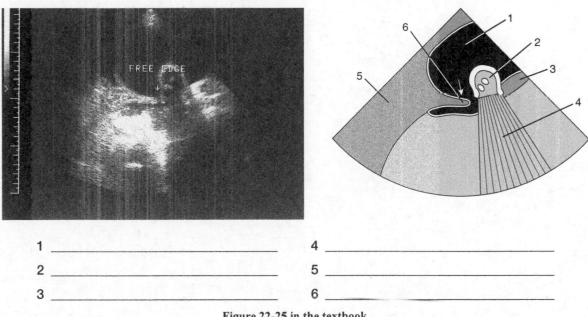

FREE EDGE

1	_____	4	_____
2	_____	5	_____
3	_____	6	_____

Figure 22-25 in the textbook

V. CHAPTER SUBHEADINGS EXERCISE

Directions to Students:

1. Convert each chapter subheading into a question; for example, change "Development of Fetal Membranes" to "How do the fetal membranes develop?" Write the answer to each question in a short paragraph in your notebook.

2. Exchange answers with your lab partner and check each other's work. Refer back to the textbook for further information and explanations.

3. What questions do you still have about the chapter? Write your questions in your notebook.

VI. CHAPTER EVALUATION EXERCISE

Directions to Students: Use a fresh sheet of notebook paper. Based on your work with the chapter and its accompanying laboratory assignments, identify three concepts you believe are the most important. You may draw from any of the assignments you've already completed in the previous pages including learning objectives, anatomy and physiology, images, or chapter subheadings. Include a detailed rationale in your answers.

Answer the questions below. Refer to page 383 for the answers.

Multiple Choice

1. What aids in maintaining the proper temperature for the embryo?
   a. Corpus luteum
   b. Chorionic villi
   c. Amnion
   d. Amniotic fluid

2. What is the maximum size of a normal yolk sac?
   a. 5 mm
   b. 6 mm
   c. 7 mm
   d. 8 mm

3. What hormone is produced by the corpus luteum to prepare for pregnancy?
   a. Progesterone
   b. Follicle-stimulating hormone
   c. Estrogen
   d. a and c

4. What parameter is not used to determine fetal risk for aneuploidy?
   a. Maternal serum screen
   b. Fetal age
   c. Maternal age
   d. Nuchal translucency

5. At which gestational age will you likely see the double bleb sign?
   a. 3 weeks, 2 days
   b. 4 weeks, 4 days
   c. 6 weeks, 0 days
   d. 1 week, 6 days

6. At what hCG level should a gestational sac be seen?
   a. 1000
   b. 2000
   c. 3000
   d. 4000

7. Which hormone causes ovulation to occur when increased?
   a. Human chorionic gonadotropin
   b. Progesterone
   c. Follicle stimulating hormone
   d. Luteinizing hormone

8. Where does fertilization usually take place?
   a. Ovary
   b. Adnexa
   c. Uterus
   d. Fallopian tube

9. Which of these is associated with ectopic pregnancy?
   a. Double sac sign
   b. Double yolk sac
   c. Gestational sac in the fundus or midportion of the uterus
   d. Pseudo-gestational sac

10. What part of the embryonic brain forms the cerebellum?
   a. Prosencephalon
   b. Midbrain
   c. Rhombencephalon
   d. None of the above

Second and Third Trimester Obstetrics 23

I. MEMORIZATION EXERCISE

Directions to Students: Write the key words in your notebook or on note cards. Write the words on one side of the notepaper and then write the definitions on the opposite side of the page or on the back of the paper. If using note cards, write the key word on the front and the definition on the back. *This step should be completed before the lab session begins.*

Memorize the key word definitions silently for 5 minutes, then work with a lab partner and identify the words you still need help with. List the words here. Add additional rows if needed.

II. COMPREHENSION EXERCISE

Directions to Students: Work with a lab partner to complete this exercise. You will need to write in your notebook. First, change each objective into a question.

> *Example: "Describe the sonographic appearance of the placenta and its role in supporting gestation" becomes "What is the sonographic appearance of the placenta, and what is its role in supporting gestation?"*

Next, write a short answer to the question just created.

> *Example: "The placenta can be visualized as early as 10 weeks as hyperechoic tissue surrounding a portion of the gestational sac. The purpose of the placenta is to provide a large circulatory surface for exchange of fetal nutrients and waste."*

Highlight or circle any part of your answers about which you are unsure, and check the answers in your textbook. If you are still unsure of the answers, put a question mark next to the answer(s) for the review session of the lab.

III. APPLICATION OF ANATOMY AND PHYSIOLOGY EXERCISE

Directions to Students: Work on the following with your lab partner.
1. In your notebook, draw the different grades of the placenta.

2. Label as many structures as you can in each of the drawings. Ask your lab partner to critique your work. What did you miss? Check your drawing using the sketches in your textbook, and complete any missing structures from your drawing.

3. Below your drawing, write two or three summary sentences on the development of the second and third trimester fetus. Ask your lab partner to check your work. Now check your work against the physiology section in the textbook. What else can you add to your description?

IV. IMAGE ANALYSIS EXERCISE

Directions to Students: Work on the following figures with your lab partner. It's your choice! You can label all the sketches at once, then go back and label each image with your lab partner, or label an image and its accompanying sketch at the same time. Either way, the goal is to label all of the sketches correctly and carefully compare the sketch with the sonographic image.

For each image, your assessment should include (1) the view of each major structure (axial or longitudinal; note: these are not the scanning planes) and (2) structures identified in the image with the correct sonographic appearance, description, and measurements if shown (see Chapter 7 in the textbook for information on how to write a technical observation).

For each sonographic image, write a very brief observation that could be presented to your instructor, the clinical sonographer, or the sonologist. Your observation will be based on Chapter 7 in the textbook, which describes how to write a technical observation. Please go back and review that chapter if needed.

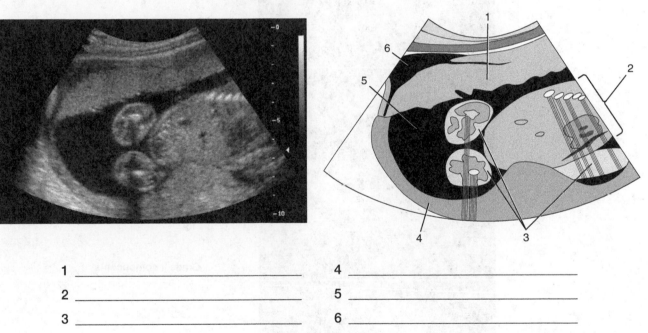

1 _____   4 _____

2 _____   5 _____

3 _____   6 _____

Figure 23-1 in the textbook

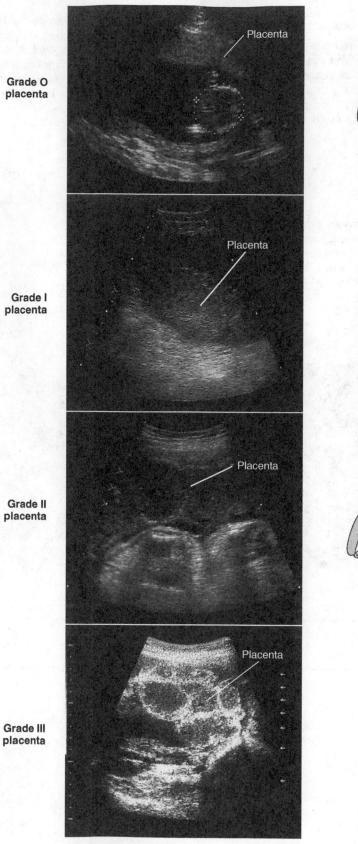

Grade O
placenta

Placenta

Grade I
placenta

Placenta

Grade II
placenta

Placenta

Grade III
placenta

Placenta

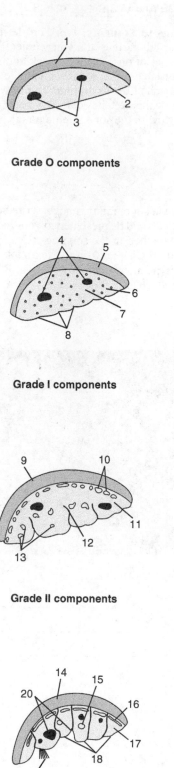

Grade O components

Grade I components

Grade II components

Grade III components

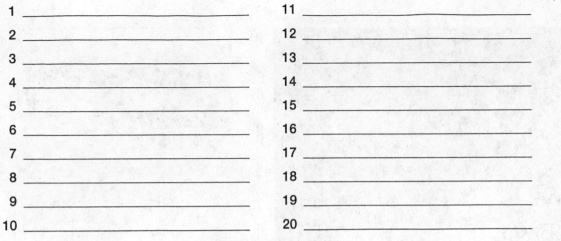

1 _____   11 _____

2 _____   12 _____

3 _____   13 _____

4 _____   14 _____

5 _____   15 _____

6 _____   16 _____

7 _____   17 _____

8 _____   18 _____

9 _____   19 _____

10 _____   20 _____

Figure 23-3 in the textbook

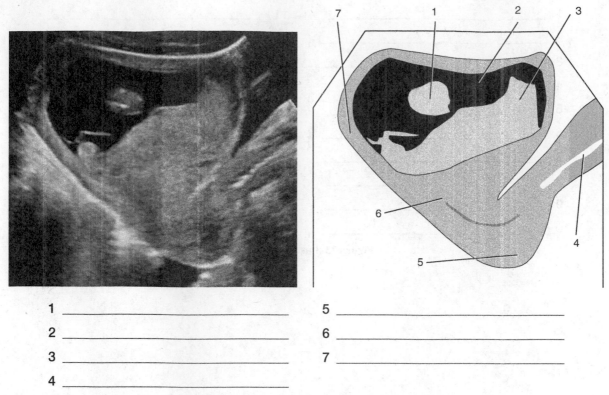

1 _____   5 _____

2 _____   6 _____

3 _____   7 _____

4 _____

Figure 23-4 in the textbook

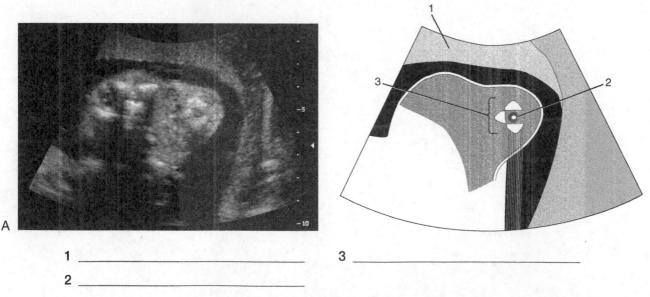

A

1 _____   3 _____

2 _____

Figure 23-6A in the textbook

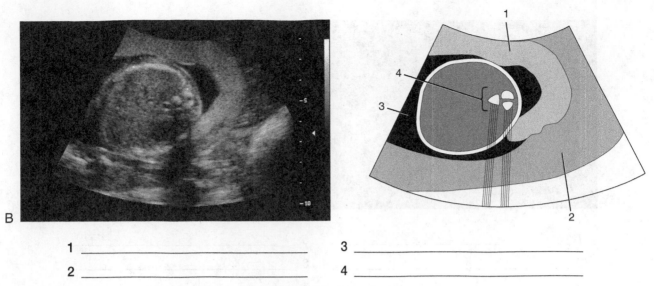

B

1 _____   3 _____

2 _____   4 _____

Figure 23-6B in the textbook

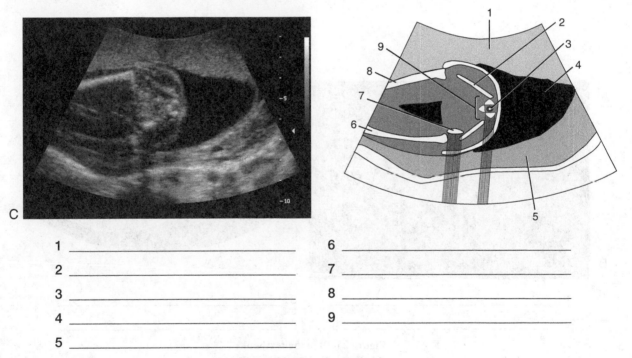

C

1 _____   6 _____

2 _____   7 _____

3 _____   8 _____

4 _____   9 _____

5 _____

Figure 23-6C in the textbook

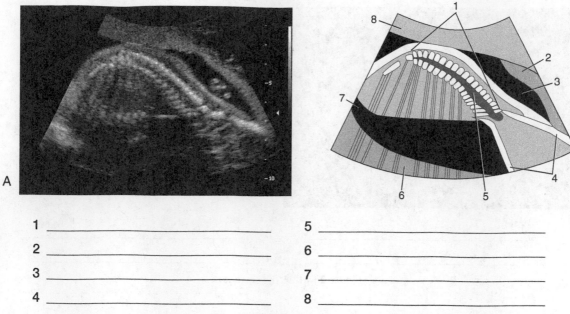

A

1 _____   5 _____

2 _____   6 _____

3 _____   7 _____

4 _____   8 _____

Figure 23-7A in the textbook

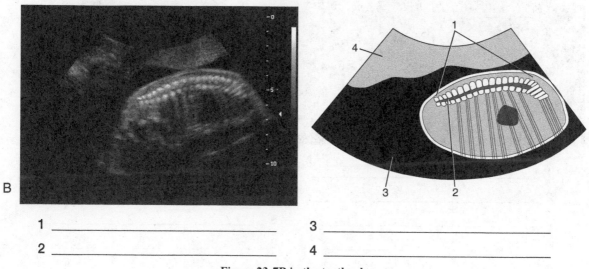

B

1 _____   3 _____

2 _____   4 _____

Figure 23-7B in the textbook

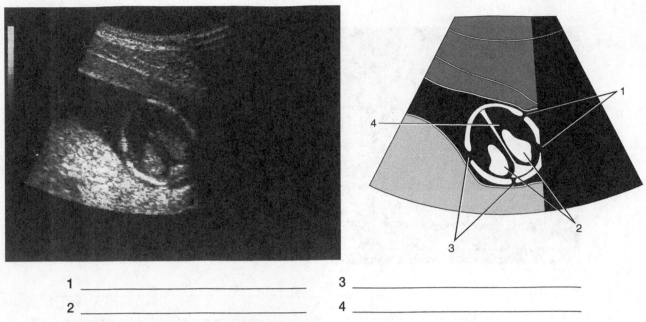

1 _____   3 _____

2 _____   4 _____

Figure 23-8 in the textbook

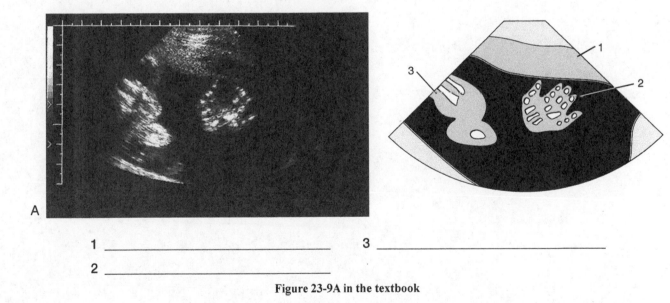

1 _____   3 _____

2 _____

Figure 23-9A in the textbook

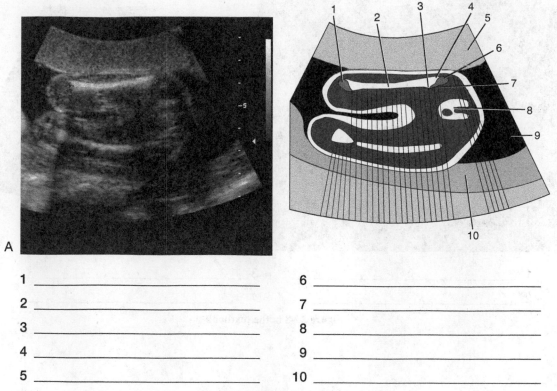

A

1 _____   6 _____
2 _____   7 _____
3 _____   8 _____
4 _____   9 _____
5 _____   10 _____

Figure 23-10A in the textbook

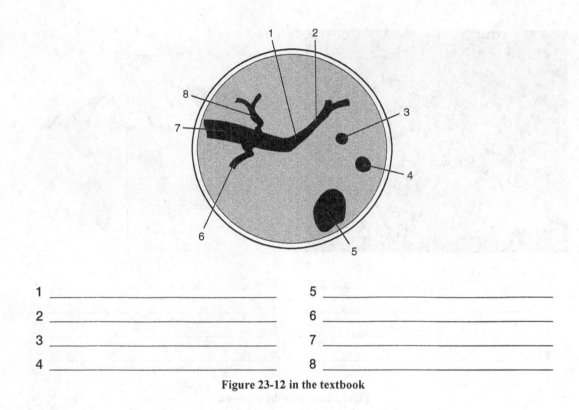

1	_____	5	_____
2	_____	6	_____
3	_____	7	_____
4	_____	8	_____

Figure 23-12 in the textbook

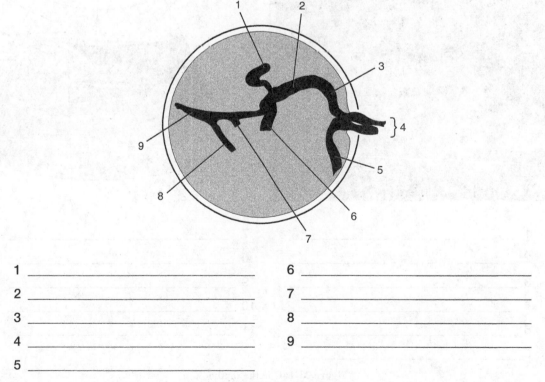

1	_____	6	_____
2	_____	7	_____
3	_____	8	_____
4	_____	9	_____
5	_____		

Figure 23-13 in the textbook

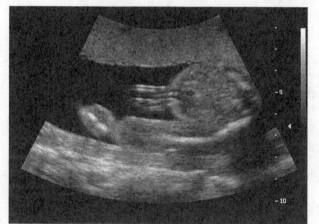

B

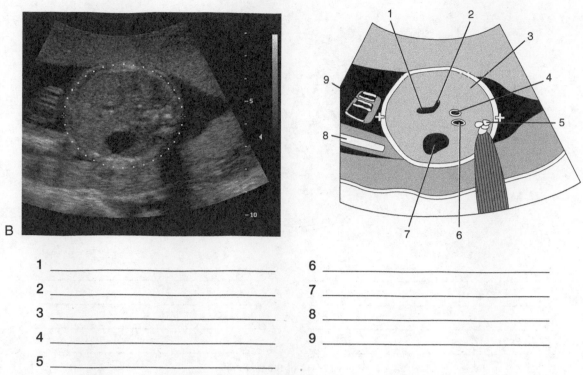

1 _____   6 _____
2 _____   7 _____
3 _____   8 _____
4 _____   9 _____
5 _____

Figure 23-14B in the textbook

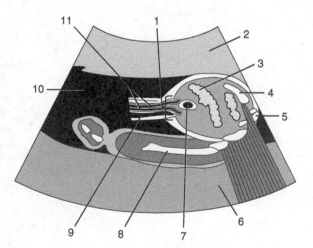

C

1 _____   7 _____
2 _____   8 _____
3 _____   9 _____
4 _____   10 _____
5 _____   11 _____
6 _____

Figure 23-14C in the textbook

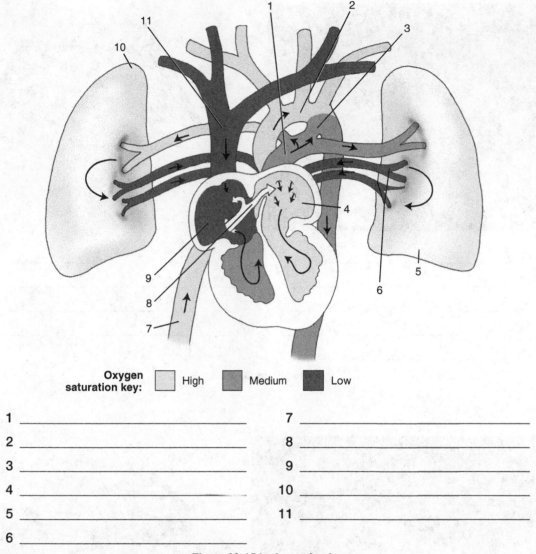

Oxygen saturation key: □ High ▨ Medium ■ Low

1 _____   7 _____
2 _____   8 _____
3 _____   9 _____
4 _____   10 _____
5 _____   11 _____
6 _____

Figure 23-15 in the textbook

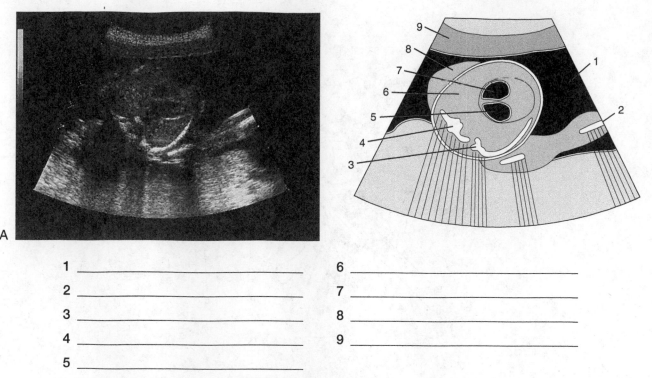

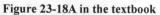

1	_____	6	_____
2	_____	7	_____
3	_____	8	_____
4	_____	9	_____
5	_____		

Figure 23-18A in the textbook

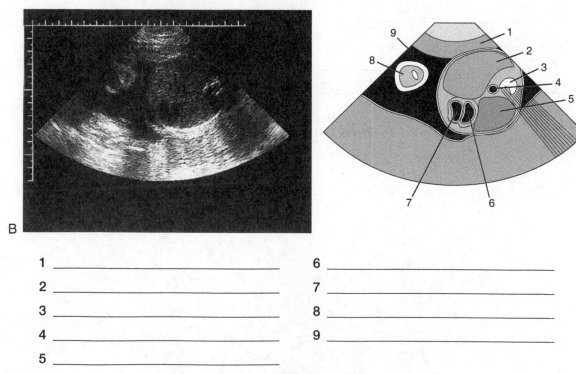

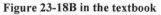

1	_____	6	_____
2	_____	7	_____
3	_____	8	_____
4	_____	9	_____
5	_____		

Figure 23-18B in the textbook

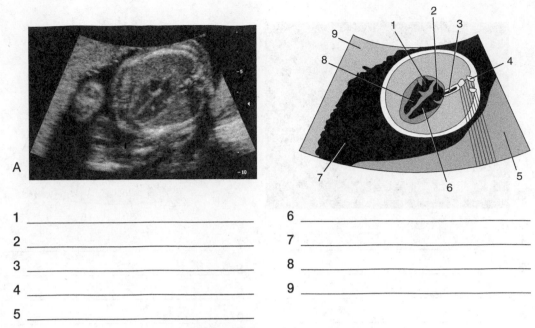

1	_____	6	_____
2	_____	7	_____
3	_____	8	_____
4	_____	9	_____
5	_____		

Figure 23-19A in the textbook

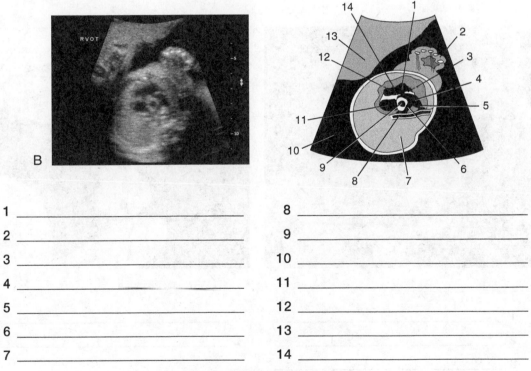

1	_____	8	_____
2	_____	9	_____
3	_____	10	_____
4	_____	11	_____
5	_____	12	_____
6	_____	13	_____
7	_____	14	_____

Figure 23-19B in the textbook

Chapter **23** **Second and Third Trimester Obstetrics**

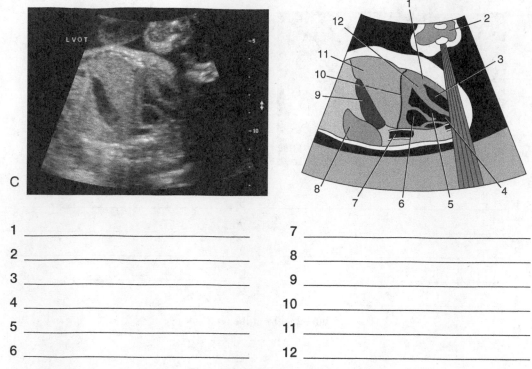

1	_____	7	_____
2	_____	8	_____
3	_____	9	_____
4	_____	10	_____
5	_____	11	_____
6	_____	12	_____

Figure 23-19C in the textbook

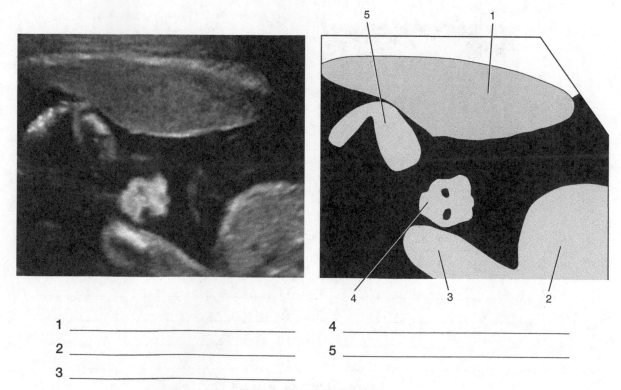

1	_____	4	_____
2	_____	5	_____
3	_____		

Figure 23-20 in the textbook

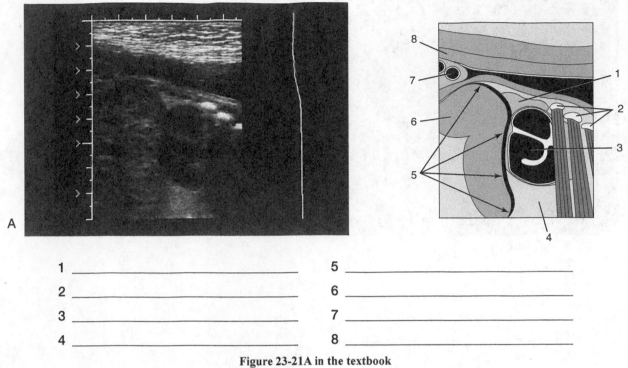

A

1 _____ 5 _____

2 _____ 6 _____

3 _____ 7 _____

4 _____ 8 _____

Figure 23-21A in the textbook

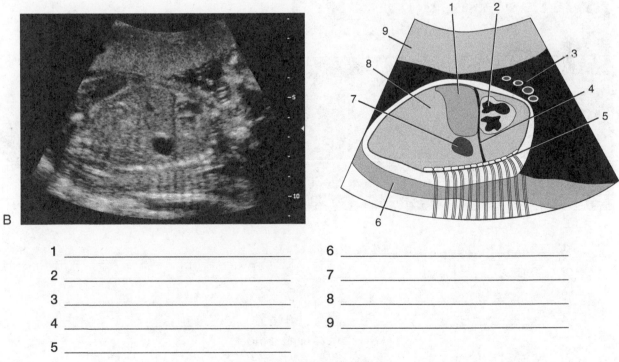

B

1 _____ 6 _____

2 _____ 7 _____

3 _____ 8 _____

4 _____ 9 _____

5 _____

Figure 23-21B in the textbook

Chapter **23** **Second and Third Trimester Obstetrics**

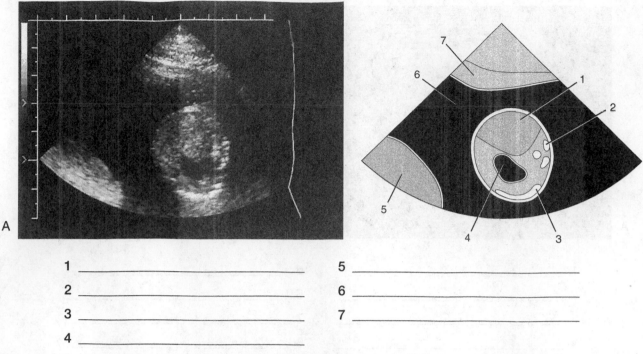

A

1	_____	5	_____
2	_____	6	_____
3	_____	7	_____
4	_____		

Figure 23-22A in the textbook

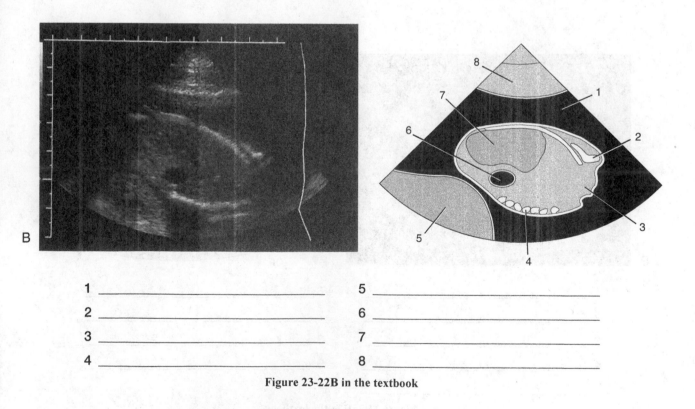

B

1	_____	5	_____
2	_____	6	_____
3	_____	7	_____
4	_____	8	_____

Figure 23-22B in the textbook

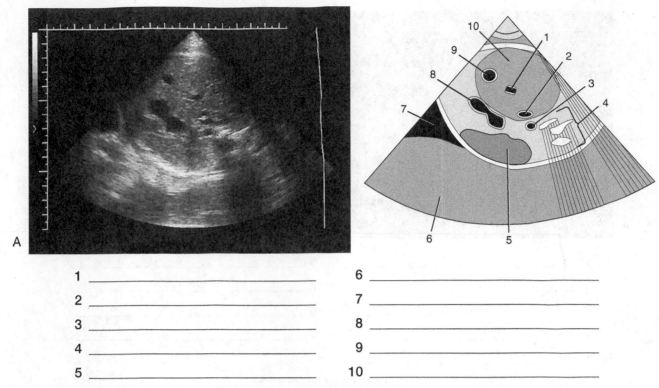

1	_____	6	_____
2	_____	7	_____
3	_____	8	_____
4	_____	9	_____
5	_____	10	_____

Figure 23-23A in the textbook

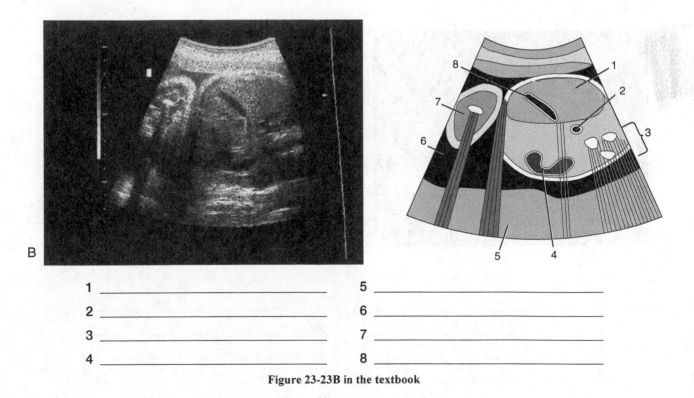

1	_____	5	_____
2	_____	6	_____
3	_____	7	_____
4	_____	8	_____

Figure 23-23B in the textbook

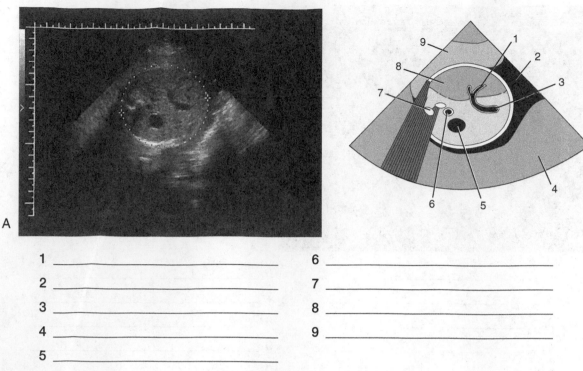

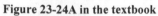

1 _____   6 _____
2 _____   7 _____
3 _____   8 _____
4 _____   9 _____
5 _____

Figure 23-24A in the textbook

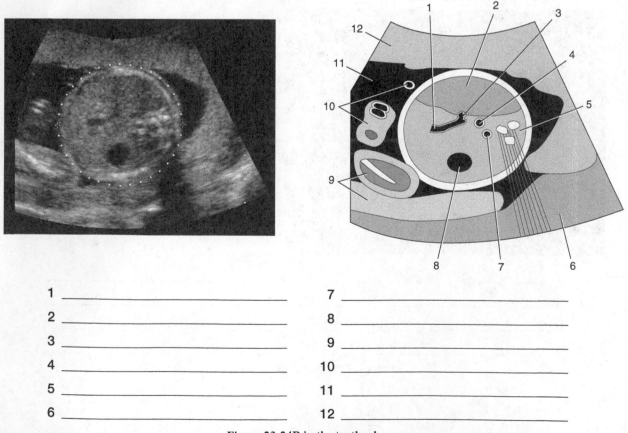

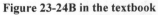

1 _____   7 _____
2 _____   8 _____
3 _____   9 _____
4 _____   10 _____
5 _____   11 _____
6 _____   12 _____

Figure 23-24B in the textbook

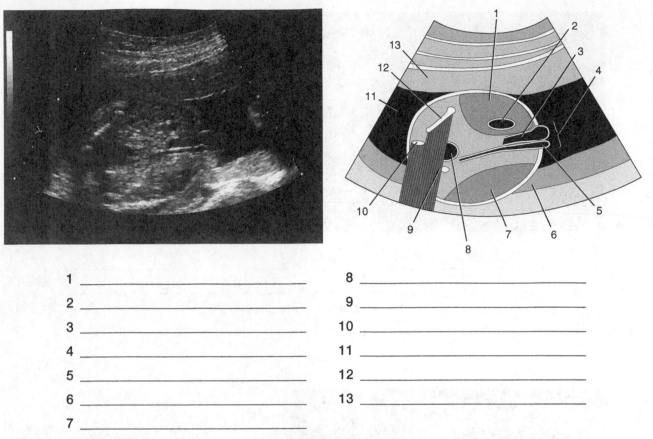

1 _____   8 _____

2 _____   9 _____

3 _____   10 _____

4 _____   11 _____

5 _____   12 _____

6 _____   13 _____

7 _____

Figure 23-25 in the textbook

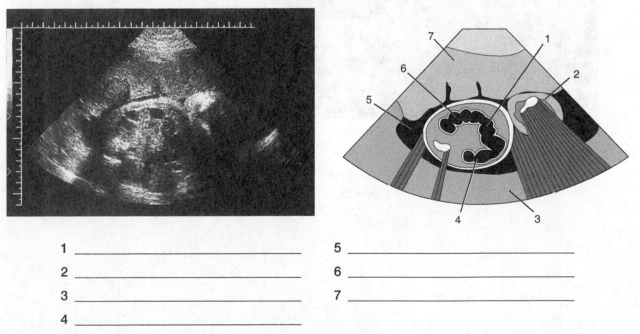

1 _____   5 _____

2 _____   6 _____

3 _____   7 _____

4 _____

Figure 23-26 in the textbook

251

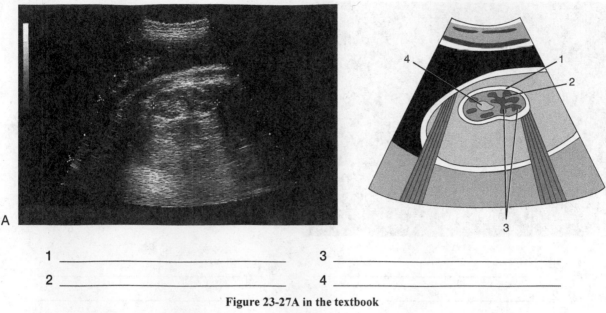

1 _____	3 _____
2 _____	4 _____

Figure 23-27A in the textbook

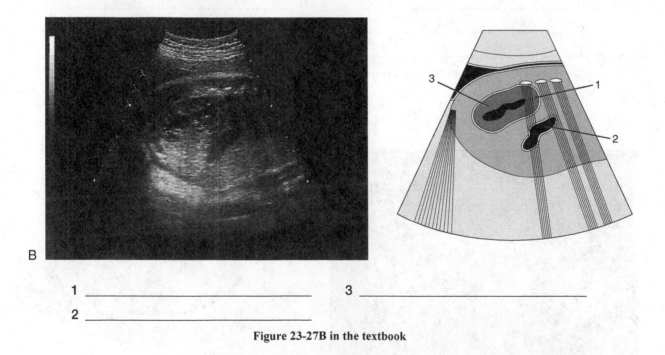

1 _____	3 _____
2 _____	

Figure 23-27B in the textbook

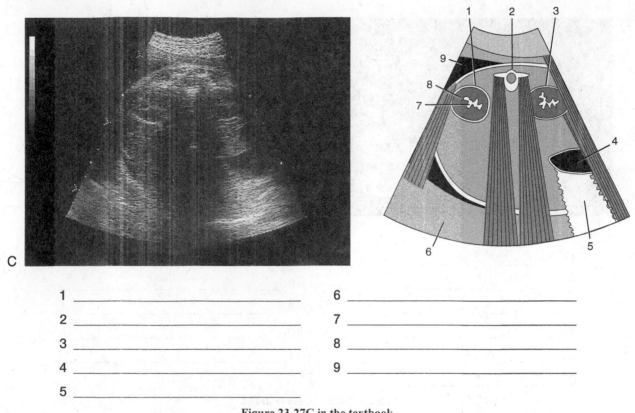

C

1 _____	6 _____
2 _____	7 _____
3 _____	8 _____
4 _____	9 _____
5 _____	

Figure 23-27C in the textbook

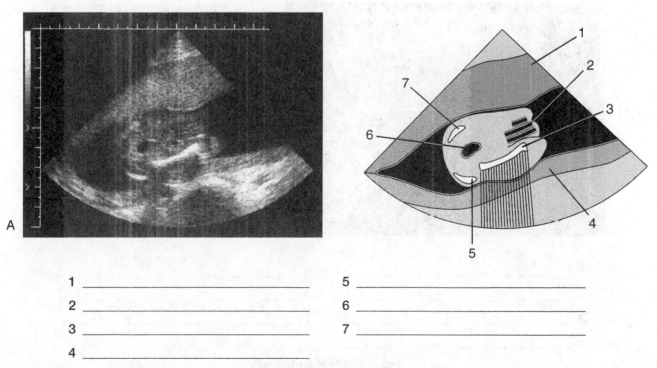

A

1 _____	5 _____
2 _____	6 _____
3 _____	7 _____
4 _____	

Figure 23-28A in the textbook

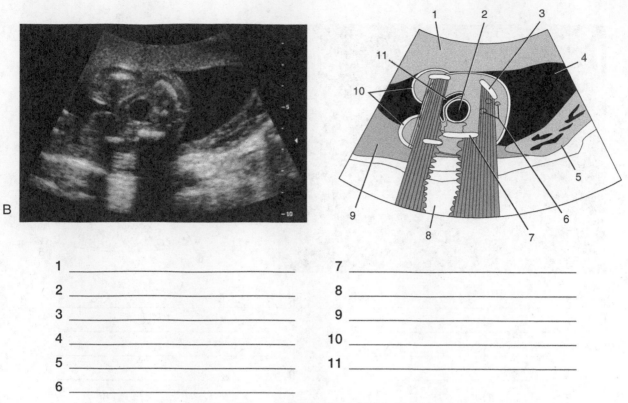

1	_____	7	_____
2	_____	8	_____
3	_____	9	_____
4	_____	10	_____
5	_____	11	_____
6	_____		

Figure 23-28B in the textbook

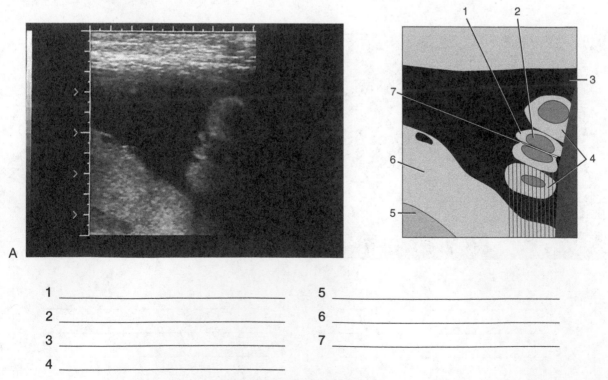

1	_____	5	_____
2	_____	6	_____
3	_____	7	_____
4	_____		

Figure 23-29A in the textbook

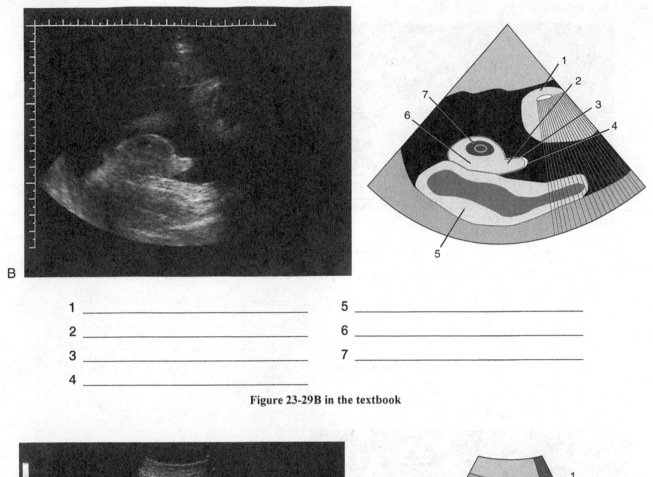

1	_____	5	_____
2	_____	6	_____
3	_____	7	_____
4	_____		

Figure 23-29B in the textbook

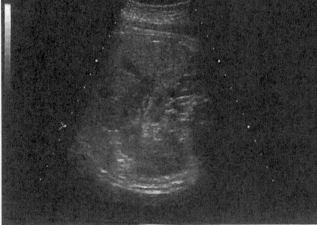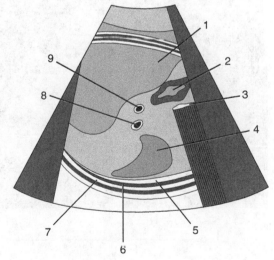

1	_____	6	_____
2	_____	7	_____
3	_____	8	_____
4	_____	9	_____
5	_____		

Figure 23-30 in the textbook

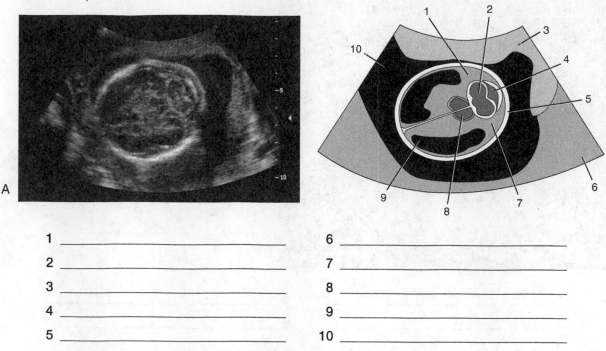

A

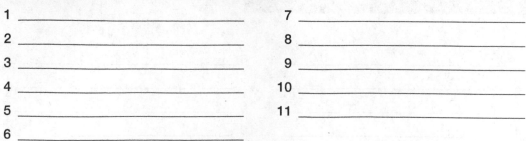

1	_____	6	_____
2	_____	7	_____
3	_____	8	_____
4	_____	9	_____
5	_____	10	_____

Figure 23-31A in the textbook

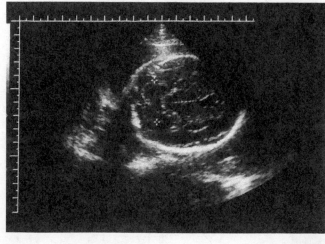

B

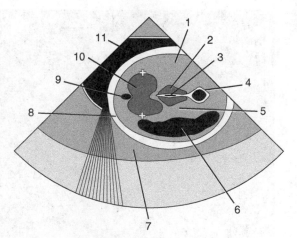

1	_____	7	_____
2	_____	8	_____
3	_____	9	_____
4	_____	10	_____
5	_____	11	_____
6	_____		

Figure 23-31B in the textbook

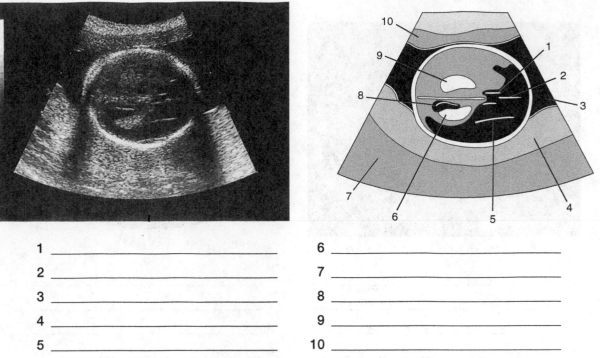

1 _____   6 _____
2 _____   7 _____
3 _____   8 _____
4 _____   9 _____
5 _____   10 _____

Figure 23-32 in the textbook

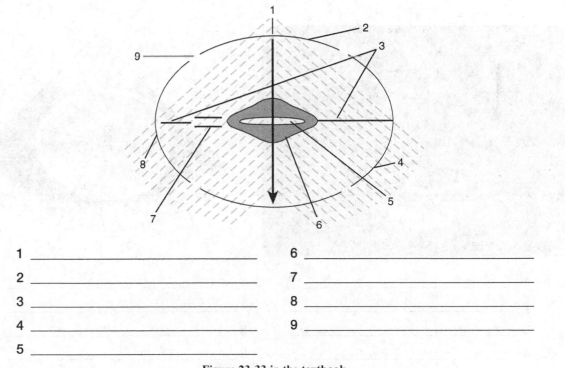

1 _____   6 _____
2 _____   7 _____
3 _____   8 _____
4 _____   9 _____
5 _____

Figure 23-33 in the textbook

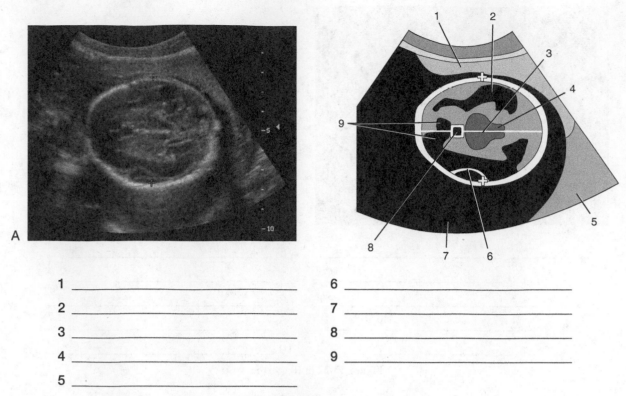

A

Figure 23-34A in the textbook

1 _____   6 _____
2 _____   7 _____
3 _____   8 _____
4 _____   9 _____
5 _____

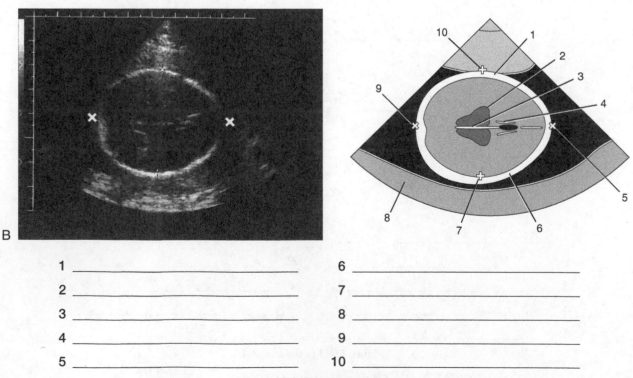

B

Figure 23-34B in the textbook

1 _____   6 _____
2 _____   7 _____
3 _____   8 _____
4 _____   9 _____
5 _____   10 _____

Chapter **23** **Second and Third Trimester Obstetrics**

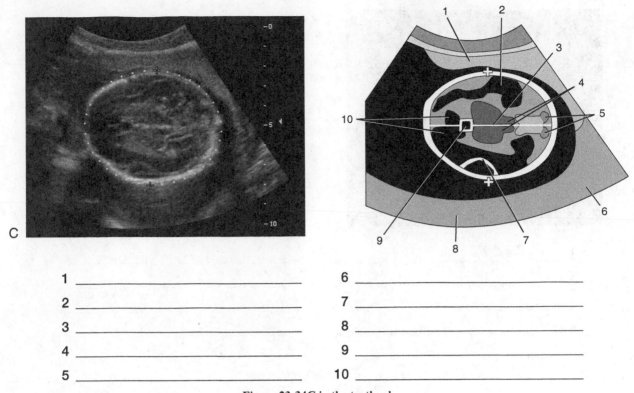

C

1	_____	6	_____
2	_____	7	_____
3	_____	8	_____
4	_____	9	_____
5	_____	10	_____

Figure 23-34C in the textbook

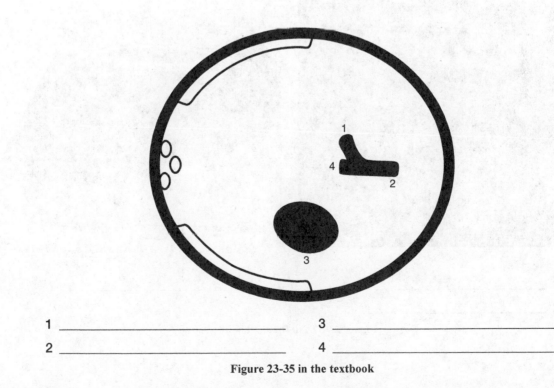

| 1 | _____ | 3 | _____ |
| 2 | _____ | 4 | _____ |

Figure 23-35 in the textbook

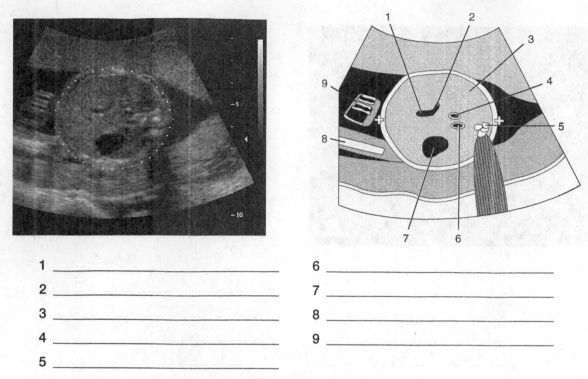

1 _____ 6 _____

2 _____ 7 _____

3 _____ 8 _____

4 _____ 9 _____

5 _____

Figure 23-36 in the textbook

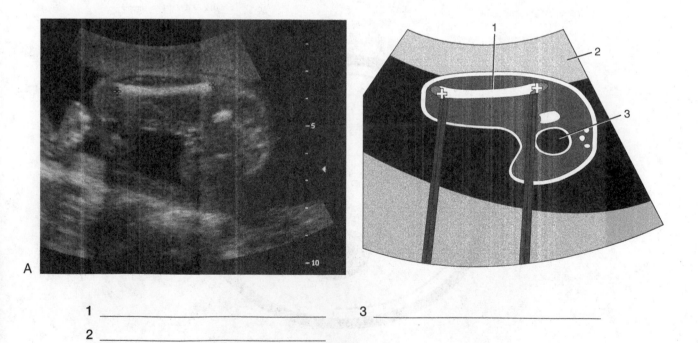

A

1 _____ 3 _____

2 _____

Figure 23-37A in the textbook

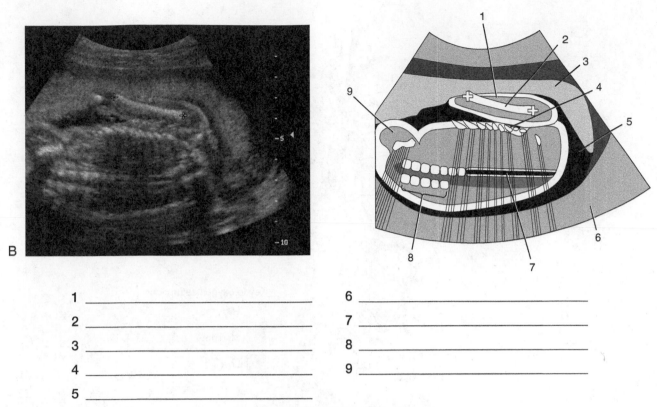

B

1 _____   6 _____
2 _____   7 _____
3 _____   8 _____
4 _____   9 _____
5 _____

Figure 23-37B in the textbook

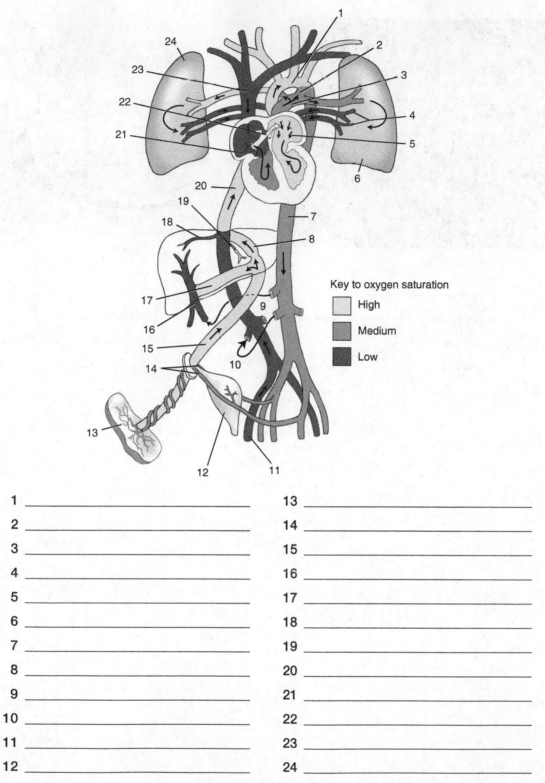

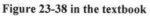

Figure 23-38 in the textbook

1 _____	13 _____
2 _____	14 _____
3 _____	15 _____
4 _____	16 _____
5 _____	17 _____
6 _____	18 _____
7 _____	19 _____
8 _____	20 _____
9 _____	21 _____
10 _____	22 _____
11 _____	23 _____
12 _____	24 _____

V. CHAPTER SUBHEADINGS EXERCISE

Directions to Students:

1. Convert each chapter subheading into a question; for example, change "The Fetal Organ Systems" to "How do the fetal organs appear on ultrasound?" Write the answer to each question in a short paragraph in your notebook.

2. Exchange answers with your lab partner and check each other's work. Refer back to the textbook for further information and explanations.

3. What questions do you still have about the chapter? Write your questions in your notebook.

VI. CHAPTER EVALUATION EXERCISE

Directions to Students: Use a fresh sheet of notebook paper. Based on your work with the chapter and its accompanying laboratory assignments, identify three concepts you believe are the most important. You may draw from any of the assignments you've already completed in the previous pages including learning objectives, anatomy and physiology, images, or chapter subheadings. Include a detailed rationale in your answers.

Answer the questions below. Refer to page 383 for the answers.

Multiple Choice

1. When is the placenta usually visible sonographically?
   a. 5 weeks
   b. 7 weeks
   c. 8 weeks
   d. 10 weeks

2. What occurs when any portion of the internal cervical os is covered by part of the placenta?
   a. Preeclampsia
   b. Oligohydramnios
   c. Placenta previa
   d. Polyhydramnios

3. What is vernix?
   a. Stool
   b. Urine
   c. Skin and hair
   d. Mucus

4. What structure in the liver does the umbilical vein become after closing?
   a. Reidel's lobe
   b. Ligamentum teres
   c. Ligamentum venosum
   d. Right portal vein

5. What allows blood to move from the pulmonary artery to the aorta?
   a. Foramen ovale
   b. Right ventricular outflow tract
   c. Ductus arteriosus
   d. Ductus venosus

True/False

6. Meconium is fetal waste that accumulates in the cecum.

7. A partial or incomplete placenta previa occurs when a portion of the cervical os is obstructed by the overlying placenta.

8. If the single largest pocket of amniotic fluid measures <3 cm, oligohydramnios is indicated.

9. Placenta previa usually requires a cesarean delivery.

10. A grade II placenta should not be seen before 36 weeks.

High-Risk Obstetric Sonography 24

I. MEMORIZATION EXERCISE

Directions to Students: Write the key words in your notebook or on note cards. Write the words on one side of the notepaper and then write the definitions on the opposite side of the page or on the back of the paper. If using note cards, write the key word on the front and the definition on the back. *This step should be completed before the lab session begins.*

Memorize the key word definitions silently for 5 minutes, then work with a lab partner and identify the words you still need help with. List the words here. Add additional rows if needed.

II. COMPREHENSION EXERCISE

Directions to Students: Work with a lab partner to complete this exercise. You will need to write in your notebook. First, change each objective into a question.

> *Example: "Describe the indications for a biophysical profile" becomes "What are the indications of a biophysical profile?"*

Next, write a short answer to the question just created.

> *Example: "The biophysical profile is used to determine fetal well-being. It consists of fetal heart rate, fetal body movements, fetal tone, fetal breathing movements, amniotic fluid volume, and placental grading."*

Highlight or circle any part of your answers about which you are unsure, and check the answers in your textbook. If you are still unsure of the answers, put a question mark next to the answer(s) for the review session of the lab.

III. APPLICATION OF ANATOMY AND PHYSIOLOGY EXERCISE

Directions to Students: Work on the following with your lab partner.
1. In your notebook, draw the development of monozygotic and dizygotic twins including placentation.

2. Label as many structures as you can in each of the drawings. Ask your lab partner to critique your work. What did you miss? Check your drawing using the sketches in your textbook, and complete any missing structures from your drawing.

3. Below your drawing, write two or three summary sentences about the use of ultrasound in high-risk pregnancy. Ask your lab partner to check your work. What else can you add to your description?

IV. IMAGE ANALYSIS EXERCISE

Directions to Students: Work on the following figures with your lab partner. It's your choice! You can label all the sketches at once, then go back and label each image with your lab partner, or label an image and its accompanying sketch at the same time. Either way, the goal is to label all of the sketches correctly and carefully compare the sketch with the sonographic image.

For each sonographic image, write a very brief observation that could be presented to your instructor, the clinical sonographer, or the sonologist. Your observation will be based on Chapter 7 in the textbook, which describes how to write a technical observation. Please go back and review that chapter if needed.

For each image, your assessment should include (1) the view of each major structure (axial or longitudinal; note: these are not the scanning planes) and (2) structures identified in the image with the correct sonographic appearance, description, and measurements if shown (see Chapter 7 in the textbook for information on how to write a technical observation).

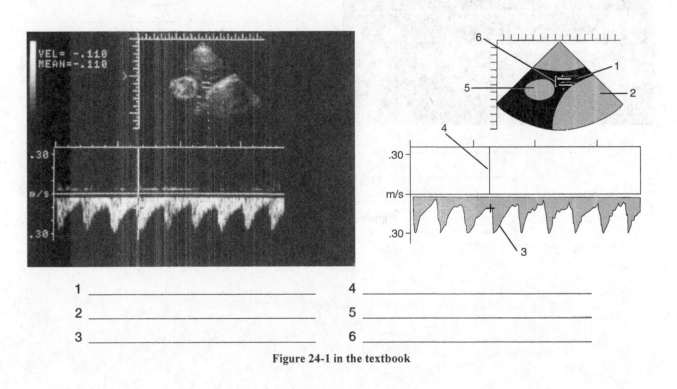

1 _____   4 _____

2 _____   5 _____

3 _____   6 _____

Figure 24-1 in the textbook

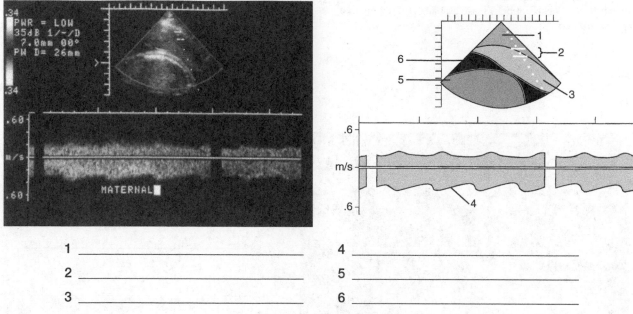

1 _____   4 _____

2 _____   5 _____

3 _____   6 _____

Figure 24-2 in the textbook

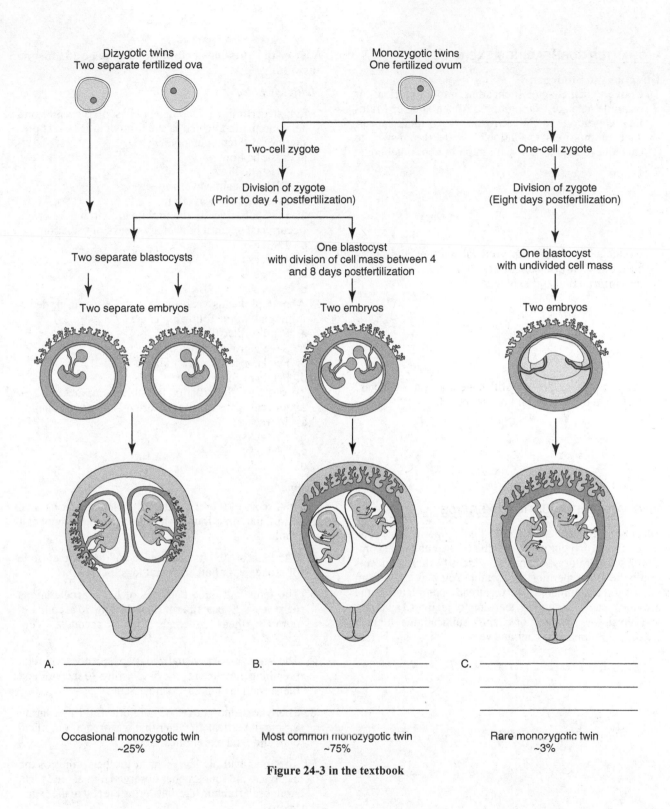

Dizygotic twins
Two separate fertilized ova

Monozygotic twins
One fertilized ovum

Two-cell zygote

One-cell zygote

Division of zygote
(Prior to day 4 postfertilization)

Division of zygote
(Eight days postfertilization)

Two separate blastocysts

One blastocyst
with division of cell mass between 4
and 8 days postfertilization

One blastocyst
with undivided cell mass

Two separate embryos

Two embryos

Two embryos

A. _____
_____
_____

B. _____
_____
_____

C. _____
_____
_____

Occasional monozygotic twin
~25%

Most common monozygotic twin
~75%

Rare monozygotic twin
~3%

Figure 24-3 in the textbook

V. CHAPTER SUBHEADINGS EXERCISE

Directions to Students:

1. Convert each chapter subheading into a question; for example, change "Sonographic Appearance of Multifetal Gestation" to "What is the sonographic appearance of multifetal gestation?" Write the answer to each question in a short paragraph in your notebook.

2. Exchange answers with your lab partner and check each other's work. Refer back to the textbook for further information and explanations.

3. What questions do you still have about the chapter? Write your questions in your notebook.

VI. CHAPTER EVALUATION EXERCISE

Directions to Students: Use a fresh sheet of notebook paper. Based on your work with the chapter and its accompanying laboratory assignments, identify three concepts you believe are the most important. You may draw from any of the assignments you've already completed in the previous pages including learning objectives, anatomy and physiology, images, or chapter subheadings. Include a detailed rationale in your answers.

Answer the questions below. Refer to page 383 for the answers.

Multiple Choice

1. When performing Doppler studies of placental and fetal circulation, which of the following is best at predicting poor fetal outcome?
   a. Systolic flow
   b. Diastolic flow
   c. High resistant waveform
   d. Low resistant waveform

2. Venous pulsations in the umbilical vein are a normal occurrence up until how many weeks of gestation?
   a. 15 weeks
   b. 18 weeks
   c. 21 weeks
   d. 24 weeks

3. Abnormal ductus venosus velocity is useful in determining all of the following except
   a. Fetal cardiac disease
   b. Severe growth restriction
   c. Fetal congestive heart failure
   d. Fetal anemia

4. To decrease the risk for possible complications, an amniocentesis is ideally performed no earlier than
   a. 14 weeks
   b. 16 weeks
   c. 18 weeks
   d. 20 weeks

Completion

Assign a score of 0 or 2 for the following scenarios seen in a 30-minute time frame while performing a biophysical profile.

5. The fetus arched its back twice and had one episode of movement of all arms and legs. Score _____

6. The fetus had three episodes of heart accelerations of at least 22 beats per minute lasting 17 seconds in duration, then 15 seconds, then 20 seconds. Score _____

7. The sonographer visualized two episodes of fetal breathing movements, the first lasting 30 seconds and the second lasting 25 seconds. Score _____

8. There was one pocket of amniotic fluid measuring 2.5 cm in vertical diameter that was free of umbilical cord and fetal extremities. Score _____

9. The fetus had his legs bent at the beginning of the exam and the sonographer observed him extend them straight and remain like that during the rest of the exam. Score _____

10. The fetus was observed opening and closing his hand. Score _____

25 Fetal Echocardiography

I. MEMORIZATION EXERCISE

Directions to Students: Write the key words in your notebook or on note cards. Write the words on one side of the notepaper and then write the definitions on the opposite side of the page or on the back of the paper. If using note cards, write the key word on the front and the definition on the back. *This step should be completed before the lab session begins.*

Memorize the key word definitions silently for 5 minutes, then work with a lab partner and identify the words you still need help with. List the words here. Add additional rows if needed.

II. COMPREHENSION EXERCISE

Directions to Students: Work with a lab partner to complete this exercise. You will need to write in your notebook. First, change each objective into a question.

> *Example: "Describe the location and size of the heart in the fetus" becomes "What is the location and size of the heart in the fetus?"*

Next, write a short answer to the question just created.

> *Example: "The fetal heart is located in the anterior half of the chest with the base of the heart, the atria, in the middle of the chest. The apex of the heart, the tip of the ventricles, is to the left of the midline. The fetal heart is about the size of a quarter at 20 weeks' gestational age."*

Highlight or circle any part of your answers about which you are unsure, and check the answers in your textbook. If you are still unsure of the answers, put a question mark next to the answer(s) for the review session of the lab.

III. APPLICATION OF ANATOMY AND PHYSIOLOGY EXERCISE

Directions to Students: Work on the following with your lab partner.

1. In your notebook, draw the blood flow of the fetal heart and include the following structures: four-chamber fetal heart, ductus arteriosus, foramen ovale, inferior vena cava, descending aorta, main pulmonary artery, and right and left lungs.

2. Label as many structures as you can in each of the drawings. Ask your lab partner to critique your work. What did you miss?

3. Below your drawing, write two or three summary sentences about the physiology of the fetal heart. Ask your lab partner to check your work. Now check your work against the physiology section in the textbook. What else can you add to your description?

IV. IMAGE ANALYSIS EXERCISE

Directions to Students: Work on the following figures with your lab partner. It's your choice! You can label all the sketches at once, then go back and label each image with your lab partner, or label an image and its accompanying sketch at the same time. Either way, the goal is to label all of the sketches correctly and carefully compare the sketch with the sonographic image.

For each sonographic image, write a very brief observation that could be presented to your instructor, the clinical sonographer, or the sonologist. Your observation will be based on Chapter 7 in the textbook, which describes how to write a technical observation. Please go back and review that chapter if needed.

For each image, your assessment should include (1) the view of each major structure (axial or longitudinal; note: these are not the scanning planes) and (2) structures identified in the image with the correct sonographic appearance, description, and measurements if shown (see Chapter 7 in the textbook for information on how to write a technical observation).

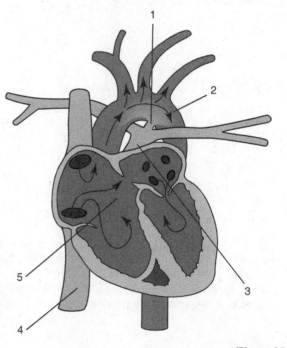

1 _____

2 _____

3 _____

4 _____

5 _____

Figure 25-1 in the textbook

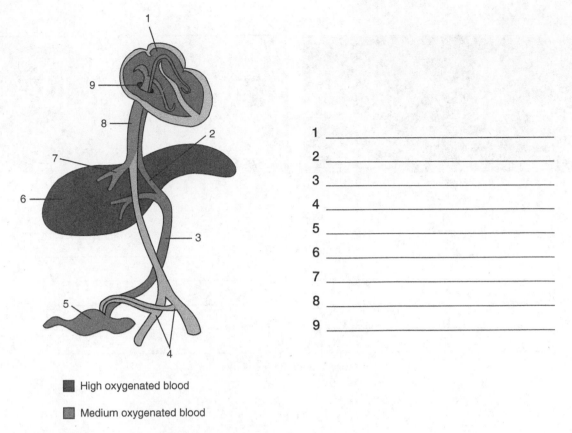

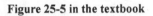

1 _____
2 _____
3 _____
4 _____
5 _____
6 _____
7 _____
8 _____
9 _____

■ High oxygenated blood

■ Medium oxygenated blood

■ Low oxygenated blood

Figure 25-5 in the textbook

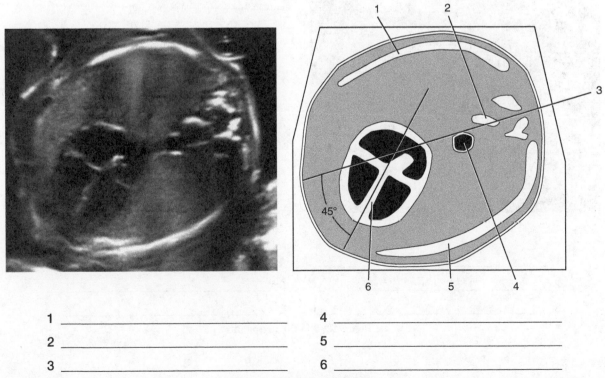

1 _____   4 _____
2 _____   5 _____
3 _____   6 _____

Figure 25-6 in the textbook

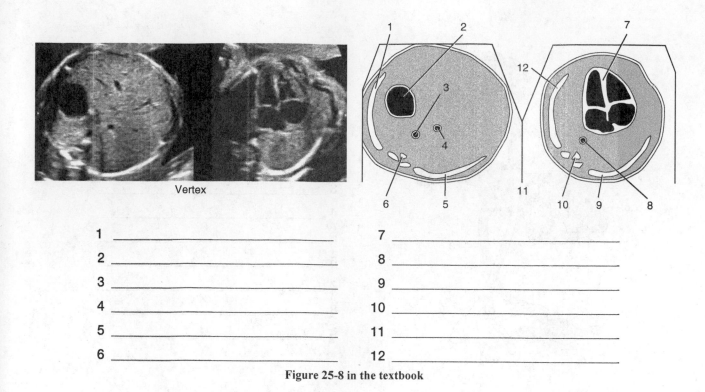

Vertex

1 _____	7 _____
2 _____	8 _____
3 _____	9 _____
4 _____	10 _____
5 _____	11 _____
6 _____	12 _____

Figure 25-8 in the textbook

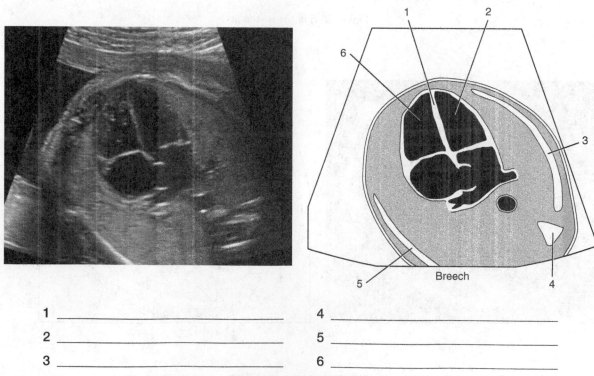

Breech

1 _____	4 _____
2 _____	5 _____
3 _____	6 _____

Figure 25-9 in the textbook

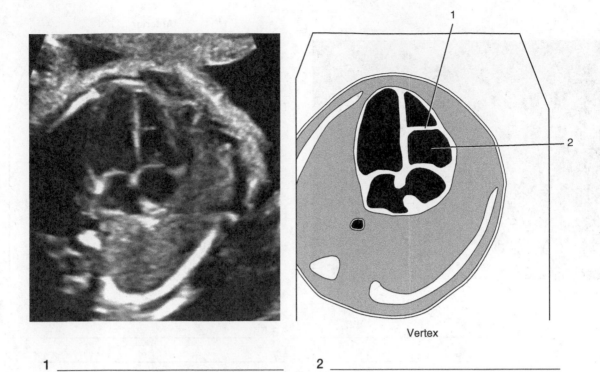

1 _____ 2 _____

Figure 25-11 in the textbook

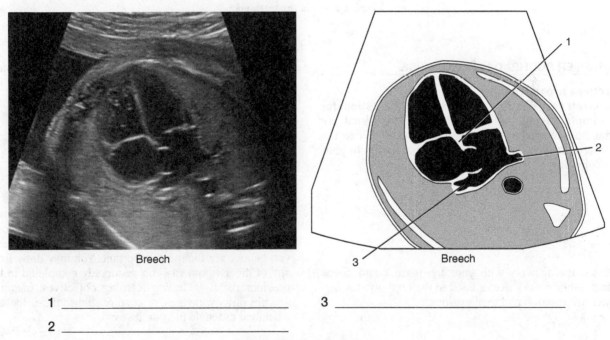

Breech

Breech

1 _____ 3 _____

2 _____

Figure 25-13 in the textbook

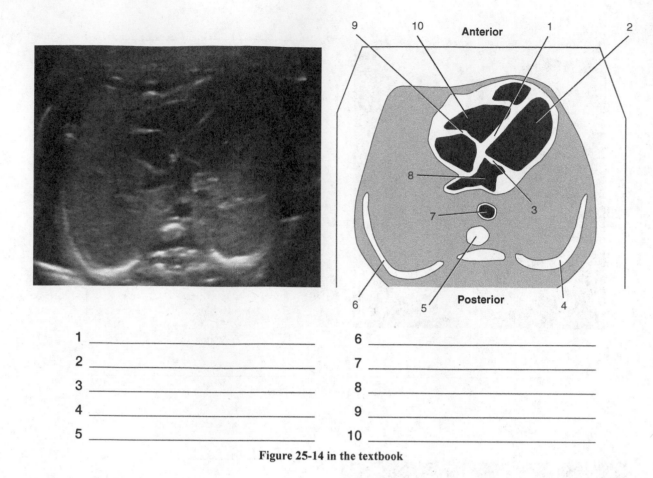

1	_____	6	_____
2	_____	7	_____
3	_____	8	_____
4	_____	9	_____
5	_____	10	_____

Figure 25-14 in the textbook

V. CHAPTER SUBHEADINGS EXERCISE

Directions to Students:

1. Convert each chapter subheading into a question; for example, change "Normal Variants" to "What are the normal variants of the fetal heart?" Write the answer to each question in a short paragraph in your notebook.

2. Exchange answers with your lab partner and check each other's work. Refer back to the textbook for further information and explanations.

3. What questions do you still have about the chapter? Write your questions in your notebook.

VI. CHAPTER EVALUATION EXERCISE

Directions to Students: Use a fresh sheet of notebook paper. Based on your work with the chapter and its accompanying laboratory assignments, identify three concepts you believe are the most important. You may draw from any of the assignments you've already completed in the previous pages including learning objectives, anatomy and physiology, images, or chapter subheadings. Include a detailed rationale in your answers.

Answer the questions below. Refer to page 383 for the answers.

Multiple Choice

1. How many views are necessary for screening of the fetal heart?
   a. Three
   b. Four
   c. Five
   d. Six

2. The normal axis of the heart is 45 degrees to the left of the midsagittal plane. Which structure in the heart is examined to see that this angle is correct?
   a. The descending aorta
   b. The moderator band
   c. The atrioventricular valves
   d. The interventricular septum

3. Which of the following would NOT be helpful adjustments to aid in visualizing the fetal heart?
   a. Increasing the contrast
   b. Magnifying the heart
   c. Using a low frame rate
   d. Increasing the transducer frequency

4. What are the three shunts in fetal circulation?
   a. Ductus venosus, eustachian valve, ductus arteriosus
   b. Eustachian valve, fossa ovalis, coronary sinus
   c. Ductus arteriosus, fossa ovalis, ductus venosus
   d. Coronary sinus, ductus arteriosus, eustachian valve

5. What is the normal heart rate range in the second trimester?
   a. 120–160 bpm
   b. 110–150 bpm
   c. 150–180 bpm
   d. 100–140 bpm

True/False

6. The ductus arteriosus is a shunt in the fetal heart between the main pulmonary artery and the ascending aorta.

7. A technically correct four-chamber view is necessary for the cephalad sweep into the left ventricular outflow tract and right ventricular outflow tract to be adequately obtained.

8. The ventricular chambers should be similar in size; however, it is normal for the right ventricle to be up to 20% larger than the left ventricle.

9. The different types of four-chamber views that may be necessary to show all of the elements needed to be identified are the apical, basal, and short-axis four-chamber views.

10. In the three vessels and trachea view, the structure seen furthest to the left is the superior vena cava.

The Neonatal Brain 26

I. MEMORIZATION EXERCISE

Directions to Students: Write the key words in your notebook or on note cards. Write the words on one side of the notepaper and then write the definitions on the opposite side of the page or on the back of the paper. If using note cards, write the key word on the front and the definition on the back. *This step should be completed before the lab session begins.*

Memorize the key word definitions silently for 5 minutes, then work with a lab partner and identify the words you still need help with. List the words here. Add additional rows if needed.

II. COMPREHENSION EXERCISE

Directions to Students: Work with a lab partner to complete this exercise. You will need to write in your notebook. First, change each objective into a question.

Example: "Identify the major structures in the neonatal brain" becomes "What are the major structures in the neonatal brain?"

Next, write a short answer to the question just created.

Example: "The brain has four major regions: cerebral hemispheres, diencephalon, brain stem, and cerebellum. The cerebral hemispheres are further divided into frontal, parietal, temporal, and occipital lobes. The diencephalon, also called the interbrain, rests superior to the brain stem, is enclosed by the cerebral hemispheres, and comprises the thalamus, hypothalamus, and epithalamus. The brain stem comprises the midbrain, pons, and medulla oblongata. The cerebellum is located anterior to the brain stem."

Highlight or circle any part of your answers about which you are unsure, and check the answers in your textbook. If you are still unsure of the answers, put a question mark next to the answer(s) for the review session of the lab.

III. APPLICATION OF ANATOMY AND PHYSIOLOGY EXERCISE

Directions to Students: Work on the following with your lab partner.

1. In your notebook, draw the brain lobes from memory.

2. Label the brain and lobes; include each structure's orientation in the body (either vertical, horizontal, vertical oblique, or horizontal oblique). Ask your lab partner to critique your work. What did you miss?

3. Below your drawing, write two or three summary sentences about the physiology of the neonatal brain. Ask your lab partner to check your work. Now check your work against the physiology section in the textbook. What else can you add to your description?

IV. IMAGE ANALYSIS EXERCISE

Directions to Students: Work on the following figures with your lab partner. It's your choice! You can label all the sketches at once, then go back and label each image with your lab partner, or you can label an image and its accompanying sketch at the same time. Either way, the goal is to label correctly all of the sketches and carefully compare the sketch with the sonographic image.

For each image, your assessment should include (1) the view of each major structure (axial or longitudinal; note: these are not the scanning planes) and (2) structures identified in the image with correct sonographic appearance description and measurements if shown (see Chapter 7 in the textbook for information on how to write a technical observation).

For each sonographic image, write a brief observation that could be "presented" to your instructor, a clinical sonographer, or a sonologist. Your observation should be based on Chapter 7 in the textbook, which describes how to write a technical observation. Please go back and review that chapter if necessary.

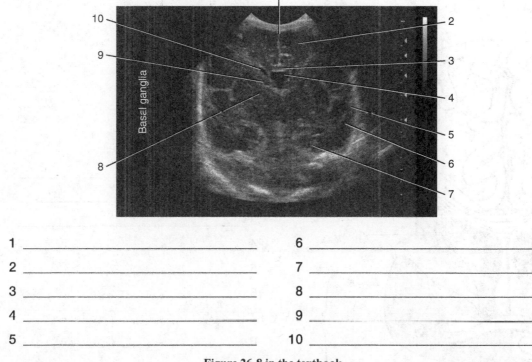

1 _____   6 _____

2 _____   7 _____

3 _____   8 _____

4 _____   9 _____

5 _____   10 _____

Figure 26-8 in the textbook

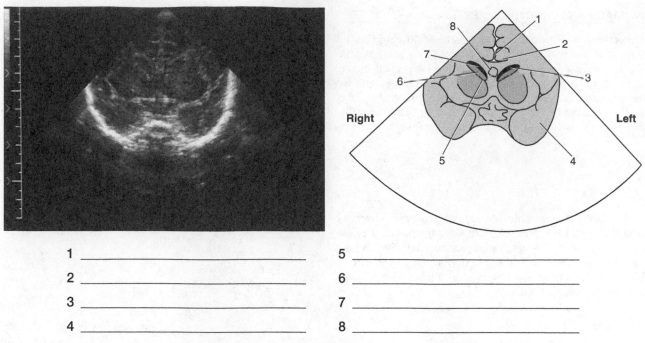

Right   Left

1 _____   5 _____

2 _____   6 _____

3 _____   7 _____

4 _____   8 _____

Figure 26-9 in the textbook

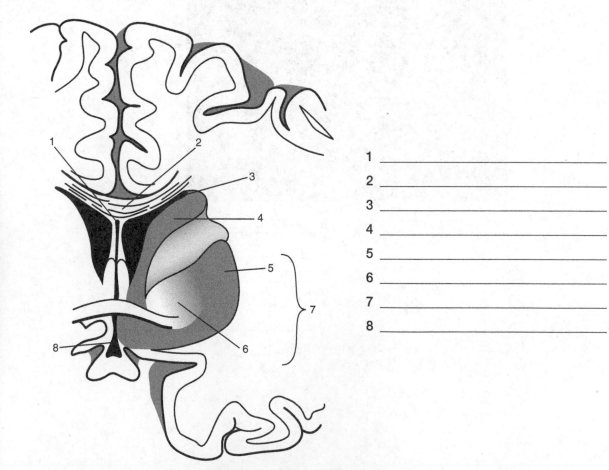

1 _____

2 _____

3 _____

4 _____

5 _____

6 _____

7 _____

8 _____

Figure 26-10 in the textbook

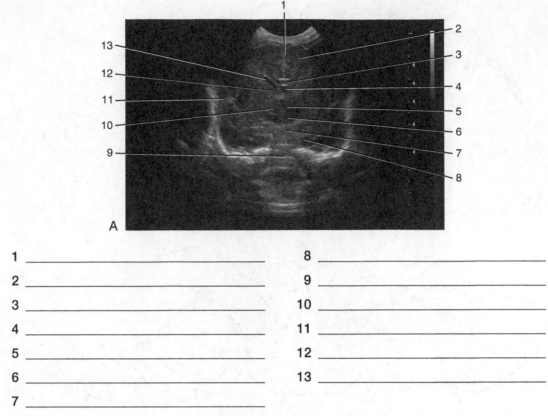

A

1 _____	8 _____
2 _____	9 _____
3 _____	10 _____
4 _____	11 _____
5 _____	12 _____
6 _____	13 _____
7 _____	

Figure 26-11A in the textbook

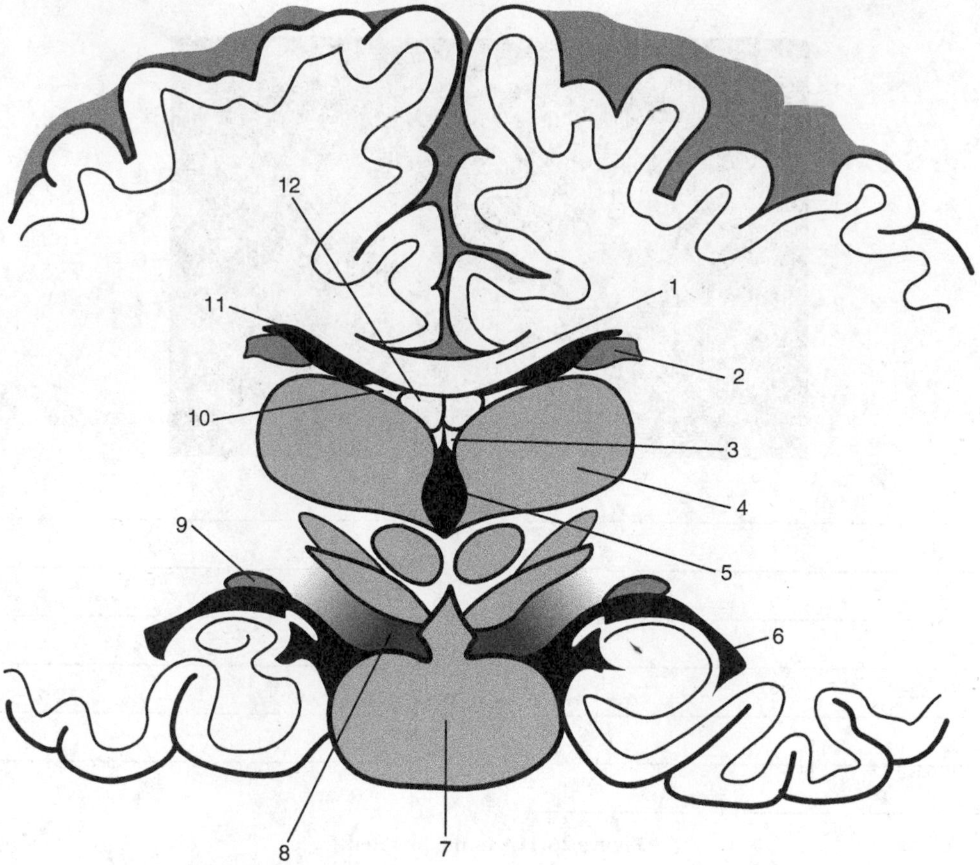

1 _____   7 _____

2 _____   8 _____

3 _____   9 _____

4 _____   10 _____

5 _____   11 _____

6 _____   12 _____

Figure 26-12 in the textbook

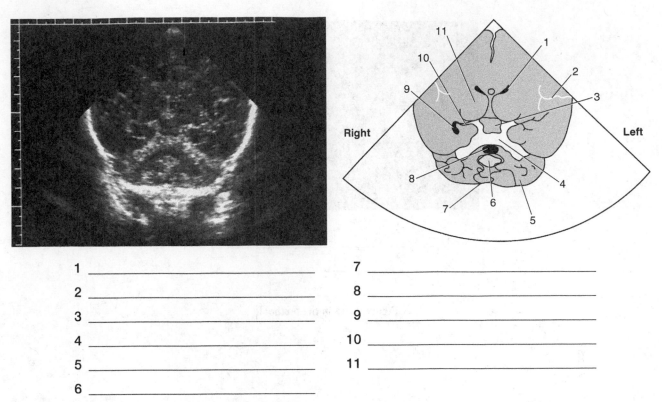

1 _____   7 _____

2 _____   8 _____

3 _____   9 _____

4 _____   10 _____

5 _____   11 _____

6 _____

Figure 26-13 in the textbook

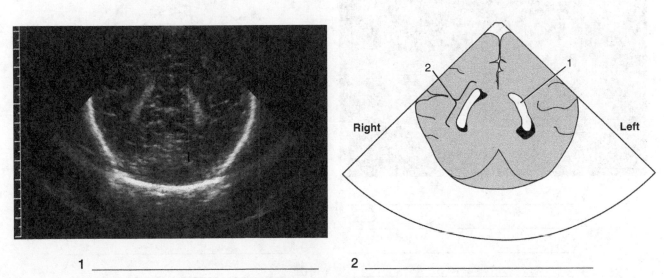

1 _____   2 _____

Figure 26-14 in the textbook

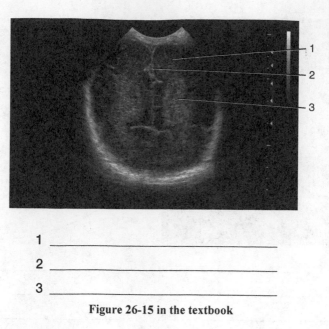

1 _____

2 _____

3 _____

Figure 26-15 in the textbook

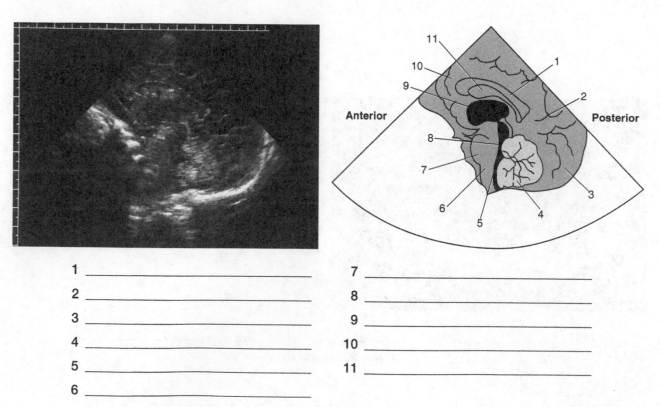

1 _____   7 _____

2 _____   8 _____

3 _____   9 _____

4 _____   10 _____

5 _____   11 _____

6 _____

Figure 26-17 in the textbook

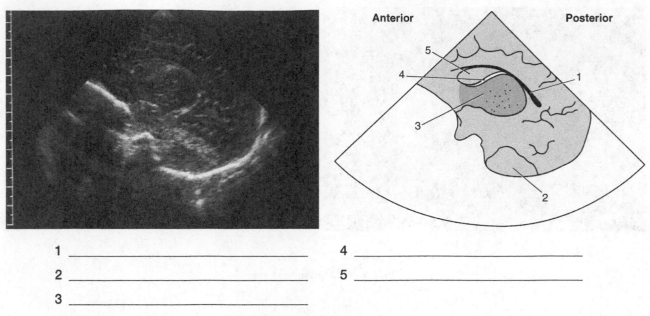

1 _____	4 _____
2 _____	5 _____
3 _____	

Figure 26-18 in the textbook

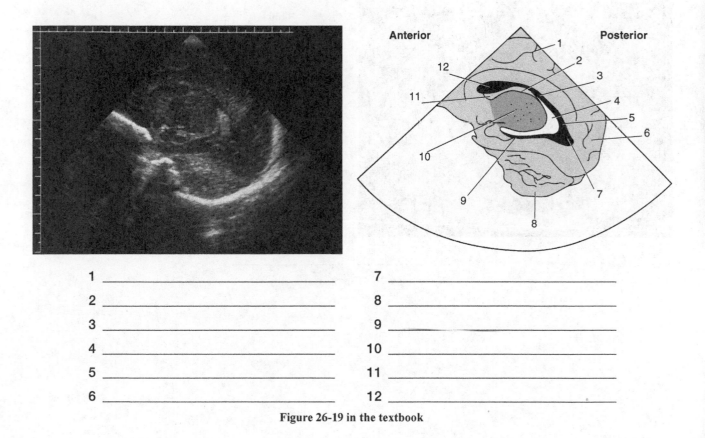

1 _____	7 _____
2 _____	8 _____
3 _____	9 _____
4 _____	10 _____
5 _____	11 _____
6 _____	12 _____

Figure 26-19 in the textbook

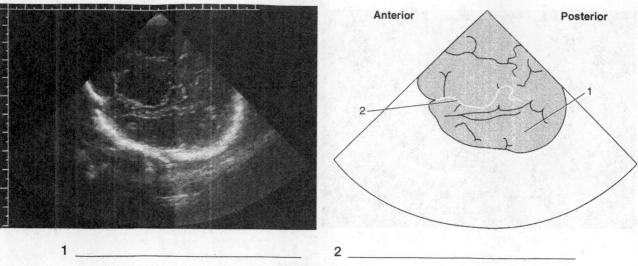

Anterior   Posterior

1 _____ 2 _____

Figure 26-20 in the textbook

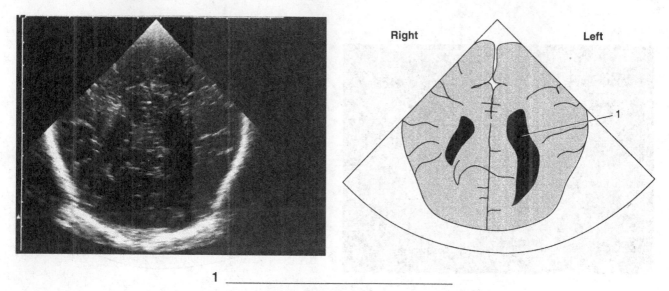

Right   Left

1 _____

Figure 26-21 in the textbook

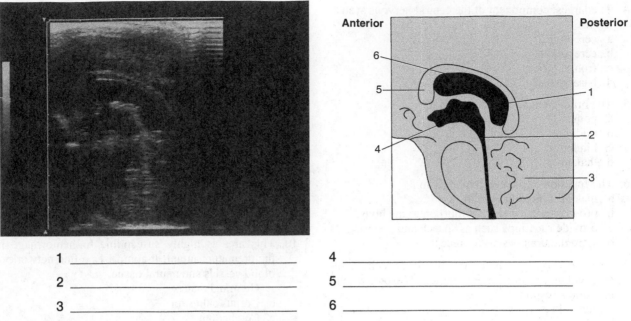

1	_____	4	_____
2	_____	5	_____
3	_____	6	_____

Figure 26-22 in the textbook

V. CHAPTER SUBHEADINGS EXERCISE

Directions to Students:

1. Convert each chapter subheading into a question; for example, change "Gross Anatomy" to "What is the gross anatomy of the neonatal brain?" Write the answer to each question in a short paragraph in your notebook.

2. Exchange answers with your lab partner and check each other's work. Refer back to the textbook for further information and explanation.

3. What questions about the chapter do you still have? Write your questions in your notebook.

VI. CHAPTER EVALUATION EXERCISE

Directions to Students: Use a fresh sheet of notebook paper. Based on your work with the chapter and its accompanying laboratory assignments, identify three concepts you believe are the most important. You may draw from any of the assignments you've already completed in the previous pages, including learning objectives, anatomy and physiology, images, or chapter subheadings. Include a detailed rationale in your answers.

Answer the questions below. Refer to page 383 for the answers.

Multiple Choice

1. The anterior fontanelle is commonly referred to as the
   a. hot spot.
   b. cold spot.
   c. soft spot.
   d. bony cover.

2. Over past decades, what has been the primary imaging method for evaluation of the neonatal brain?
   a. MRI
   b. CT
   c. Sonography
   d. Nuclear medicine

3. _____ are the cells that create brain activity.
   a. Protons
   b. Neurons
   c. Neutrons
   d. Gyri

4. The largest component of the central nervous system is the
   a. cerebrum.
   b. cerebellum.
   c. frontal lobe.
   d. basal ganglia.

5. The brain stem is also known as the
   a. pons.
   b. midbrain.
   c. hindbrain.
   d. thalami.

6. The function of the cerebellum is to
   a. make cerebrospinal fluid.
   b. provide balance and equilibrium to the body.
   c. provide functions such as speech and memory.
   d. store the brain's sensory receptors.

7. The _____ is responsible for speech, memory, voluntary movement, logical reasoning, and emotional response.
   a. cerebellum
   b. cerebrum
   c. brain stem
   d. choroid plexus

8. Which of the following is NOT a normal variant of the premature neonatal brain?
   a. Asymmetry of the lateral ventricles is a common variant.
   b. The lateral ventricles can measure any size and be normal.
   c. The left ventricle is generally larger than the right ventricle.
   d. Ventricular size can vary among infants.

9. This is an anechoic, fluid-filled space between the anterior horns of the lateral ventricles.
   a. Cavum septum vergae
   b. Cavum septum pellucidum
   c. Posterior ventricle
   d. Fourth ventricle

10. This area is highly susceptible to hemorrhage in the premature infant. It comprises a fine network of blood vessels and neural tissue.
    a. Germinal matrix
    b. Corpus callosum
    c. Cerebellum
    d. Periventricular white matter

27 The Thyroid and Parathyroid Glands

I. MEMORIZATION EXERCISE

Directions to Students: Write the key words in your notebook or on note cards. Write the words on one side of the notepaper and then write the definitions on the opposite side of the page or on the back of the paper. If using note cards, write the key word on the front and the definition on the back. *This step should be completed before the lab session begins.*

Memorize the key word definitions silently for 5 minutes, then work with a lab partner and identify the words you still need help with. List the words here. Add additional rows if needed.

II. COMPREHENSION EXERCISE

Directions to Students: Work with a lab partner to complete this exercise. You will need to write in your notebook. First, change each objective into a question.

> *Example: "Describe the physiology of the thyroid and parathyroid glands" becomes "What is the physiology of the thyroid and parathyroid glands?"*

Next, write a short answer to the question just created.

> *Example: "The thyroid is essential to normal growth and development, and regulates basal metabolism, including blood calcium concentrations, through three hormones—triiodothyronine (T_3), thyroxine (T_4), and calcitonin. The parathyroids are four small glands embedded in the thyroid, two on each side, that also help maintain blood calcium concentrations."*

Highlight or circle any part of your answers about which you are unsure, and check the answers in your textbook. If you are still unsure of the answers, put a question mark next to the answer(s) for the review session of the lab.

III. APPLICATION OF ANATOMY AND PHYSIOLOGY EXERCISE

Directions to Students: Work on the following with your lab partner.

1. In your notebook, draw the thyroid, parathyroid, and adjacent anatomy from memory.

2. Label the thyroid, parathyroid, and surrounding structures; include each structure's orientation in the body (either vertical, horizontal, vertical oblique, or horizontal oblique). Ask your lab partner to critique your work. What did you miss?

3. Below your drawing, write two or three summary sentences about the physiology of the thyroid and parathyroid. Ask your lab partner to check your work. Now check your work against the physiology section in the textbook. What else can you add to your description?

287

IV. IMAGE ANALYSIS EXERCISE

Directions to Students: Work on the following figures with your lab partner. It's your choice! You can label all the sketches at once, then go back and label each image with your lab partner, or you can label an image and its accompanying sketch at the same time. Either way, the goal is to label correctly all of the sketches and carefully compare the sketch with the sonographic image.

For each sonographic image, write a brief observation that could be "presented" to your instructor, a clinical sonographer, or a sonologist. Your observation should be based on Chapter 7 in the textbook, which describes how to write a technical observation. Please go back and review that chapter if necessary.

For each image, your assessment should include (1) the view of each major structure (axial or longitudinal; note: these are not the scanning planes) and (2) structures identified in the image with correct sonographic appearance description and measurements if shown (see Chapter 7 in the textbook for information on how to write a technical observation).

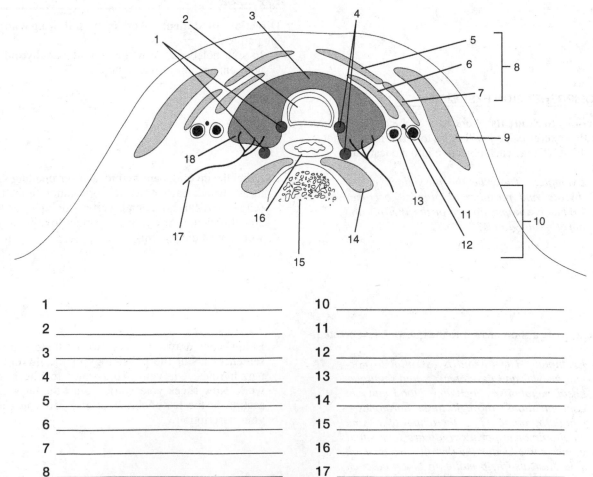

1 _____	10 _____
2 _____	11 _____
3 _____	12 _____
4 _____	13 _____
5 _____	14 _____
6 _____	15 _____
7 _____	16 _____
8 _____	17 _____
9 _____	18 _____

Figure 27-1 in the textbook

Chapter **27** **The Thyroid and Parathyroid Glands**

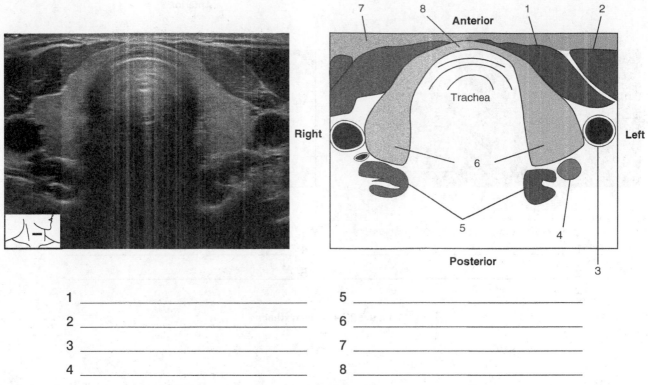

1 _____   5 _____

2 _____   6 _____

3 _____   7 _____

4 _____   8 _____

Figure 27-2 in the textbook

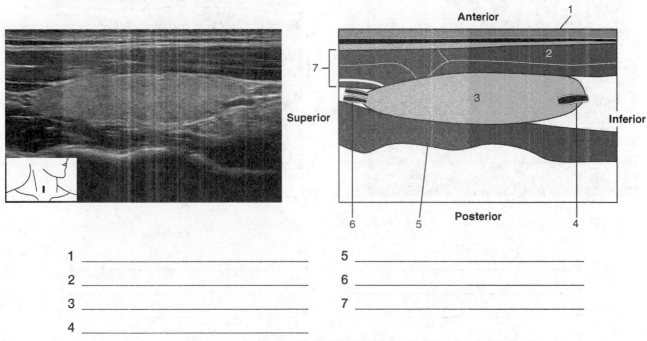

1 _____   5 _____

2 _____   6 _____

3 _____   7 _____

4 _____

Figure 27-3 in the textbook

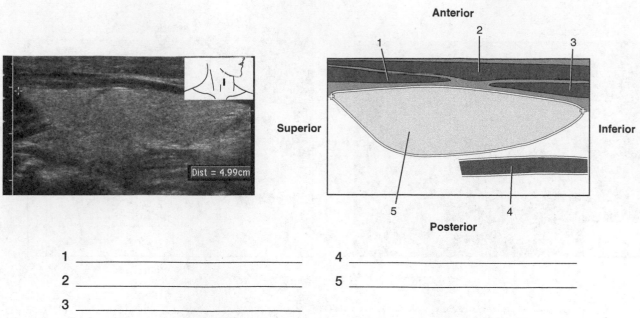

1 _____   4 _____

2 _____   5 _____

3 _____

Figure 27-4 in the textbook

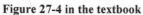

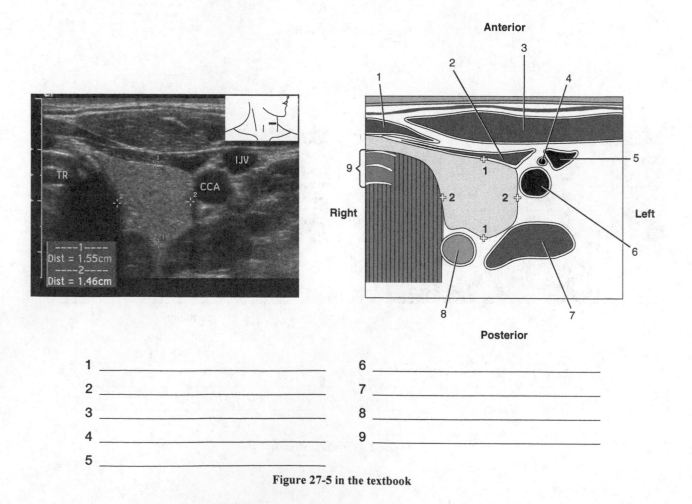

1 _____   6 _____

2 _____   7 _____

3 _____   8 _____

4 _____   9 _____

5 _____

Figure 27-5 in the textbook

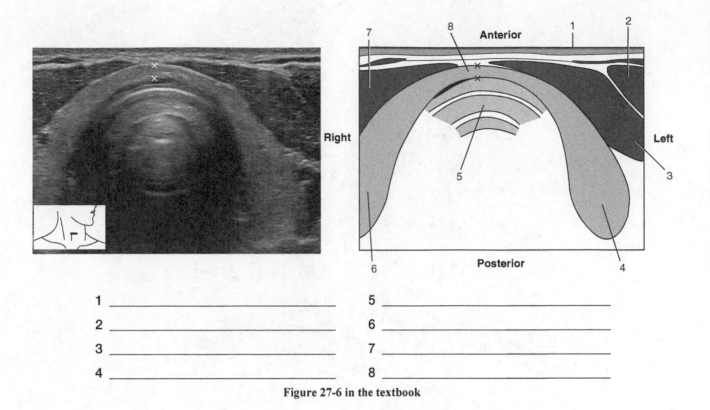

Figure 27-6 in the textbook

1 _____   5 _____
2 _____   6 _____
3 _____   7 _____
4 _____   8 _____

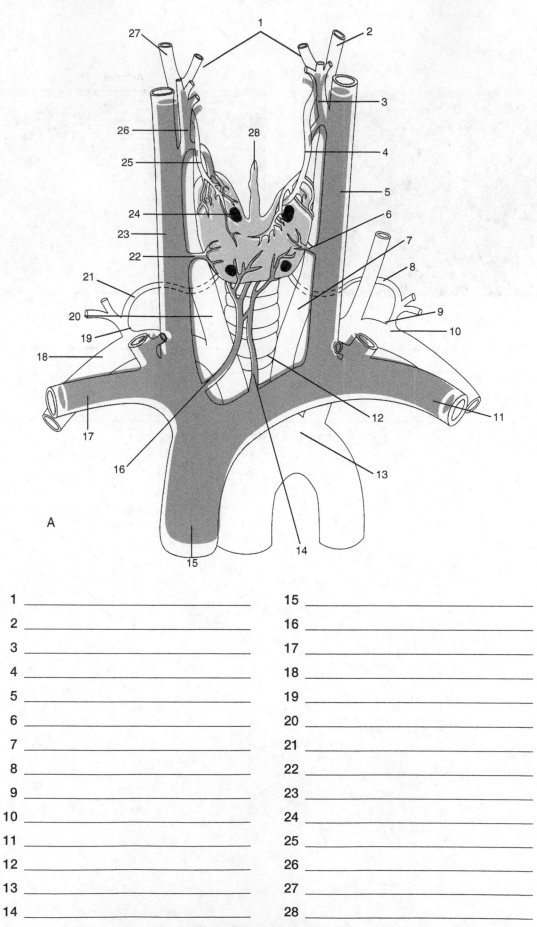

1 _____	15 _____
2 _____	16 _____
3 _____	17 _____
4 _____	18 _____
5 _____	19 _____
6 _____	20 _____
7 _____	21 _____
8 _____	22 _____
9 _____	23 _____
10 _____	24 _____
11 _____	25 _____
12 _____	26 _____
13 _____	27 _____
14 _____	28 _____

Figure 27-7A in the textbook

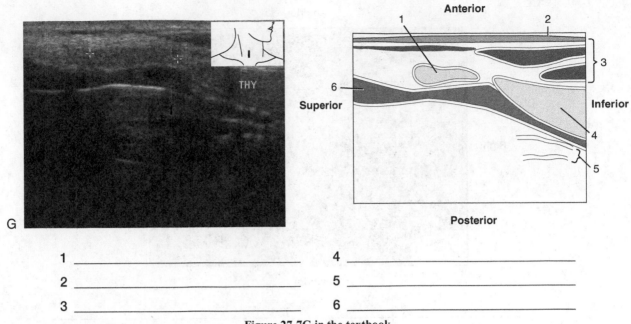

1 _____	4 _____
2 _____	5 _____
3 _____	6 _____

Figure 27-7G in the textbook

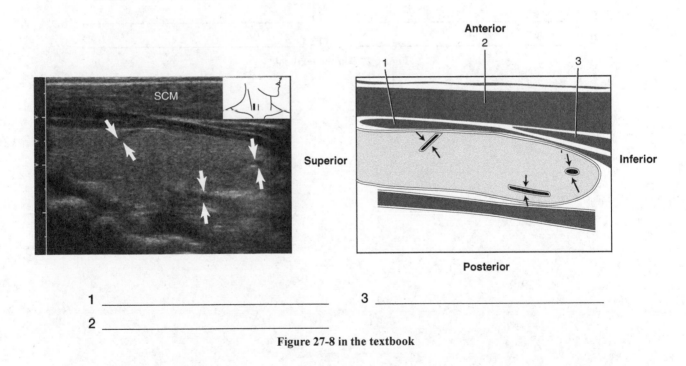

| 1 _____ | 3 _____ |
| 2 _____ | |

Figure 27-8 in the textbook

Chapter **27** **The Thyroid and Parathyroid Glands**

Anterior

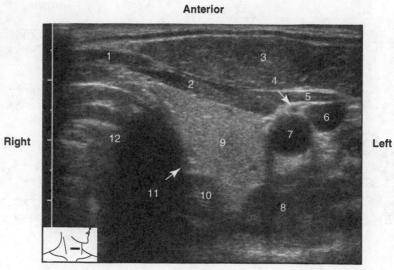

Right

Left

Posterior

1 _____   7 _____

2 _____   8 _____

3 _____   9 _____

4 _____   10 _____

5 _____   11 _____

6 _____   12 _____

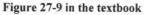

Figure 27-9 in the textbook

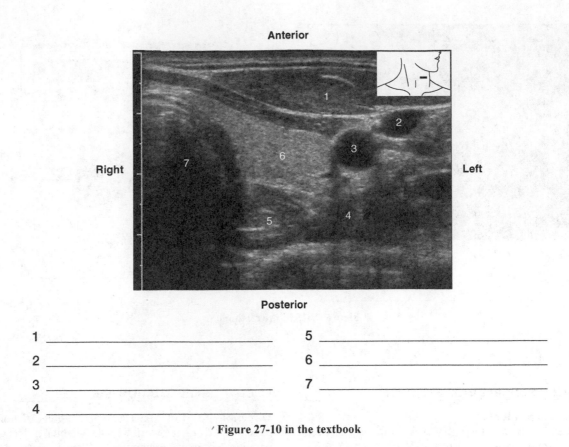

Anterior

Right   Left

Posterior

1 _____   5 _____

2 _____   6 _____

3 _____   7 _____

4 _____

Figure 27-10 in the textbook

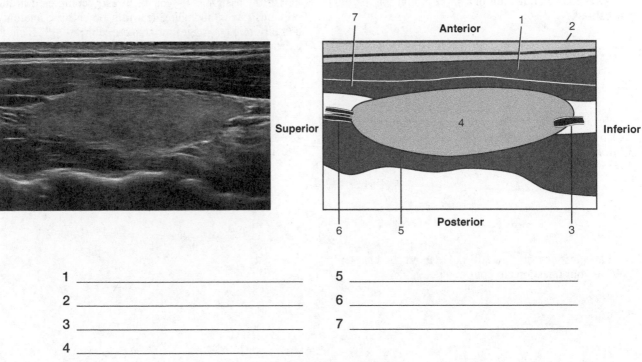

1 _____   5 _____

2 _____   6 _____

3 _____   7 _____

4 _____

Figure 27-11 in the textbook

295

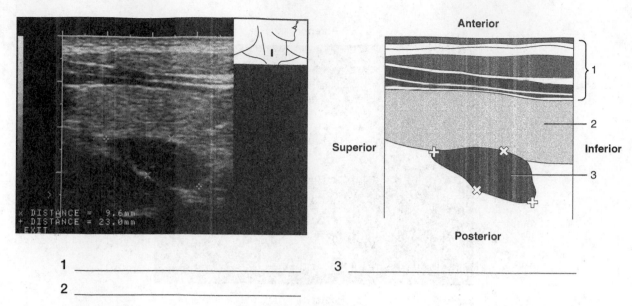

1 _____   3 _____

2 _____

Figure 27-15 in the textbook

V. CHAPTER SUBHEADINGS EXERCISE

Directions to Students:

1. Convert each chapter subheading into a question; for example, change "Normal Variants" to "What are the normal variants of the fetal heart?" Write the answer to each question in a short paragraph in your notebook.

2. Exchange answers with your lab partner and check each other's work. Refer back to the textbook for further information and explanation.

3. What questions do you still have about the chapter? Write your questions in your notebook.

VI. CHAPTER EVALUATION EXERCISE

Directions to Students: Use a fresh sheet of notebook paper. Based on your work with the chapter and its accompanying laboratory assignments, identify three concepts you believe are the most important. You may draw from any of the assignments you've already completed in the previous pages, including learning objectives, anatomy and physiology, images, or chapter subheadings. Include a detailed rationale in your answers.

Answer the questions below. Refer to page 384 for the answers.

Multiple Choice

1. Which of the following muscles does not comprise the strap muscles?
   a. infrahyoid
   b. sternocleidomastoid
   c. sternohyoid
   d. omohyoid

2. Which statement is NOT true about the thyroid gland?
   a. It is located below the larsynx.
   b. It is a gland with low vascularity.
   c. A pyramidal lobe is present in approximately 10% of the population.
   d. It has a saddlebag appearance in cross section.

3. Which of the following falls in the normal range for the thyroid gland in the average adult?
   a. 5 cm in length, 1.5 cm in AP diameter, 2 cm in width
   b. 4 cm in length, 3 cm in AP diameter, 2 cm in width
   c. 3 cm in length, 3 cm in AP diameter, 2 cm in width
   d. 6 cm in length, 2 cm in AP diameter, 3 cm in width

4. How many lobes make up the thyroid gland?
   a. Two
   b. Four
   c. Six
   d. Eight

5. The lobes of the thyroid gland are connect by the:
   a. Pyramidal lobe
   b. Trachea
   c. Isthmus
   d. Parathyroid

6. The longus colli neck muscle(s) are located:
   a. Anterior in the neck, superficial to the larynx, trachea, and thyroid
   b. Anterolateral to the thyroid
   c. Laterally in the neck, deep to the sternocleidomastoid
   d. Posterior to the thyroid

7. All of the following increase the thyroid volume except:
   a. Increased body weight
   b. Increased amounts of iodine intake
   c. Acute hepatitis
   d. Increased age

8. The size and shape of thyroids vary, which measurement is used to determine if the thyroid is enlarged?
   a. Length
   b. Anteroposterior diameter
   c. Width
   d. Volume

9. Which of the following hormones controls the amount of thyroid secretion?
   a. TSH
   b. T3
   c. T4
   d. Calcitonin

10. Which of the following hormones prevents hypercalcemia?
    a. Thyroxine
    b. Triiodothyronine
    c. Calcitonin
    d. Thyrotropin

Breast Sonography 28

I. MEMORIZATION EXERCISE

Directions to Students: Write the key words in your notebook or on note cards. Write the words on one side of the notepaper and then write the definitions on the opposite side of the page or on the back of the paper. If using note cards, write the key word on the front and the definition on the back. *This step should be completed before the lab session begins.*

Memorize the key word definitions silently for 5 minutes, then work with a lab partner and identify the words you still need help with. List the words here. Add additional rows if needed.

II. COMPREHENSION EXERCISE

Directions to Students: Work with a lab partner to complete this exercise. You will need to write in your notebook. First, change each objective into a question.

> *Example: "Describe the location of anatomy related to the breast" becomes "Where is anatomy of the breast located?"*

Next, write a short answer to the question just created.

> *Example: "The breast is anterior to the pectoralis major, serratus, and external oblique muscles. Each breast is lateral to the sternum and medial to the axilla. The layers of the breast, moving from anterior to posterior, are skin, subcutaneous fat, glandular tissue, subcutaneous fat, and posterior muscle."*

Highlight or circle any part of your answers about which you are unsure, and check the answers in your textbook. If you are still unsure of the answers, put a question mark next to the answer(s) for the review session of the lab.

III. APPLICATION OF ANATOMY AND PHYSIOLOGY EXERCISE

Directions to Students: Work on the following with your lab partner.

1. In your notebook, draw the breast, including its layers, from memory.

2. Label the breast; include each structure's orientation in the body (either vertical, horizontal, vertical oblique, or horizontal oblique). Ask your lab partner to critique your work. What did you miss?

3. Below your drawing, write two or three summary sentences about the physiology of the breast. Ask your lab partner to check your work. Now check your work against the physiology section in the textbook. What else can you add to your description?

IV. IMAGE ANALYSIS EXERCISE

Directions to Students: Work on the following figures with your lab partner. It's your choice! You can label all the sketches at once, then go back and label each image with your lab partner, or you can label an image and its accompanying sketch at the same time. Either way, the goal is to label correctly all of the sketches and carefully compare the sketch with the sonographic image.

For each sonographic image, write a brief observation that could be "presented" to your instructor, a clinical sonographer, or a sonologist. Your observation should be based on Chapter 7 in the textbook, which describes how to write a technical observation. Please go back and review that chapter if necessary.

For each image, your assessment should include (1) the view of each major structure (axial or longitudinal; note: these are not the scanning planes) and (2) structures identified in the image with correct sonographic appearance description and measurements if shown (see Chapter 7 in the textbook for information on how to write a technical observation).

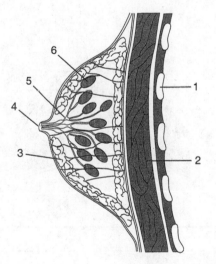

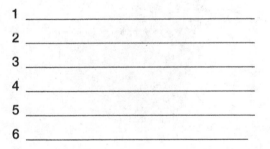

Figure 28-1 in the textbook

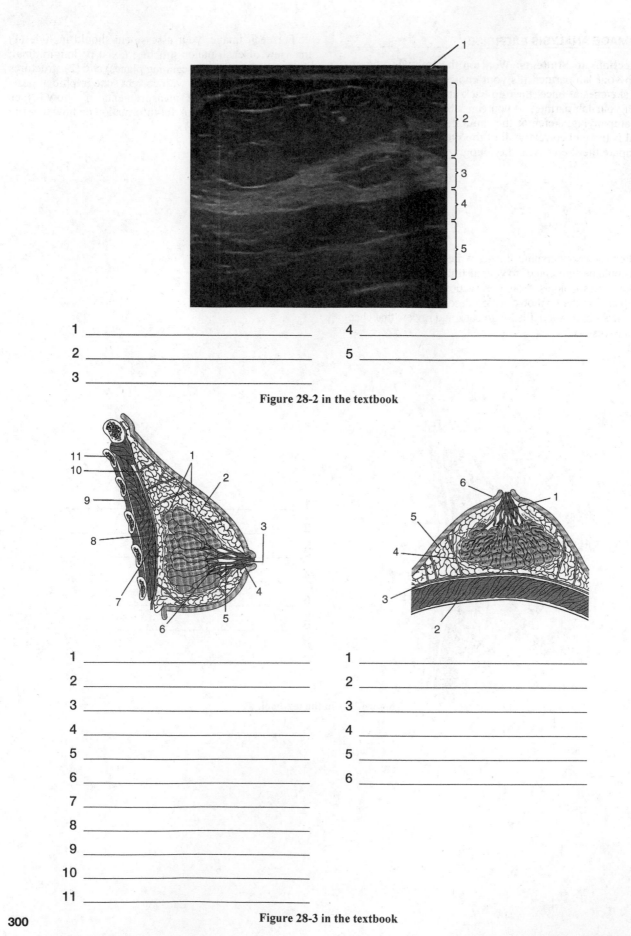

1 _____   4 _____
2 _____   5 _____
3 _____

Figure 28-2 in the textbook

1 _____   1 _____
2 _____   2 _____
3 _____   3 _____
4 _____   4 _____
5 _____   5 _____
6 _____   6 _____
7 _____
8 _____
9 _____
10 _____
11 _____

Figure 28-3 in the textbook

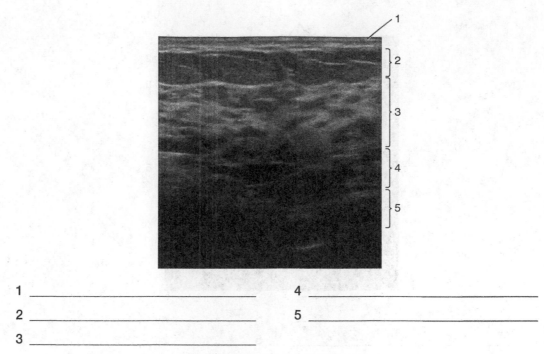

1	_____	4	_____
2	_____	5	_____
3	_____		

Figure 28-4 in the textbook

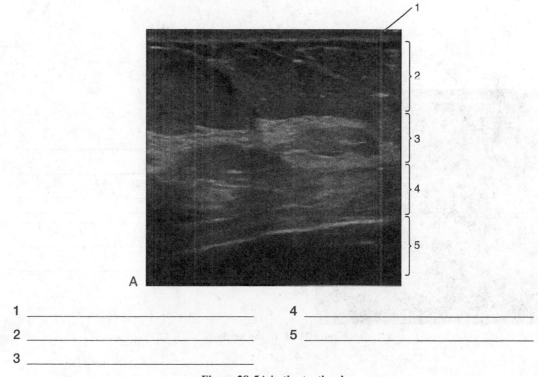

1	_____	4	_____
2	_____	5	_____
3	_____		

Figure 28-5A in the textbook

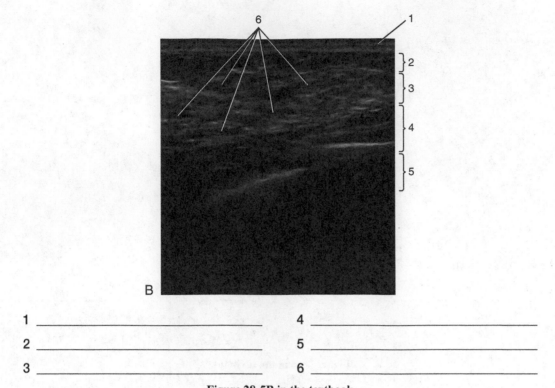

B

1 _____   4 _____

2 _____   5 _____

3 _____   6 _____

Figure 28-5B in the textbook

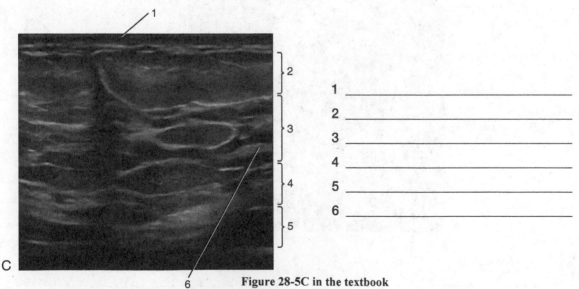

C

6

1 _____

2 _____

3 _____

4 _____

5 _____

6 _____

Figure 28-5C in the textbook

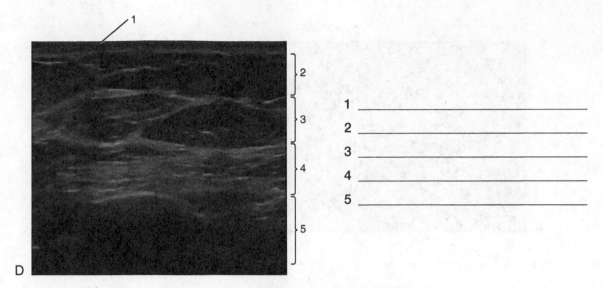

Figure 28-5D in the textbook

1 _____
2 _____
3 _____
4 _____
5 _____

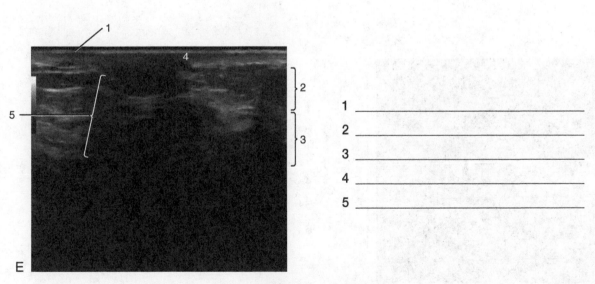

Figure 28-5E in the textbook

1 _____
2 _____
3 _____
4 _____
5 _____

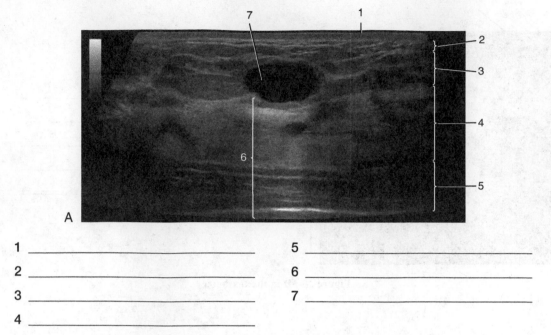

A

1	_____	5	_____
2	_____	6	_____
3	_____	7	_____
4	_____		

Figure 28-6A in the textbook

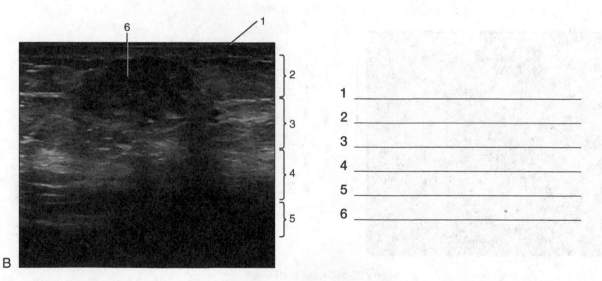

B

1	_____
2	_____
3	_____
4	_____
5	_____
6	_____

Figure 28-6B in the textbook

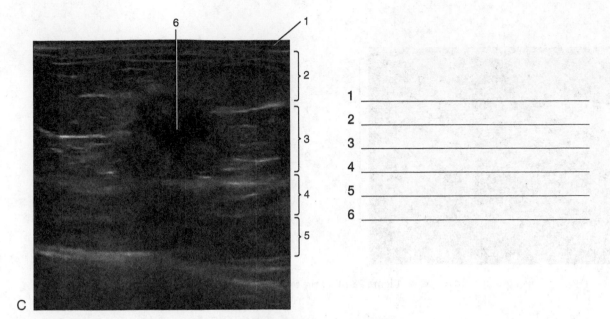

Figure 28-6C in the textbook

1 _____

2 _____

3 _____

4 _____

5 _____

6 _____

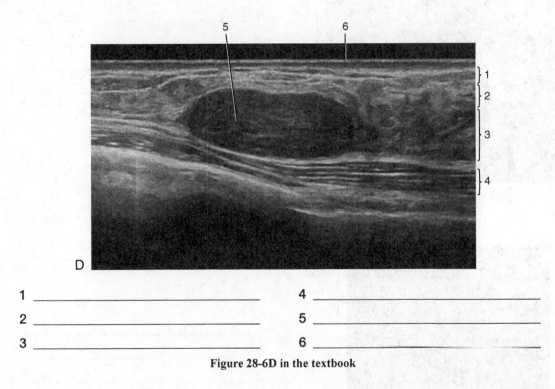

1 _____   4 _____

2 _____   5 _____

3 _____   6 _____

Figure 28-6D in the textbook

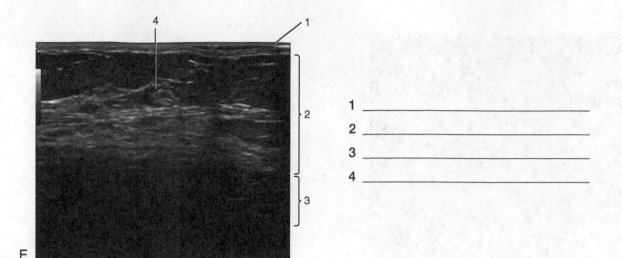

E

1 _____
2 _____
3 _____
4 _____

Figure 28-6E in the textbook

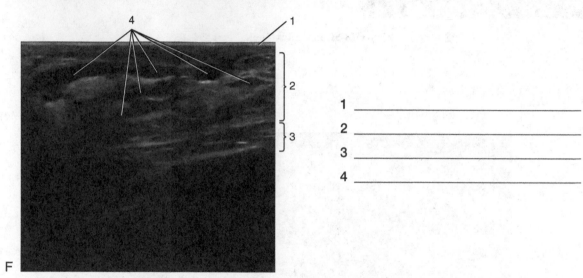

F

1 _____
2 _____
3 _____
4 _____

Figure 28-6F in the textbook

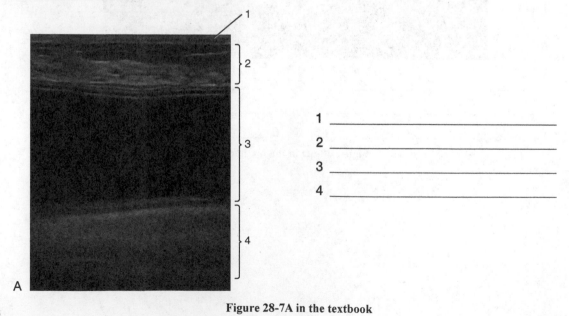

A

1 _____
2 _____
3 _____
4 _____

Figure 28-7A in the textbook

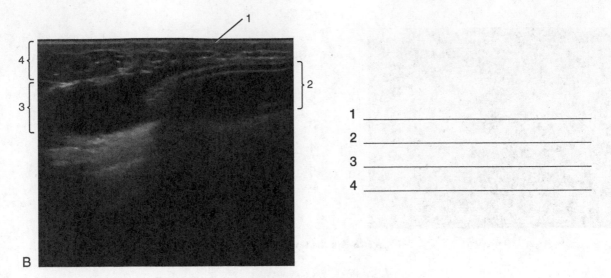

Figure 28-7B in the textbook

1 _____
2 _____
3 _____
4 _____

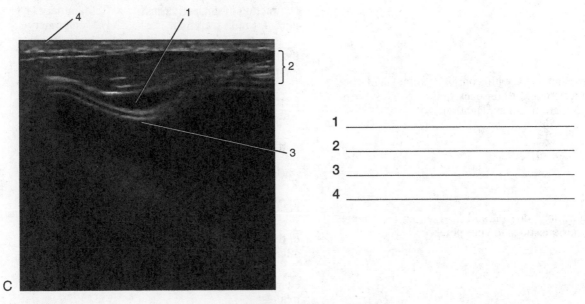

Figure 28-7C in the textbook

1 _____
2 _____
3 _____
4 _____

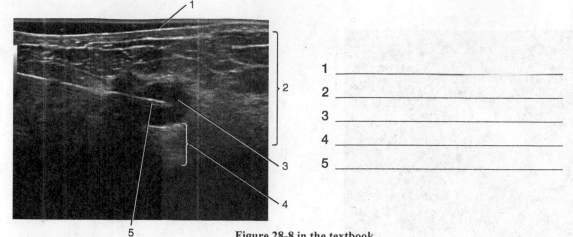

1 _____

2 _____

3 _____

4 _____

5 _____

Figure 28-8 in the textbook

V. CHAPTER SUBHEADINGS EXERCISE

Directions to Students:

1. Convert each chapter subheading into a question; for example, change "Gross Anatomy" to "What is the gross anatomy of the breast?" Write the answer to each question in a short paragraph in your notebook.

2. Exchange answers with your lab partner and check each other's work. Refer back to the textbook for further information and explanation.

3. What questions do you still have about the chapter? Write your questions in your notebook.

VI. CHAPTER EVALUATION EXERCISE

Directions to Students: Use a fresh sheet of notebook paper. Based on your work with the chapter and its accompanying laboratory assignments, identify three concepts you believe are the most important. You may draw from any of the assignments you've already completed in the previous pages, including learning objectives, anatomy and physiology, images, or chapter subheadings. Include a detailed rationale in your answers.

Answer the questions below. Refer to page 384 for the answers.

Matching

_____ 1. Contains glandular tissues, ducts, and connective tissues

_____ 2. Hormone that stimulates contraction of the lactiferous ducts for milk secretion

_____ 3. Hormone that stimulates the development of breast lobules and alveoli for lactation

_____ 4. Ampulla for each lactiferous duct near the nipple where milk can be stored

_____ 5. Grape-shaped secretory portions of a gland.

_____ 6. Contains skin and subcutaneous fat

_____ 7. Hormone that stimulates breast tissue development

_____ 8. Ducts in the parenchyma of the breast that secrete milk after pregnancy

_____ 9. Glandular tissue elements within mammary lobules

_____ 10. Contains retromammary fat, muscle, and deep connective tissues

A. Acini
B. Alveoli
C. Estrogen
D. Lactiferous ducts
E. Mammary layer
F. Montgomery's glands
G. Oxytocin
H. Progesterone
I. Retromammary layer
J. Subcutaneous layer

29 Scrotal and Penile Sonography

I. MEMORIZATION EXERCISE

Directions to Students: Write the key words in your notebook or on note cards. Write the words on one side of the notepaper and then write the definitions on the opposite side of the page or on the back of the paper. If using note cards, write the key word on the front and the definition on the back. *This step should be completed before the lab session begins*.

Memorize the key word definitions silently for 5 minutes, then work with a lab partner and identify the words you still need help with. List the words here. Add additional rows if needed.

II. COMPREHENSION EXERCISE

Directions to Students: Work with a lab partner to complete this exercise. You will need to write in your notebook. First, change each objective into a question.

> *Example: "Describe the normal size of the testicles" becomes "What is the normal size of the testicles?"*

Next, write a short answer to the question just created.

> *Example: "The normal adult testicle measures approximately 3 to 5 cm (1.5 to 2 inches) in length, 2 to 3 cm (1 inch) in anterior-to-posterior dimension, and 2 to 3 cm (1 inch) in width. The adult testicular volume is approximately 25 mL and weighs 10 to 15 g. It is only one-fifth of that volume before puberty and decreases in size with advancing age."*

Highlight or circle any part of your answers about which you are unsure, and check the answers in your textbook. If you are still unsure of the answers, put a question mark next to the answer(s) for the review session of the lab.

III. APPLICATION OF ANATOMY AND PHYSIOLOGY EXERCISE

Directions to Students: Work on the following with your lab partner.
1. In your notebook, draw the penis and scrotum from memory.

2. Label the penis and scrotum; include each structure's orientation in the body (either vertical, horizontal, vertical oblique, or horizontal oblique). Ask your lab partner to critique your work. What did you miss?

3. Below your drawing, write two or three summary sentences about the physiology of the penis and scrotum. Ask your lab partner to check your work. Now check your work against the physiology section in the textbook. What else can you add to your description?

309

IV. IMAGE ANALYSIS EXERCISE

Directions to Students: Work on the following figures with your lab partner. It's your choice! You can label all the sketches at once, then go back and label each image with your lab partner, or you can label an image and its accompanying sketch at the same time. Either way, the goal is to label correctly all of the sketches and carefully compare the sketch with the sonographic image.

For each sonographic image, write a brief observation that could be "presented" to your instructor, a clinical sonographer, or a sonologist. Your observation should be based on Chapter 7 in the textbook, which describes how to write a technical observation. Please go back and review that chapter if necessary.

For each image, your assessment should include (1) the view of each major structure (axial or longitudinal; note: these are not the scanning planes) and (2) structures identified in the image with correct sonographic appearance description and measurements if shown (see Chapter 7 in the textbook for information on how to write a technical observation).

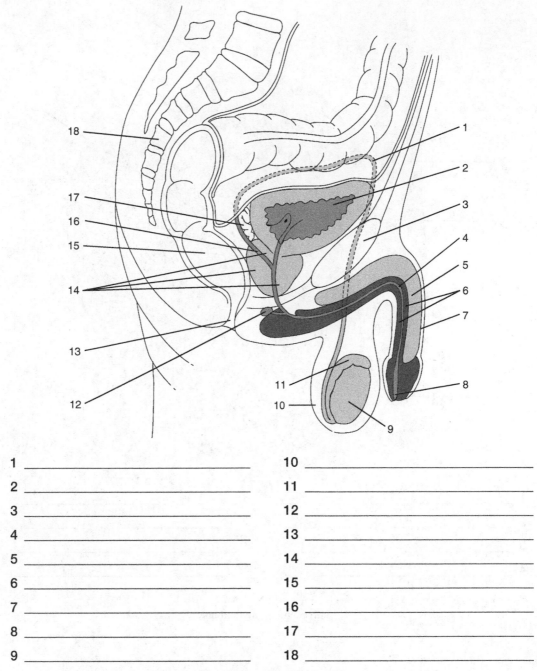

Figure 29-1 in the textbook

1 _____   10 _____
2 _____   11 _____
3 _____   12 _____
4 _____   13 _____
5 _____   14 _____
6 _____   15 _____
7 _____   16 _____
8 _____   17 _____
9 _____   18 _____

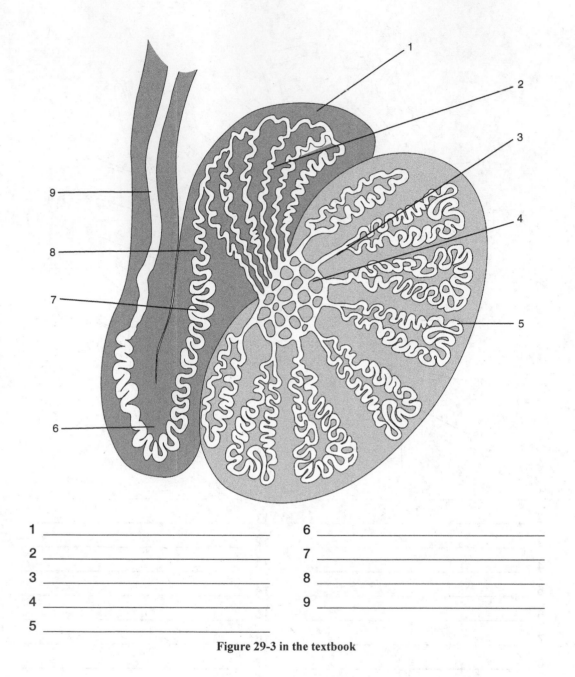

1 _____   6 _____
2 _____   7 _____
3 _____   8 _____
4 _____   9 _____
5 _____

Figure 29-3 in the textbook

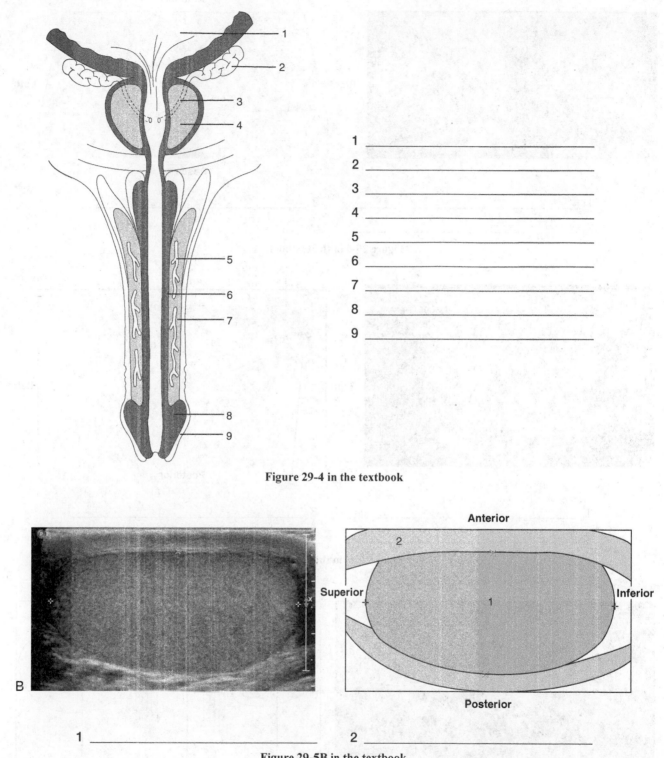

Figure 29-4 in the textbook

1 _____

2 _____

3 _____

4 _____

5 _____

6 _____

7 _____

8 _____

9 _____

Anterior

Superior   **Inferior**

Posterior

B

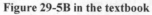

1 _____   2 _____

Figure 29-5B in the textbook

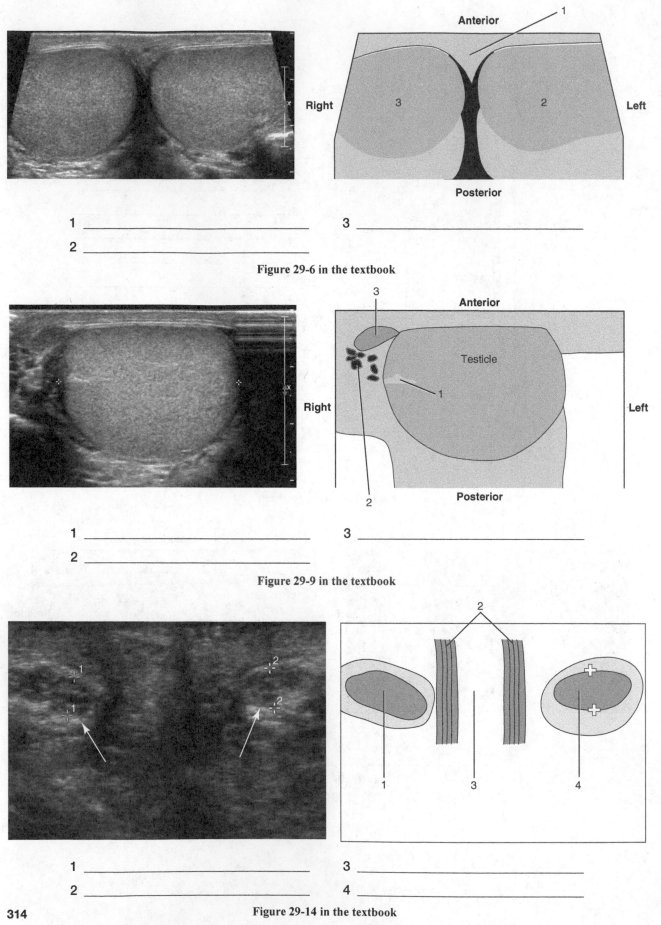

1 _____   3 _____

2 _____

Figure 29-6 in the textbook

1 _____   3 _____

2 _____

Figure 29-9 in the textbook

1 _____   3 _____

2 _____   4 _____

Chapter **29   Scrotal and Penile Sonography**

Figure 29-14 in the textbook

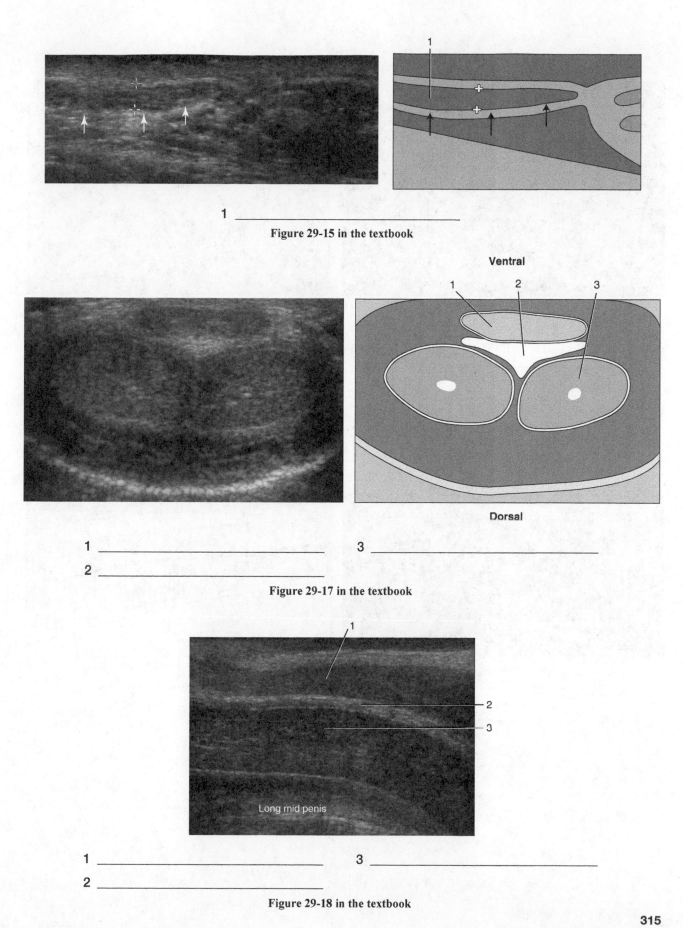

1 _____

Figure 29-15 in the textbook

Ventral

Dorsal

1 _____   3 _____

2 _____

Figure 29-17 in the textbook

Long mid penis

1 _____   3 _____

2 _____

Figure 29-18 in the textbook

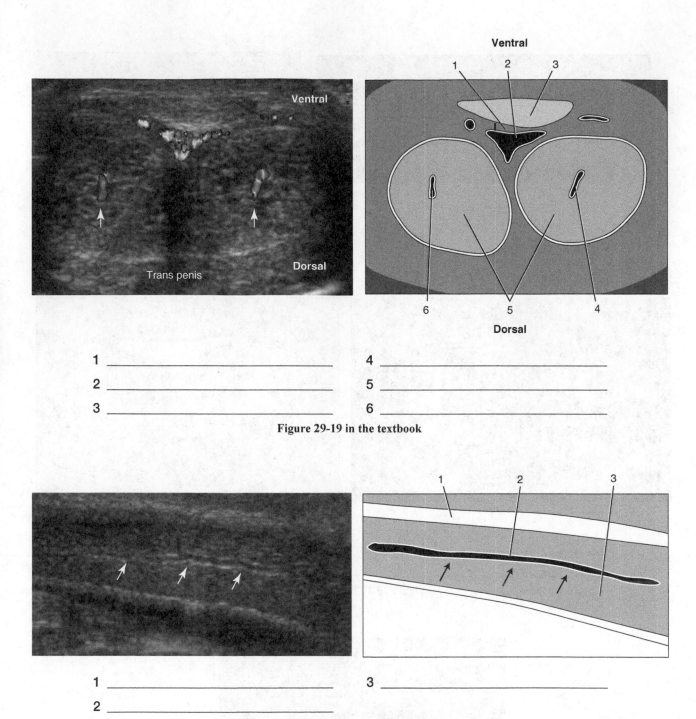

Figure 29-19 in the textbook

1 _____   4 _____

2 _____   5 _____

3 _____   6 _____

Figure 29-20 in the textbook

1 _____   3 _____

2 _____

V. CHAPTER SUBHEADINGS EXERCISE

Directions to Students:

1. Convert each chapter subheading into a question; for example, change "Gross Anatomy" to "What is the gross anatomy of the penis and scrotum?" Write the answer to each question in a short paragraph in your notebook.

2. Exchange answers with your lab partner and check each other's work. Refer back to the textbook for further information and explanation.

3. What questions do you still have about the chapter? Write your questions in your notebook.

VI. CHAPTER EVALUATION EXERCISE

Directions to Students: Use a fresh sheet of notebook paper. Based on your work with the chapter and its accompanying laboratory assignments, identify three concepts you believe are the most important. You may draw from any of the assignments you've already completed in the previous pages, including learning objectives, anatomy and physiology, images, or chapter subheadings. Include a detailed rationale in your answers.

Answer the questions below. Refer to page 384 for the answers.

Multiple Choice

1. The testes produce
   a. sperm only.
   b. testosterone only.
   c. testosterone and spermatozoa.
   d. testosterone and alkaline fluid.
2. The rete testis is located within the
   a. tunica dartos.
   b. median raphe.
   c. tunica albuginea.
   d. mediastinum testis.
3. Which scrotal tissue is continuous with the subcutaneous tissue of the abdominal wall?
   a. Buck's fascia
   b. Tunica dartos
   c. Tunica albuginea
   d. Infundibuliform fascia
4. The deep artery of the penis supplies the
   a. urethra.
   b. glans penis.
   c. corpora cavernosa.
   d. corpus spongiosum.
5. The corpora cavernosa are covered by the highly echogenic
   a. tunica dartos.
   b. tunica vaginalis.
   c. tunica albuginea.
   d. internal spermatic fascia.
6. In the sagittal scanning plane, what is represented by the parallel echogenic lines seen in the middle of the corpora cavernosa?
   a. Buck's fascia
   b. Arterial walls
   c. Mediastinum testis
   d. Pampiniform plexus
7. The spermatic cord is visualized
   a. as it courses through the median raphe.
   b. as it courses through the inguinal canal.
   c. as it courses through the corpora cavernosa.
   d. as it courses through the corpus spongiosum.

True/False

8. The echogenicity of the epididymis is equal to or slightly more than that of a normal testicle. _____

9. The ductus deferens courses superiorly and exits the scrotum through the inguinal canal. _____

10. The normal adult testicle measures approximately 6 to 7 cm in length. _____

Pediatric Echocardiography 30

I. MEMORIZATION EXERCISE

Directions to Students: Write the key words in your notebook or on note cards. Write the words on one side of the notepaper and then write the definitions on the opposite side of the page or on the back of the paper. If using note cards, write the key word on the front and the definition on the back. *This step should be completed before the lab session begins.*

Memorize the key word definitions silently for 5 minutes, then work with a lab partner and identify the words you still need help with. List the words here. Add additional rows if needed.

II. COMPREHENSION EXERCISE

Directions to Students: Work with a lab partner to complete this exercise. You will need to write in your notebook. First, change each objective into a question.

> *Example: "Name the chambers, great veins, and great arteries of the heart" becomes "What are the chambers, great veins, and great arteries of the heart?"*

Next, write a short answer to the question just created.

> *Example: "There are four chambers in the heart. The right atrium and right ventricle are connected by the tricuspid valve, which transports blood to the lungs, via a great artery—the pulmonary artery. The great veins that empty blood into the right atrium are the superior and inferior vena cavae. The left atrium and left ventricle are the remaining two chambers; they bring oxygenated blood from the lungs and ultimately to the*

> *rest of the body via the second great artery, the aorta. Oxygenated blood is returned to the left atrium via four pulmonary veins."*

Highlight or circle any part of your answers about which you are unsure, and check the answers in your textbook. If you are still unsure of the answers, put a question mark next to the answer(s) for the review session of the lab.

III. APPLICATION OF ANATOMY AND PHYSIOLOGY EXERCISE

Directions to Students: Work on the following with your lab partner.
1. In your notebook, draw the pediatric heart from memory.

2. Label the heart and its chambers and vessels; include each structure's orientation in the body (either vertical, horizontal, vertical oblique, or horizontal oblique). Ask your lab partner to critique your work. What did you miss?

3. Below your drawing, write two or three summary sentences about the physiology of the pediatric heart. Ask your lab partner to check your work. Now check your work against the physiology section in the textbook. What else can you add to your description?

IV. IMAGE ANALYSIS EXERCISE

Directions to Students: Work on the following figures with your lab partner. It's your choice! You can label all the sketches at once, then go back and label each image with your lab partner, or you can label an image and its accompanying sketch at the same time. Either way, the goal is to label correctly all of the sketches and carefully compare the sketch with the sonographic image.

For each sonographic image, write a brief observation that could be "presented" to your instructor, a clinical sonographer, or a sonologist. Your observation should be based on Chapter 7 in the textbook, which describes how to write a technical observation. Please go back and review that chapter if necessary.

For each image, your assessment should include (1) the view of each major structure (axial or longitudinal; note: these are not the scanning planes) and (2) structures identified in the image with correct sonographic appearance description and measurements if shown (see Chapter 7 in the textbook for information on how to write a technical observation).

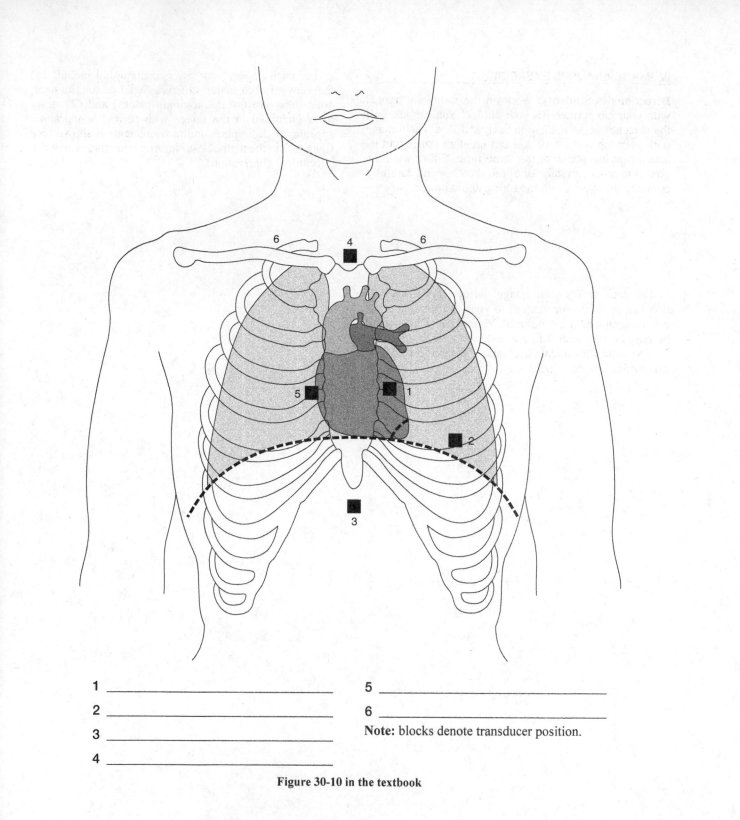

1 _____   5 _____

2 _____   6 _____

3 _____   **Note:** blocks denote transducer position.

4 _____

Figure 30-10 in the textbook

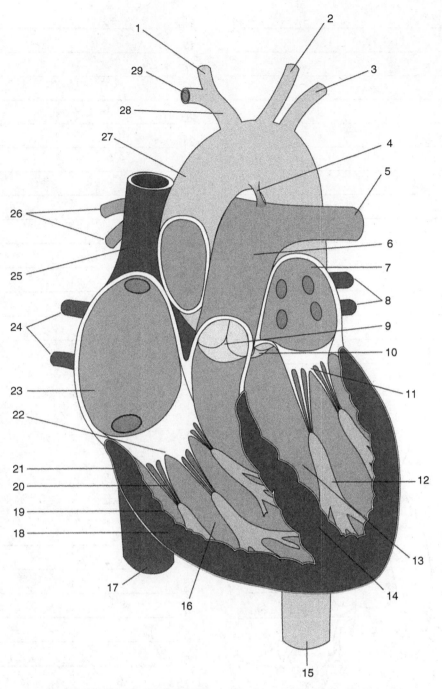

Figure 30-11 in the textbook Answer blanks are on the following page.

1 _____   16 _____

2 _____   17 _____

3 _____   18 _____

4 _____   19 _____

5 _____   20 _____

6 _____   21 _____

7 _____   22 _____

8 _____   23 _____

9 _____   24 _____

10 _____   25 _____

11 _____   26 _____

12 _____   27 _____

13 _____   28 _____

14 _____   29 _____

15 _____

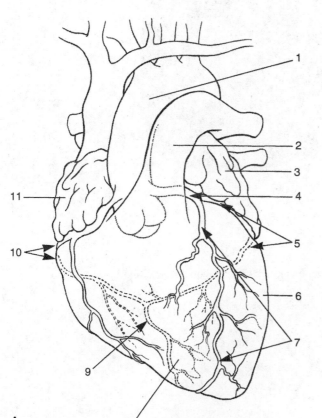

1 _____

2 _____

3 _____

4 _____

5 _____

6 _____

7 _____

8 _____

9 _____

10 _____

11 _____

A

Coronary arteries and their positions on the heart, anterior view.

Figure 30-13A in the textbook

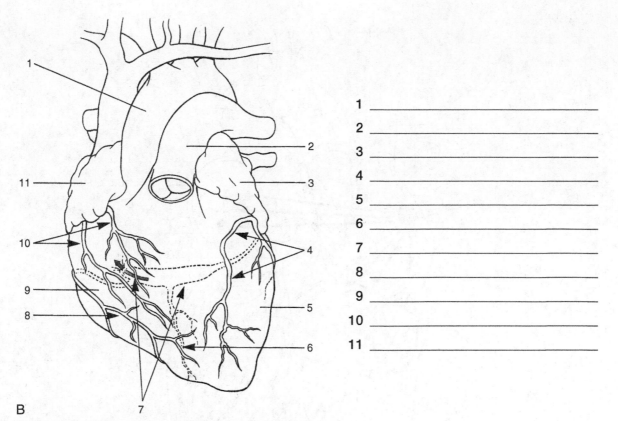

1 _____
2 _____
3 _____
4 _____
5 _____
6 _____
7 _____
8 _____
9 _____
10 _____
11 _____

B

Cardiac veins and their positions on the heart, anterior view.

Figure 30-13B in the textbook

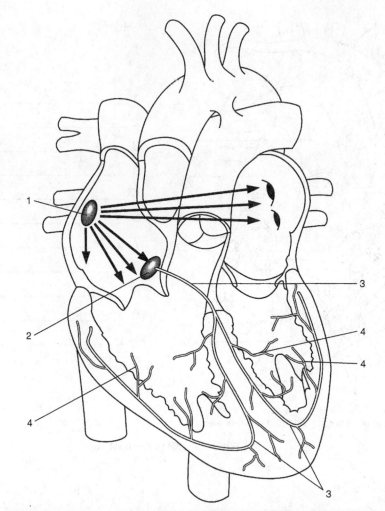

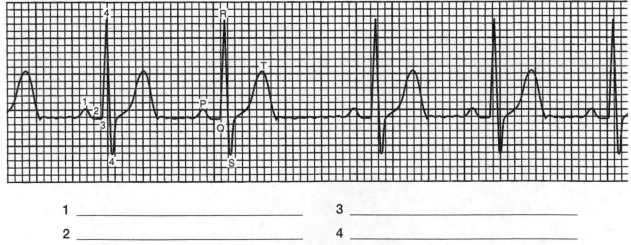

1 _____   3 _____

2 _____   4 _____

Figure 30-14 in the textbook

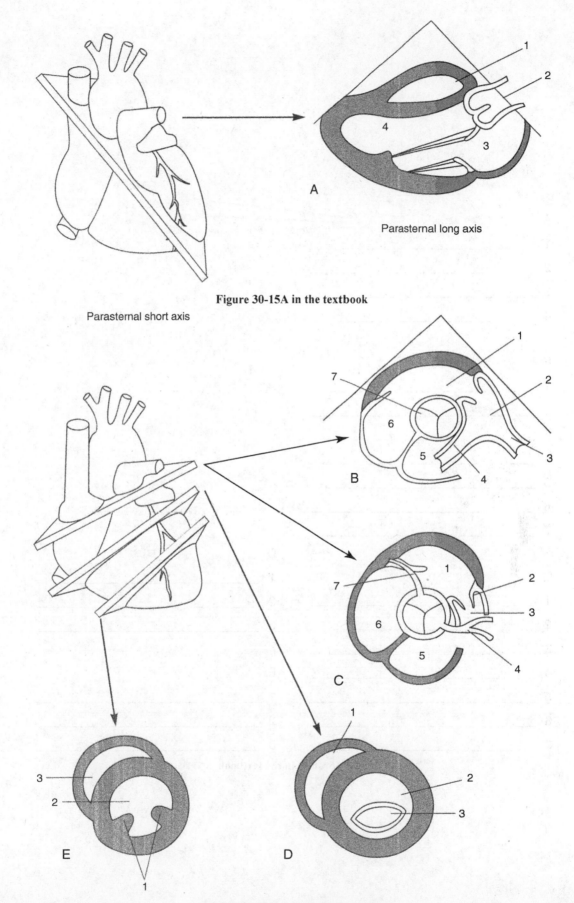

Parasternal long axis

A

Figure 30-15A in the textbook

Parasternal short axis

B

C

D

E

Figure 30-15B to E in the textbook

A

1 _____

2 _____

3 _____

4 _____

B

1 _____

2 _____

3 _____

4 _____

5 _____

6 _____

7 _____

C

1 _____

2 _____

3 _____

4 _____

5 _____

6 _____

7 _____

D

1 _____

2 _____

3 _____

E

1 _____

2 _____

3 _____

Figure 3-15A to E in the textbook

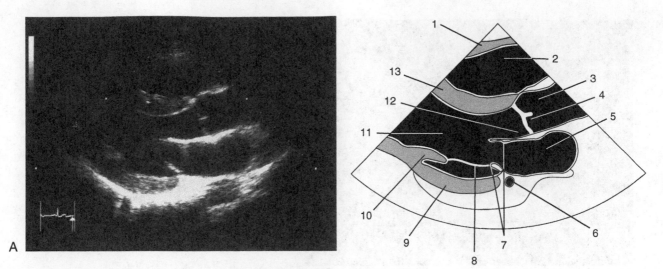

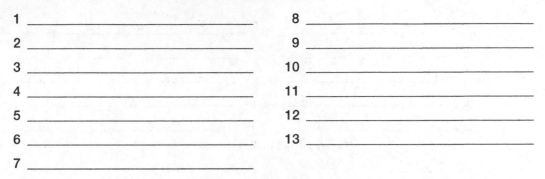

Parasternal long axis view, diastolic frame.

1	_____	8	_____
2	_____	9	_____
3	_____	10	_____
4	_____	11	_____
5	_____	12	_____
6	_____	13	_____
7	_____		

Figure 30-16A in the textbook

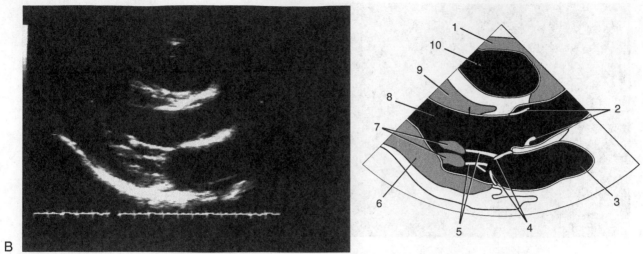

Parasternal long axis view, systolic frame.

1 _____   6 _____

2 _____   7 _____

3 _____   8 _____

4 _____   9 _____

5 _____   10 _____

Figure 30-16B in the textbook

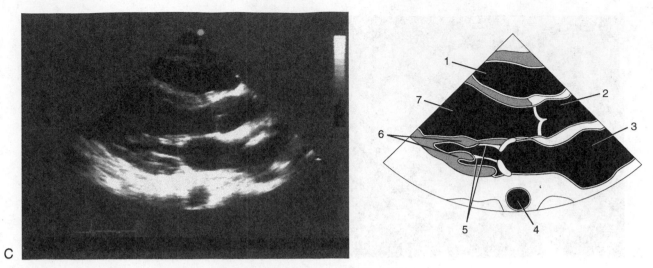

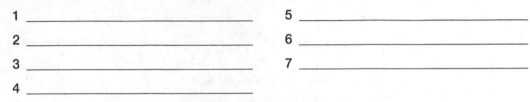

C

Parasternal long axis view, late diastolic frame.

1 _____   5 _____
2 _____   6 _____
3 _____   7 _____
4 _____

Figure 30-16C in the textbook

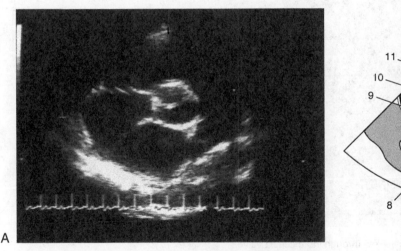

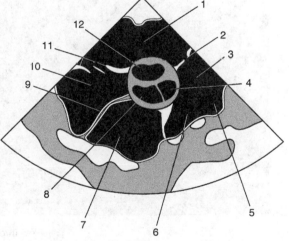

A

Closed aortic valve, parasternal short axis section.

1 _____   7 _____
2 _____   8 _____
3 _____   9 _____
4 _____   10 _____
5 _____   11 _____
6 _____   12 _____

Figure 30-21A in the textbook

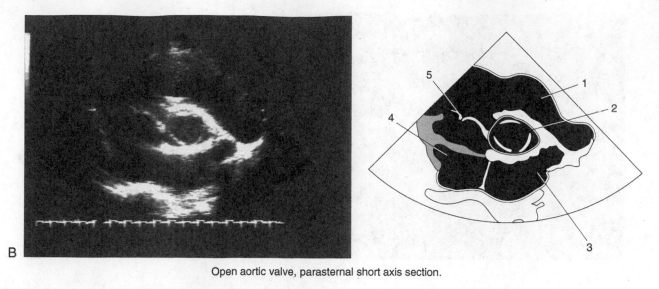

B

Open aortic valve, parasternal short axis section.

1 _____ 4 _____

2 _____ 5 _____

3 _____

Figure 30-21B in the textbook

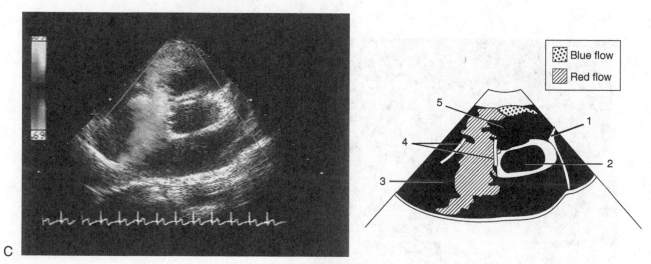

C

Flow through the tricuspid valve.

1 _____ 4 _____

2 _____ 5 _____

3 _____

Figure 30-21C in the textbook

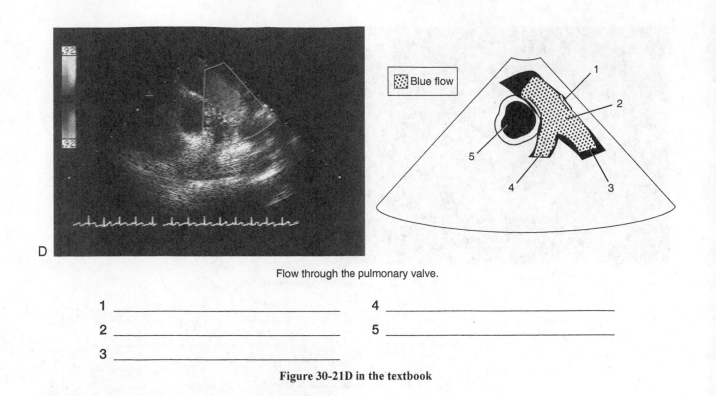

Flow through the pulmonary valve.

1 _____ 4 _____

2 _____ 5 _____

3 _____

Figure 30-21D in the textbook

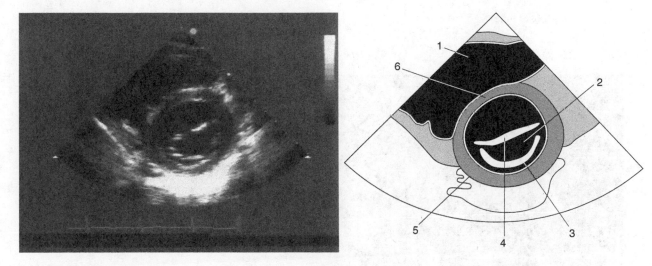

Mitral valve, short axis plane.

1 _____ 4 _____

2 _____ 5 _____

3 _____ 6 _____

Figure 30-22, top, in the textbook

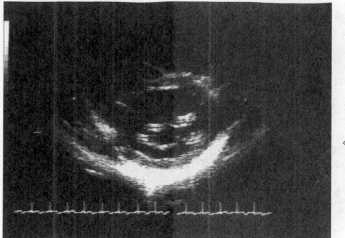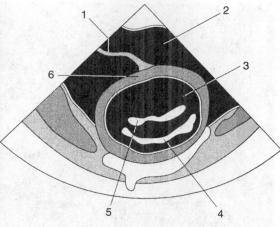

Mitral valve, short axis plane.

1 _____   4 _____
2 _____   5 _____
3 _____   6 _____

Figure 30-22, bottom, in the textbook

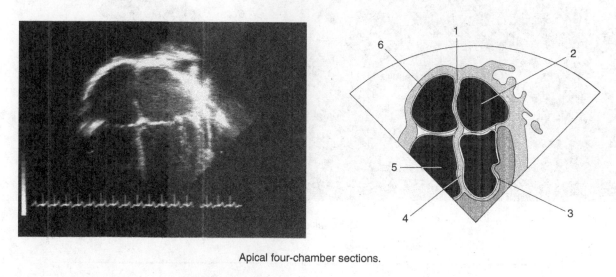

Apical four-chamber sections.

1 _____   4 _____
2 _____   5 _____
3 _____   6 _____

Figure 30-25A, top, in the textbook

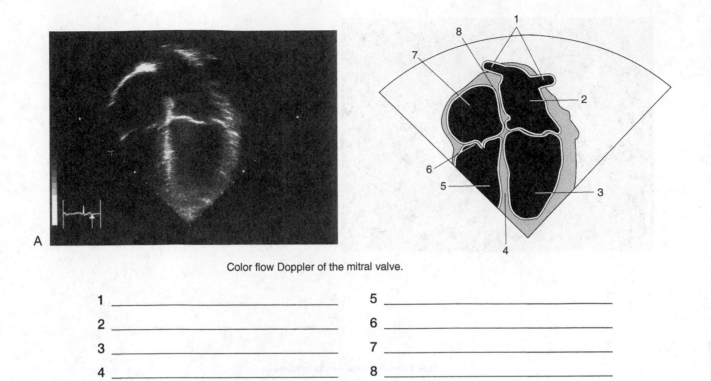

Color flow Doppler of the mitral valve.

1 _____   5 _____

2 _____   6 _____

3 _____   7 _____

4 _____   8 _____

Figure 30-25A, bottom, in the textbook

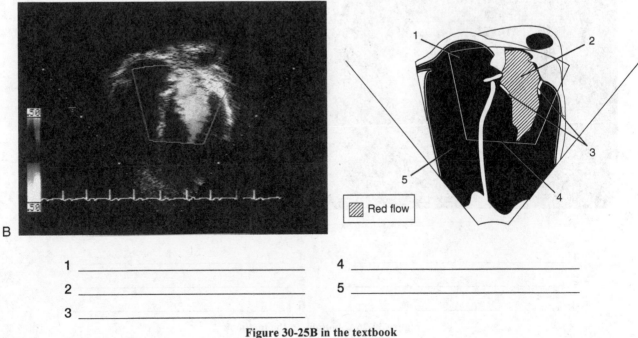

Red flow

1 _____   4 _____

2 _____   5 _____

3 _____

Figure 30-25B in the textbook

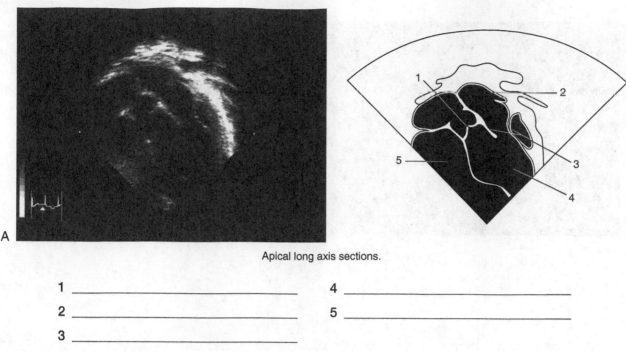

Apical long axis sections.

1 _____   4 _____

2 _____   5 _____

3 _____

Figure 30-26A, top, in the textbook

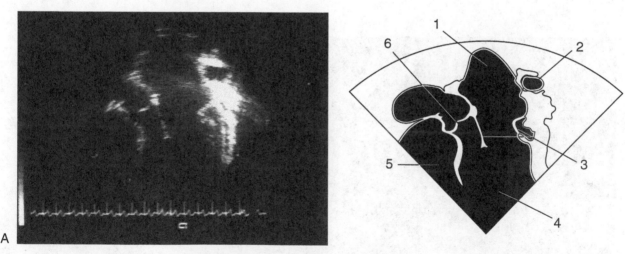

Apical long axis view with color flow.

1 _____   4 _____

2 _____   5 _____

3 _____   6 _____

Figure 30-26A, bottom, in the textbook

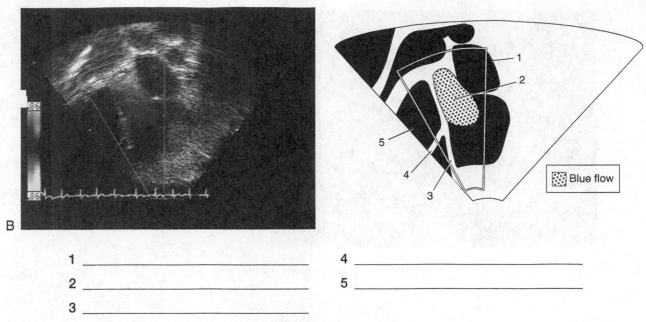

B

1	_____	4	_____
2	_____	5	_____
3	_____		

Figure 30-26B in the textbook

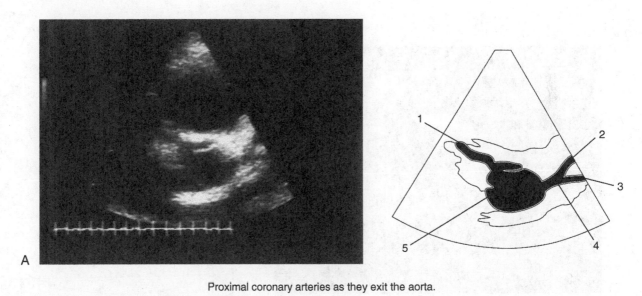

A

Proximal coronary arteries as they exit the aorta.

1	_____	4	_____
2	_____	5	_____
3	_____		

Figure 30-34A in the textbook

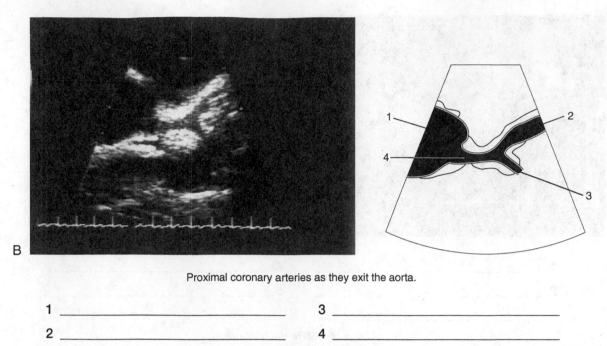

Proximal coronary arteries as they exit the aorta.

1 _____   3 _____

2 _____   4 _____

Figure 30-34B in the textbook

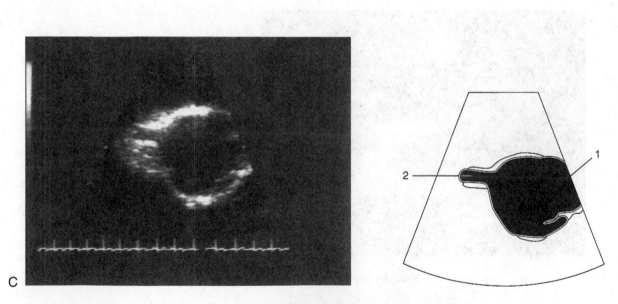

Proximal coronary artery exiting the aorta.

1 _____   2 _____

Figure 30-34C in the textbook

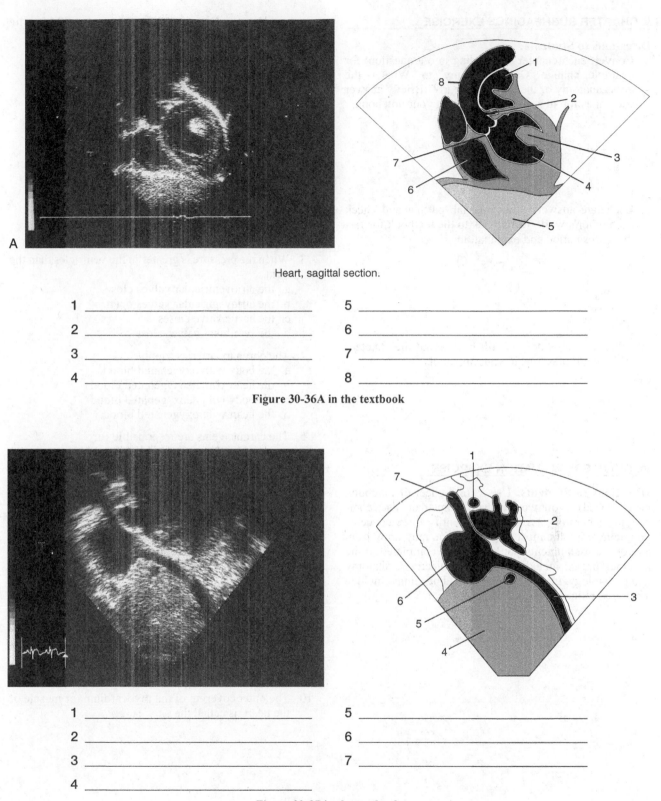

Heart, sagittal section.

1 _____	5 _____
2 _____	6 _____
3 _____	7 _____
4 _____	8 _____

Figure 30-36A in the textbook

1 _____	5 _____
2 _____	6 _____
3 _____	7 _____
4 _____	

Figure 30-37 in the textbook

V. CHAPTER SUBHEADINGS EXERCISE

Directions to Students:

1. Convert each chapter subheading into a question; for example, change "Gross Anatomy" to "What is the gross anatomy of the pediatric heart?" Briefly answer each question in a short paragraph in your notebook.

2. Exchange answers with your lab partner and check each other's work. Refer back to the textbook for further information and explanation.

3. What questions do you still have about the chapter? Write your questions in your notebook.

VI. CHAPTER EVALUATION EXERCISE

Directions to Students: Use a fresh sheet of notebook paper. Based on your work with the chapter and its accompanying laboratory assignments, identify three concepts you believe are the most important. You may draw from any of the assignments you've already completed in the previous pages, including learning objectives, anatomy and physiology, images, or chapter subheadings. Include a detailed rationale in your answers.

Answer the questions below. Refer to page 384 for the answers.

Multiple Choice

1. The eustachian valve is found in the
   a. right atria.
   b. right ventricle.
   c. left atria.
   d. left ventricle.

2. The parasternal long-axis view allows for identification of all the following EXCEPT the
   a. left ventricle.
   b. right ventricle.
   c. aorta.
   d. right atrium.

3. When the pressure is greater in the ventricles than the atria,
   a. the atrioventricular valves close.
   b. the atrioventricular valves open.
   c. the aortic valve closes.
   d. the semilunar valves close.

4. The coronary arteries supply
   a. the body with oxygenated blood.
   b. the heart with deoxygenated blood.
   c. the body with deoxygenated blood.
   d. the heart with oxygenated blood.

5. The cardiac veins are responsible for
   a. carrying deoxygenated blood to the right atria.
   b. carrying oxygenated blood to the right atria.
   c. carrying oxygenated blood to the left atria.
   d. carrying deoxygenated blood to the left atria.

Completion

6. The right and left atria are separated by the _____.

7. In the cardiac conduction system the _____ is responsible for setting the pace of the heart.

8. The inner lining of the cavities of the heart is called the _____.

9. In the fetal heart. before the foramen primum is closed, a second opening, called the _____, is formed.

10. The outer covering of the myocardium, or muscle of the heart, is called the _____.

31 Adult Echocardiography

I. MEMORIZATION EXERCISE

Directions to Students: Write the key words in your notebook or on note cards. Write the words on one side of the notepaper and then write the definitions on the opposite side of the page or on the back of the paper. If using note cards, write the key word on the front and the definition on the back. *This step should be completed before the lab session begins.*

Memorize the key word definitions silently for 5 minutes, then work with a lab partner and identify the words you still need help with. List the words here. Add additional rows if needed.

II. COMPREHENSION EXERCISE

Directions to Students: Work with a lab partner to complete this exercise. You will need to write in your notebook. First, change each objective into a question.

> *Example: "Describe the location of the heart in the chest" becomes "Where is the heart located in the chest?"*

Next, write a short answer to the question just created.

> *Example: "The heart sits within the thoracic cavity, posterior to the sternum and adjacent to the right and left lungs in the mediastinum. The heart sits within a sac called the pericardium. The heart sits at a slight angle, with its lower tip, or apex, pointed to the left of midline. The apex is more inferior and anterior than the base of the heart, where the pulmonary artery and aorta are located."*

Highlight or circle any part of your answers about which you are unsure, and check the answers in your textbook. If you are still unsure of the answers, put a question mark next to the answer(s) for the review session of the lab.

III. APPLICATION OF ANATOMY AND PHYSIOLOGY EXERCISE

Directions to Students: Work on the following with your lab partner.
1. In your notebook, draw the adult heart from memory.

2. Label the heart and its chambers and vessels; include each structure's orientation in the body (either vertical, horizontal, vertical oblique, or horizontal oblique). Ask your lab partner to critique your work. What did you miss?

3. Below your drawing, write two or three summary sentences about the physiology of the heart. Ask your lab partner to check your work. Now check your work against the physiology section in the textbook. What else can you add to your description?

IV. IMAGE ANALYSIS EXERCISE

Directions to Students: Work on the following figures with your lab partner. It's your choice! You can label all the sketches at once, then go back and label each image with your lab partner, or label an image and its accompanying sketch at the same time. Either way, the goal is to label correctly all of the sketches and carefully compare the sketch with the sonographic image.

For each sonographic image, write a brief observation that could be "presented" to your instructor, a clinical sonographer, or a sonologist. Your observation should be based on Chapter 7 in the textbook, which describes how to write a technical observation. Please go back and review that chapter if necessary.

For each image, your assessment should include (1) the view of each major structure (axial or longitudinal; note: these are not the scanning planes) and (2) structures identified in the image with correct sonographic appearance description and measurements if shown (see Chapter 7 in the textbook for information on how to write a technical observation).

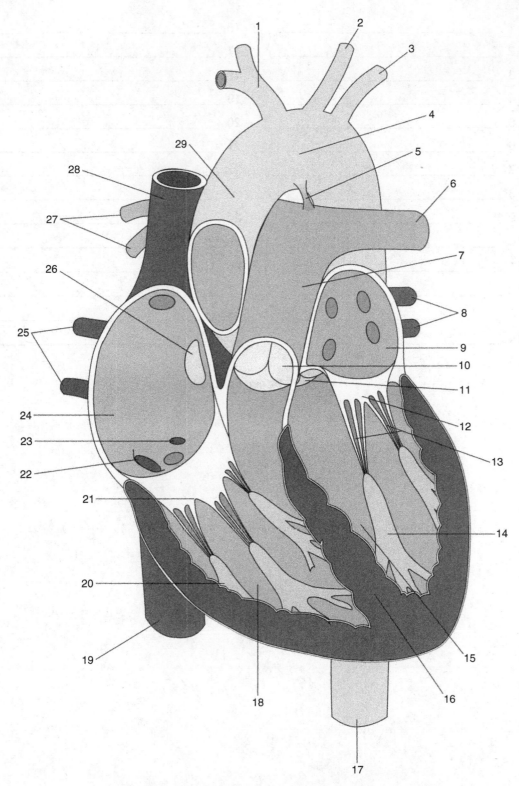

Figure 31-2 in the textbook Answer blanks are on following page.

1 _____ 16 _____

2 _____ 17 _____

3 _____ 18 _____

4 _____ 19 _____

5 _____ 20 _____

6 _____ 21 _____

7 _____ 22 _____

8 _____ 23 _____

9 _____ 24 _____

10 _____ 25 _____

11 _____ 26 _____

12 _____ 27 _____

13 _____ 28 _____

14 _____ 29 _____

15 _____

Figure 31-2 in the textbook

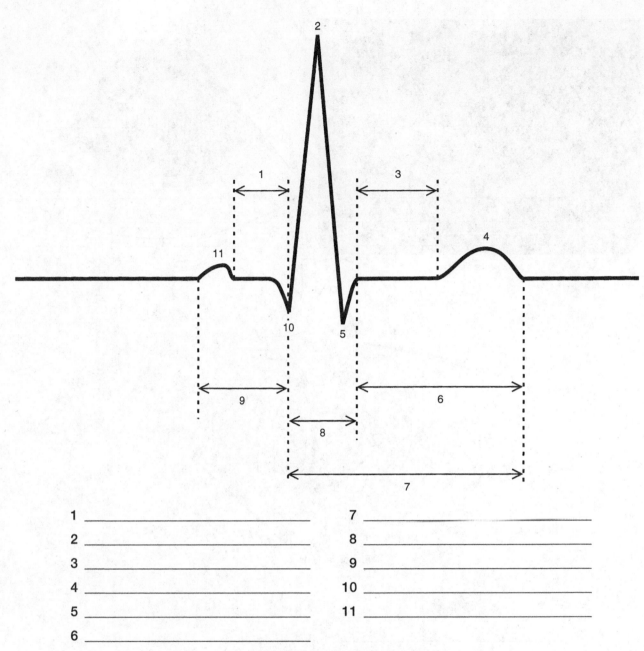

1	_____	7	_____
2	_____	8	_____
3	_____	9	_____
4	_____	10	_____
5	_____	11	_____
6	_____		

Figure 31-5 in the textbook

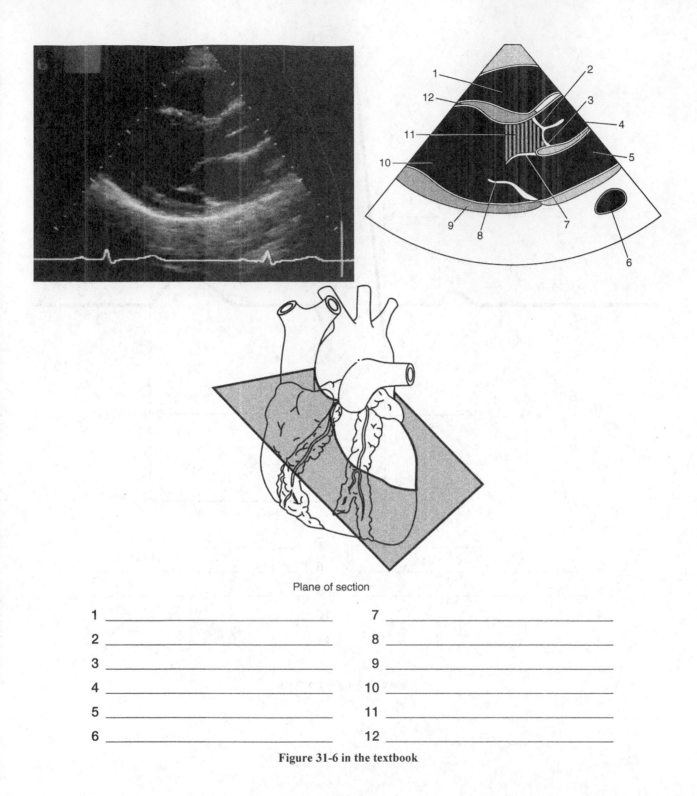

Plane of section

1 _____   7 _____

2 _____   8 _____

3 _____   9 _____

4 _____   10 _____

5 _____   11 _____

6 _____   12 _____

Figure 31-6 in the textbook

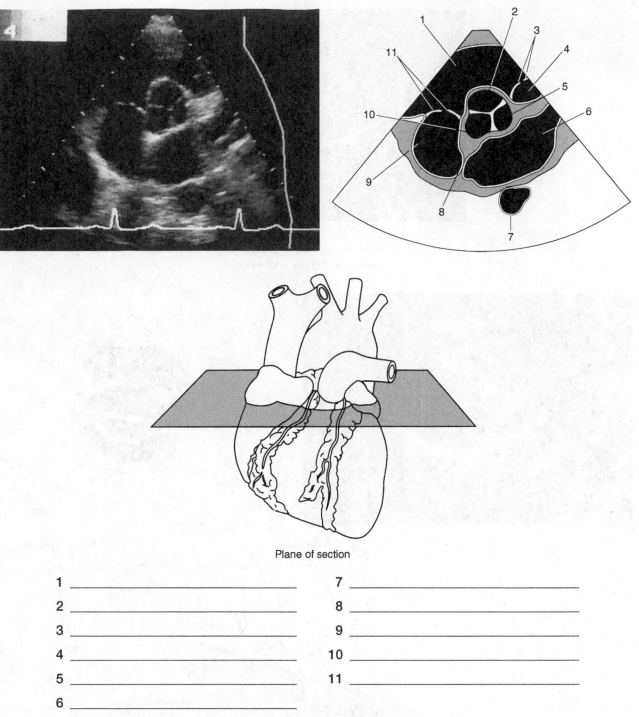

Plane of section

1 _____   7 _____

2 _____   8 _____

3 _____   9 _____

4 _____   10 _____

5 _____   11 _____

6 _____

Figure 31-8 in the textbook

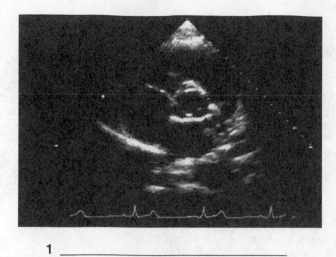

1 _____

Figure 31-9 in the textbook

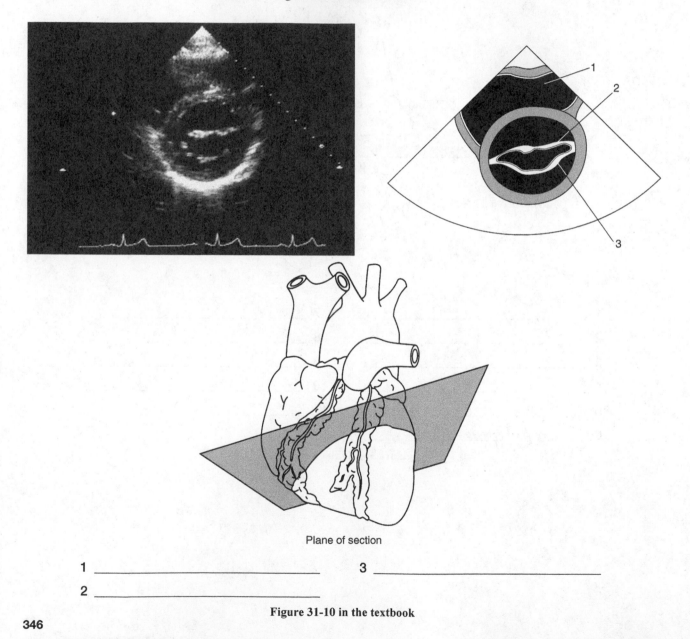

Plane of section

1 _____   3 _____

2 _____

Figure 31-10 in the textbook

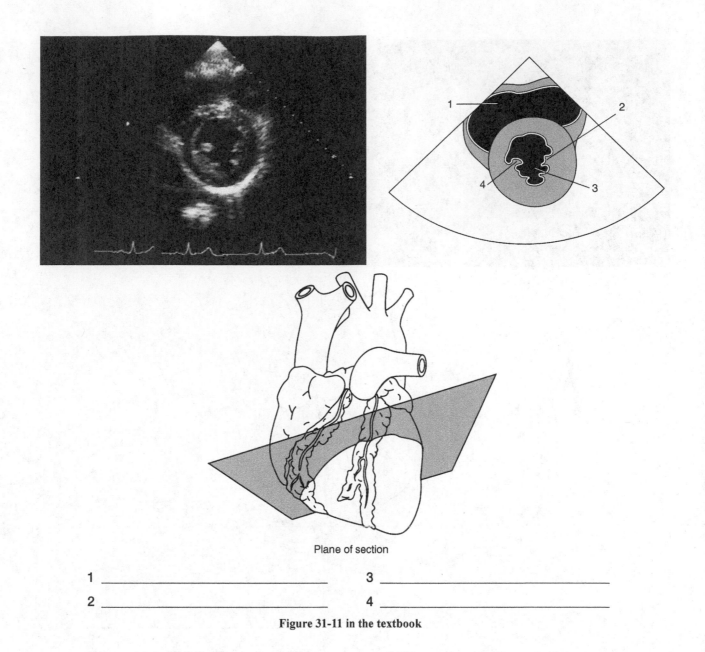

Plane of section

1 _____   3 _____

2 _____   4 _____

Figure 31-11 in the textbook

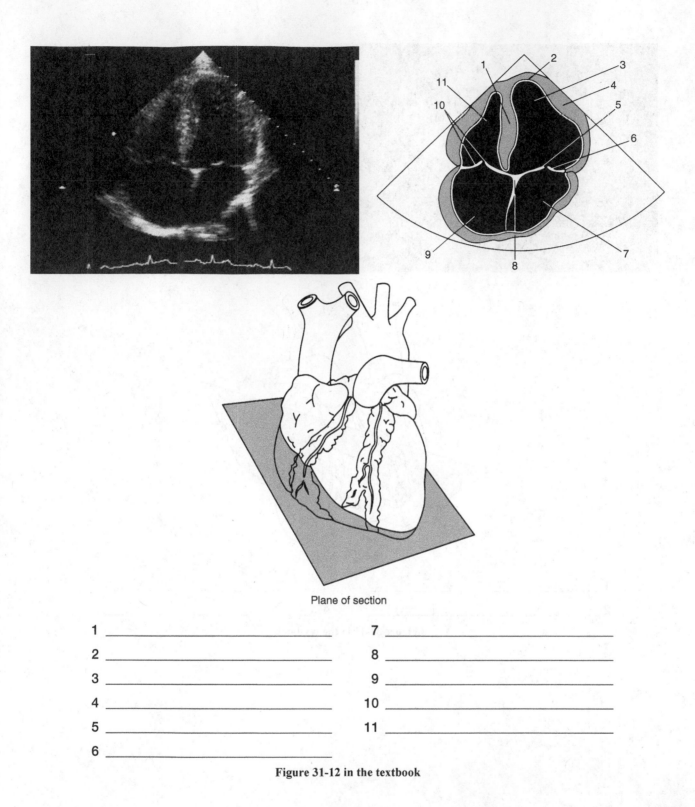

Plane of section

1 _____	7 _____
2 _____	8 _____
3 _____	9 _____
4 _____	10 _____
5 _____	11 _____
6 _____	

Figure 31-12 in the textbook

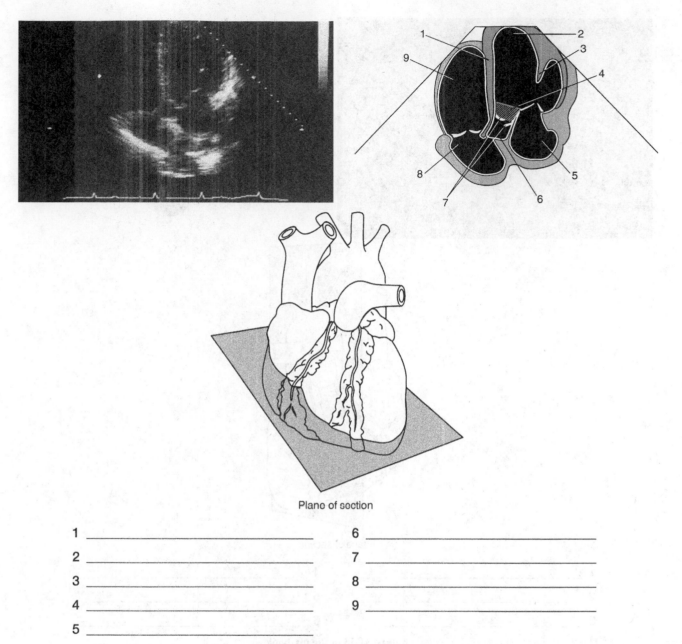

Plane of section

1 _____   6 _____
2 _____   7 _____
3 _____   8 _____
4 _____   9 _____
5 _____

Figure 31-14 in the textbook

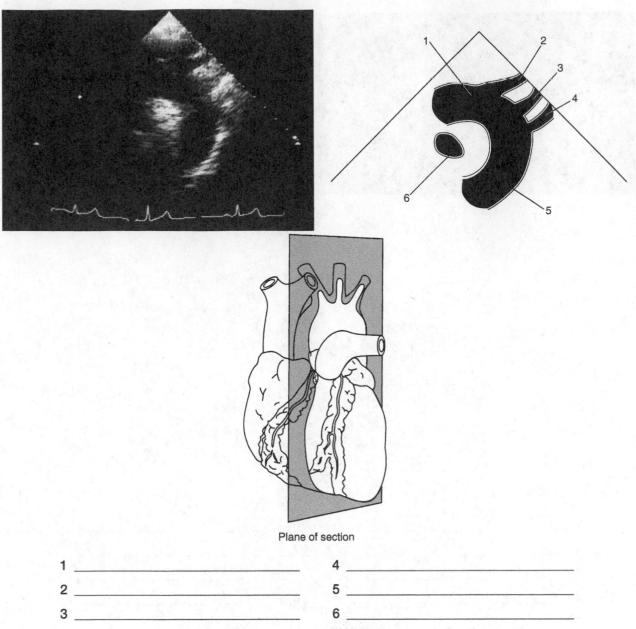

Plane of section

1 _____   4 _____

2 _____   5 _____

3 _____   6 _____

Figure 31-15 in the textbook

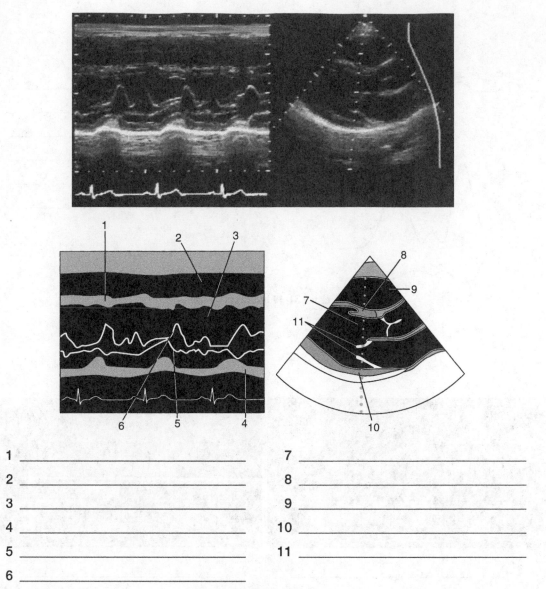

1 _____   7 _____

2 _____   8 _____

3 _____   9 _____

4 _____   10 _____

5 _____   11 _____

6 _____

Figure 31-18 in the textbook

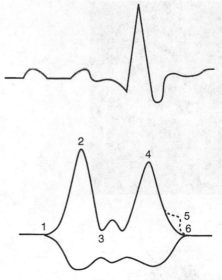
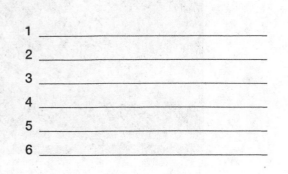

1 _____

2 _____

3 _____

4 _____

5 _____

6 _____

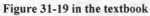

Figure 31-19 in the textbook

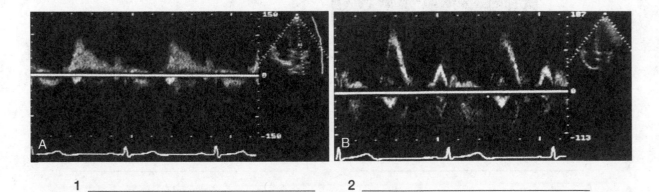

1 _____ 2 _____

Figure 31-23 in the textbook

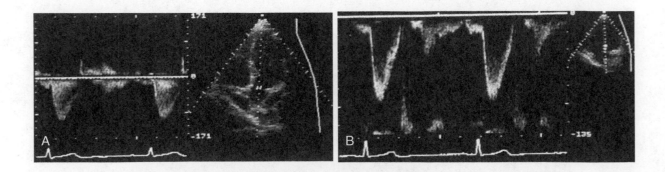

1 _____ 2 _____

Figure 31-24 in the textbook

Chapter **31** **Adult Echocardiography**

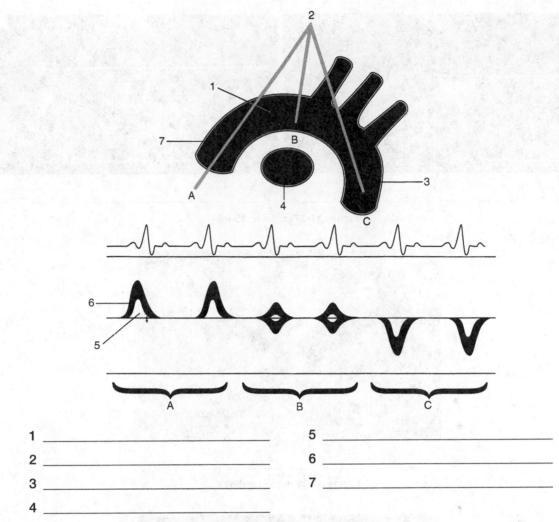

1 _____   5 _____

2 _____   6 _____

3 _____   7 _____

4 _____

Figure 31-25 in the textbook

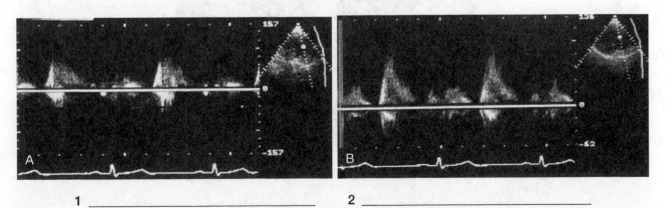

1 _____   2 _____

Figure 31-26 in the textbook

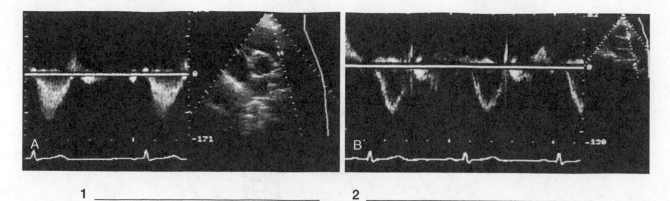

1 _____   2 _____

Figure 31-27 in the textbook

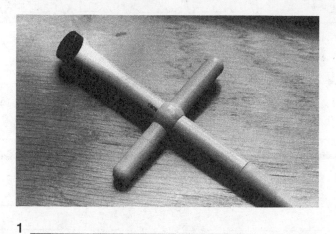

1 _____

Figure 31-28 in the textbook

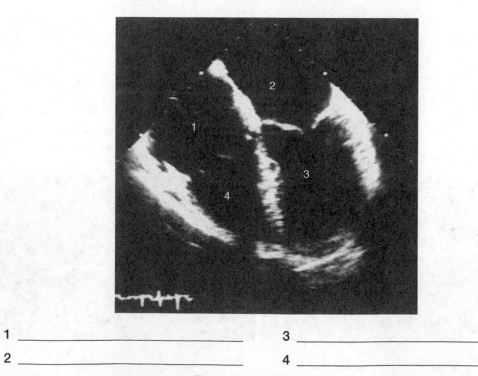

1 _____   3 _____

2 _____   4 _____

Figure 31-29 in the textbook

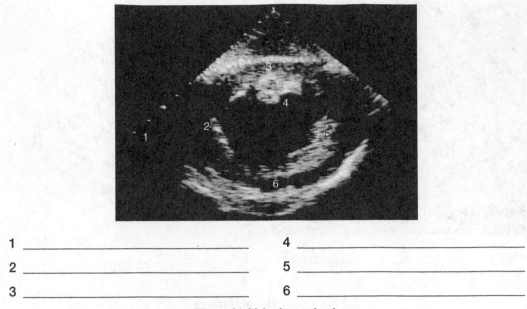

1 _____	4 _____
2 _____	5 _____
3 _____	6 _____

Figure 31-30 in the textbook

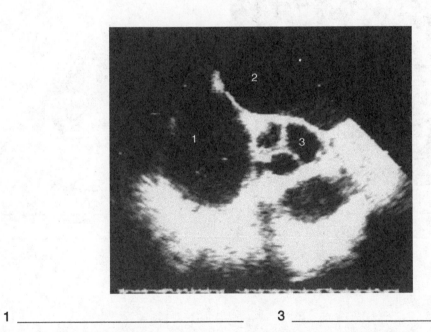

| 1 _____ | 3 _____ |
| 2 _____ | |

Figure 31-31 in the textbook

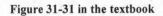

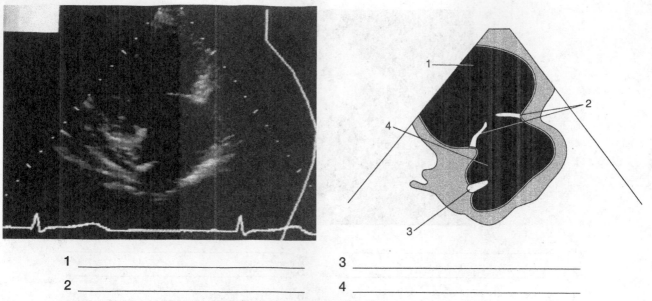

1 _____   3 _____

2 _____   4 _____

Figure 31-33 in the textbook

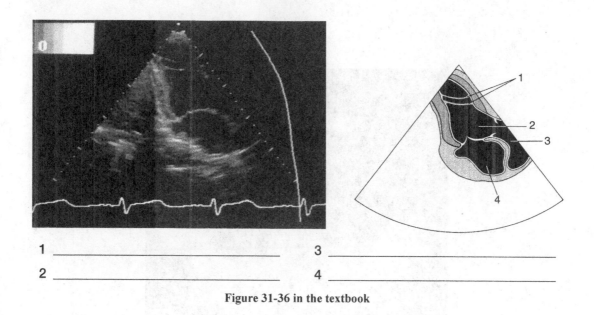

1 _____   3 _____

2 _____   4 _____

Figure 31-36 in the textbook

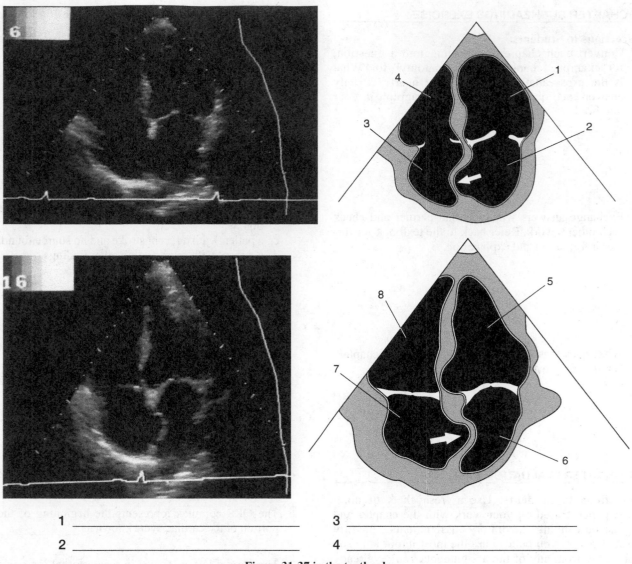

1 _____   3 _____

2 _____   4 _____

Figure 31-37 in the textbook

V. CHAPTER SUBHEADINGS EXERCISE

Directions to Students:

1. Convert each chapter subheading into a question; for example, change "Gross Anatomy" to "What is the gross anatomy of the adult heart?" Briefly answer each question in a short paragraph in your notebook.

2. Exchange answers with your lab partner and check each other's work. Refer back to the textbook for further information and explanation.

3. What questions do you still have about the chapter? Write your questions in your notebook.

VI. CHAPTER EVALUATION EXERCISE

Directions to Students: Use a fresh sheet of notebook paper. Based on your work with the chapter and its accompanying laboratory assignments, identify three concepts you believe are the most important. You may draw from any of the assignments you've already completed in the previous pages, including learning objectives, anatomy and physiology, images, or chapter subheadings. Include a detailed rationale in your answers.

Answer the questions below. Refer to page 384 for the answers.

Multiple Choice

1. Suspected aortic root dissection may be diagnosed with confidence with a
   a. TTE.
   b. chest radiograph.
   c. fast CT scan.
   d. TEE.

2. A TEE examination is indicated for
   a. a patient with a low EF by 2-dimensional echocardiography.
   b. a patient with a mild amount of mitral regurgitation.
   c. a patient with a recent stroke and no source found.
   d. a patient with fever and no other findings.

3. An exercise stress test is indicated for
   a. a 25-year-old male patient with sharp stabbing chest pain.
   b. a 75-year-old male patient with a history of CABG.
   c. a 45-year-old female patient with atypical chest pain.
   d. a 65-year-old female patient with angina and a positive family history of CAD.

Completion

4. A normal heart rate is considered to be from _____ to _____ bpm.

5. The P wave on an EKG represents atrial depolarization caused by the _____ node.

6. The QRS complex represents the beginning of the portion of the cardiac cycle known as _____ _____.

7. The normal left atrial size in a parasternal long-axis view is less than _____ cm.

8. The normal left ventricular ejection fraction is _____.

9. The most common indication for a TEE is evaluation for a cardiac source of _____.

10. The mitral valve comprises the _____ and _____ leaflets.

32 Vascular Technology

I. MEMORIZATION EXERCISE

Directions to Students: Write the key words in your notebook or on note cards. Write the words on one side of the notepaper and then write the definitions on the opposite side of the page or on the back of the paper. If using note cards, write the key word on the front and the definition on the back. *This step should be completed before the lab session begins.*

Memorize the key word definitions silently for 5 minutes, then work with a lab partner and identify the words you still need help with. List the words here. Add additional rows if needed.

II. COMPREHENSION EXERCISE

Directions to Students: Work with a lab partner to complete this exercise. You will need to write in your notebook. First, change each objective into a question.

Example: "Describe the role of indirect and direct noninvasive techniques used for the evaluation of vascular disease" becomes "What are the roles of indirect and direct noninvasive techniques used for the evaluation of vascular disease?"

Next, write a short answer to the question just created.

Example: "Noninvasive tests are divided into two categories: indirect and direct. Indirect tests are physiologic tests designed to show whether there is significant occlusive disease by demonstrating volume changes downstream from the area of disease. Direct noninvasive tests use B-mode imaging, Doppler spectral analysis, and Doppler color flow imaging to examine frequency shifts in determining the degree of occlusive disease, if any, in the arterial and venous vascular systems."

Highlight or circle any part of your answers about which you are unsure, and check the answers in your textbook. If you are still unsure of the answers, put a question mark next to the answer(s) for the review session of the lab.

III. APPLICATION OF ANATOMY AND PHYSIOLOGY EXERCISE

Directions to Students: Work on the following with your lab partner.
1. In your notebook, draw as many major arteries and veins of the head and extremities as you can from memory.

2. Label the arteries and veins, and include each structure's orientation in the body (either vertical, horizontal, vertical oblique, or horizontal oblique). Ask your lab partner to critique your work. What did you miss?

3. Below your drawing, write two or three summary sentences about the physiology of the vasculature. Ask your lab partner to check your work. Now check your work against the physiology section in the textbook. What else can you add to your description?

IV. IMAGE ANALYSIS EXERCISE

Directions to Students: Work on the following figures with your lab partner. It's your choice! You can label all the sketches at once, then go back and label each image with your lab partner, or you can label an image and its accompanying sketch at the same time. Either way, the goal is to label correctly all of the sketches and carefully compare the sketch with the sonographic image.

For each sonographic image, write a brief observation that could be "presented" to your instructor, a clinical sonographer, or a sonologist. Your observation should be based on Chapter 7 in the textbook, which describes how to write a technical observation. Please go back and review that chapter if necessary.

For each image, your assessment should include (1) the view of each major structure (axial or longitudinal; note: these are not the scanning planes) and (2) structures identified in the image with correct sonographic appearance description and measurements if shown (see Chapter 7 in the textbook for information on how to write a technical observation).

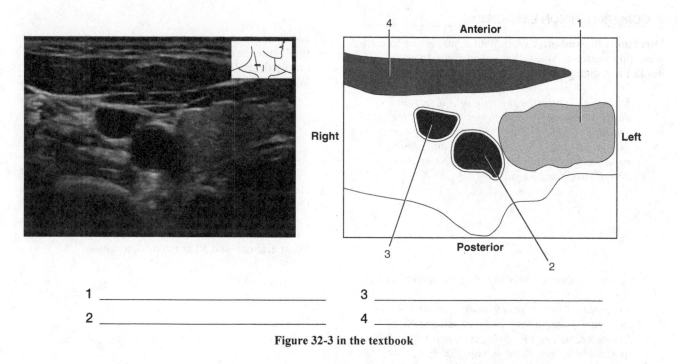

1 _____   3 _____

2 _____   4 _____

Figure 32-3 in the textbook

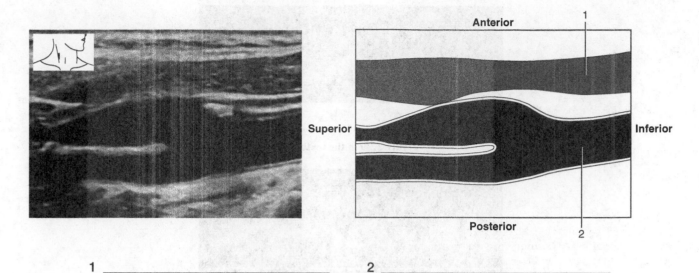

Anterior

1

Superior

Inferior

Posterior

2

1 _____   2 _____

Figure 32-4 in the textbook

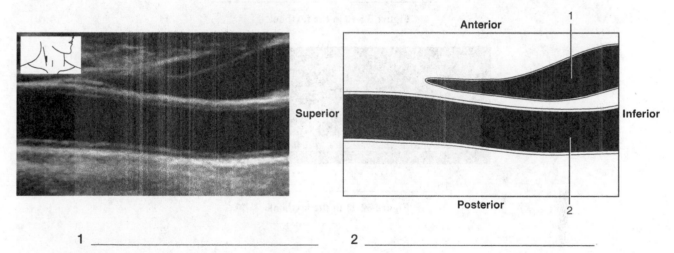

Anterior

1

Superior

Inferior

Posterior

2

1 _____   2 _____

Figure 32-5 in the textbook

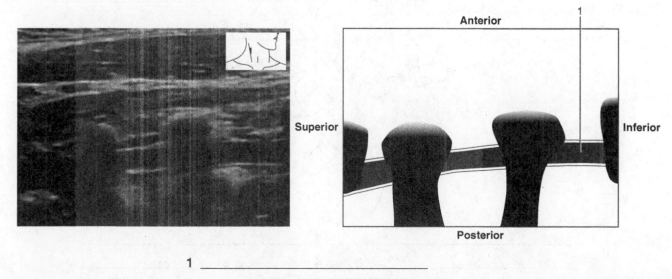

Anterior

1

Superior

Inferior

Posterior

1 _____

Figure 32-6 in the textbook

361

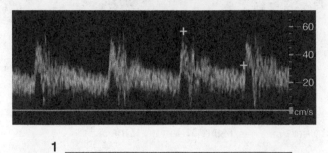

1 _____

Figure 32-9 in the textbook

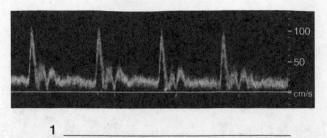

1 _____

Figure 32-10 in the textbook

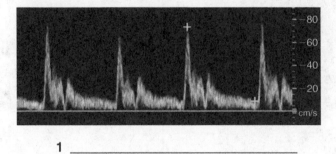

1 _____

Figure 32-11 in the textbook

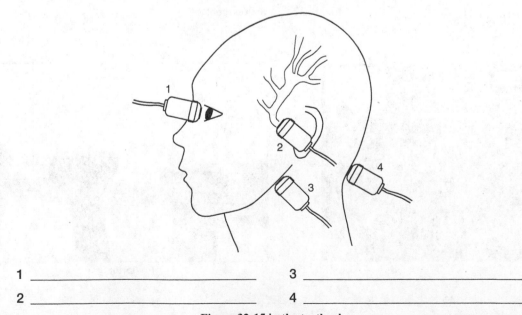

1 _____   3 _____

2 _____   4 _____

Figure 32-15 in the textbook

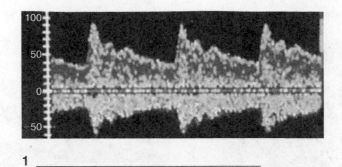

1 _____

Figure 32-16 in the textbook

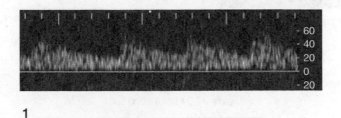

1 _____

Figure 32-17 in the textbook

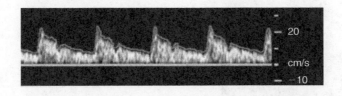

1 _____

Figure 32-18 in the textbook

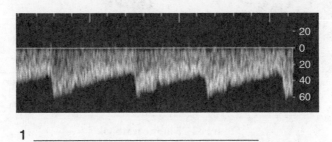

1 _____

Figure 32-19 in the textbook

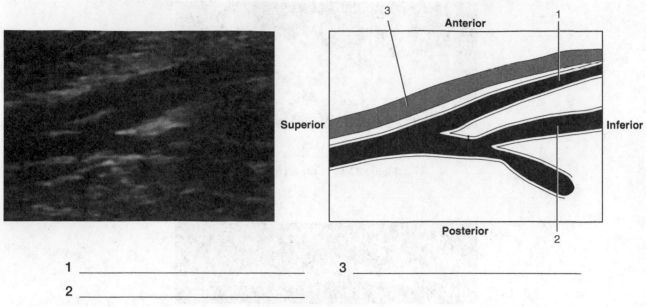

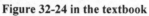

1 _____ 3 _____

2 _____

Figure 32-24 in the textbook

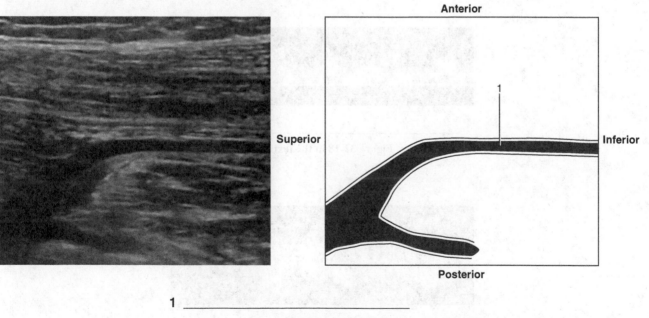

1 _____

Figure 32-25 in the textbook

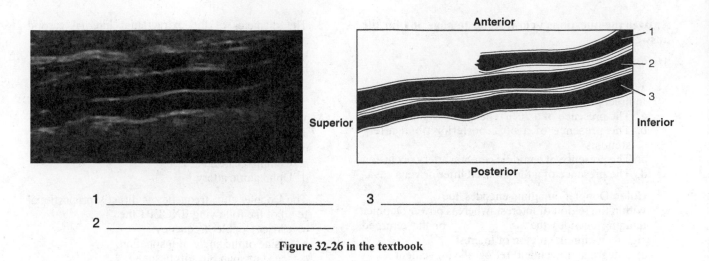

Anterior

Superior

Inferior

Posterior

1 _____

2 _____

3 _____

Figure 32-26 in the textbook

V. CHAPTER SUBHEADINGS EXERCISE

Directions to Students:

1. Convert each chapter subheading into a question; for example, change "The Lower Extremity Arterial System" to "What is the lower extremity arterial system?" Briefly answer each question in a short paragraph in your notebook.

2. Exchange answers with your lab partner and check each other's work. Refer back to the textbook for further information and explanation.

3. What questions do you still have about the chapter? Write your questions in your notebook.

VI. CHAPTER EVALUATION EXERCISE

Directions to Students: Use a fresh sheet of notebook paper. Based on your work with the chapter and its accompanying laboratory assignments, identify three concepts you believe are the most important. You may draw from any of the assignments you've already completed in the previous pages, including learning objectives, anatomy and physiology, images, or chapter subheadings. Include a detailed rationale in your answers.

Answer the questions below. Refer to page 384 for the answers.

Multiple Choice

1. Which of the following could be determined using indirect physiologic test procedures?
   a. The presence of a 70% renal artery stenosis
   b. The presence of a 60% posterior tibial artery stenosis
   c. The presence of a middle cerebral artery occlusion
   d. The presence of a thrombosed inferior vena cava

2. Color Doppler imaging encodes the _____ within the region of interest, whereas power Doppler imaging encodes the _____ of the returned signals within the region of interest.
   a. antegrade movement; retrograde movement
   b. number of pixels; volume of blood cells
   c. velocity; amplitude
   d. frequency shifts; intensity

3. All of the following arteries normally arise from the aortic arch EXCEPT the
   a. left common carotid artery.
   b. innominate artery.
   c. right common carotid artery.
   d. left subclavian artery.

4. The carotid siphon is part of the _____ segment of the internal carotid artery.
   a. cervical
   b. cerebral
   c. cavernous
   d. petrous

5. The diameter of the extracranial internal carotid artery approximates
   a. 1 to 2 mm.
   b. 2 to 3 mm.
   c. 3 to 4 mm.
   d. 4 to 5 mm.

6. Which of the following is a high-resistance vessel?
   a. Common femoral artery
   b. Middle cerebral artery
   c. Common carotid artery
   d. Ophthalmic artery

7. The Doppler shift frequency is directly proportional to all of the following EXCEPT the
   a. carrier Doppler frequency.
   b. cosine of the angle of insonation.
   c. speed of sound in soft tissue.
   d. velocity of blood flow.

8. If the Doppler shifted frequency doubles, the velocity
   a. doubles.
   b. remains the same.
   c. is halved.
   d. increases fourfold.

9. The peak systolic velocity range in the common carotid artery is normally
   a. <30 cm/s.
   b. 40 to 60 cm/s.
   c. 30 to 110 cm/s.
   d. 40 to 125 cm/s.

10. A reverse flow pattern is normally found in the
    a. CCA.
    b. bulb.
    c. ICA.
    d. vertebra.

33 3-D/4-D Sonography

I. MEMORIZATION EXERCISE

Directions to Students: Write the key words in your notebook or on note cards. Write the words on one side of the notepaper and then write the definitions on the opposite side of the page or on the back of the paper. If using note cards, write the key word on the front and the definition on the back. *This step should be completed before the lab session begins.*

Memorize the key word definitions silently for 5 minutes, then work with a lab partner and identify the words you still need help with. List the words here. Add additional rows if needed.

II. COMPREHENSION EXERCISE

Directions to Students: Work with a lab partner to complete this exercise. You will need to write in your notebook. First, change each objective into a question.

> *Example: "Define three-dimensional (3-D) sonography" becomes "What is three-dimensional (3-D) sonography?"*

Next, write a short answer to the question just created.

> *Example: "Three-dimensional sonography is an evolving technology that allows images to be viewed in three dimensions instead of the traditional two-dimensional viewing. It can be divided into three steps: volume acquisition, multiplanar display, and three-dimensional rendering. Real-time three-dimensional sonography is sometimes called four-dimensional sonography, where the fourth dimension is time."*

Highlight or circle any part of your answers about which you are unsure, and check the answers in your textbook. If you are still unsure of the answers, put a question mark next to the answer(s) for the review session of the lab.

III. APPLICATION OF ANATOMY AND PHYSIOLOGY EXERCISE

Directions to Students: Work on the following with your lab partner.

1. Using a piece of paper or clay, creat a three-dimensional structure of the kidney.

2. Label the kidney; include the structure's orientation in the body (either vertical, horizontal, vertical oblique, or horizontal oblique). Ask your lab partner to critique your work. What did you miss?

3. Check your model using the three-dimensional images in your textbook and complete any structures missing from your model.

4. In your notebook, write two or three summary sentences about three-dimensional imaging. Ask your lab partner to check your work. What else can you add to your description?

IV. IMAGE ANALYSIS EXERCISE

Directions to Students: Work on the following figures with your lab partner. It's your choice! You can label all the sketches at once, then go back and label each image with your lab partner, or you can label an image and its accompanying sketch at the same time. Either way, the goal is to label correctly all of the sketches and carefully compare the sketch with the sonographic image.

For each sonographic image, write a brief observation that could be "presented" to your instructor, a clinical sonographer, or a sonologist. Your observation should be based on Chapter 7 in the textbook, which describes how to write a technical observation. Please go back and review that chapter if necessary.

For each image, your assessment should include (1) the view of each major structure (axial or longitudinal; note: these are not the scanning planes) and (2) structures identified in the image with correct sonographic appearance description and measurements if shown (see Chapter 7 in the textbook for information on how to write a technical observation).

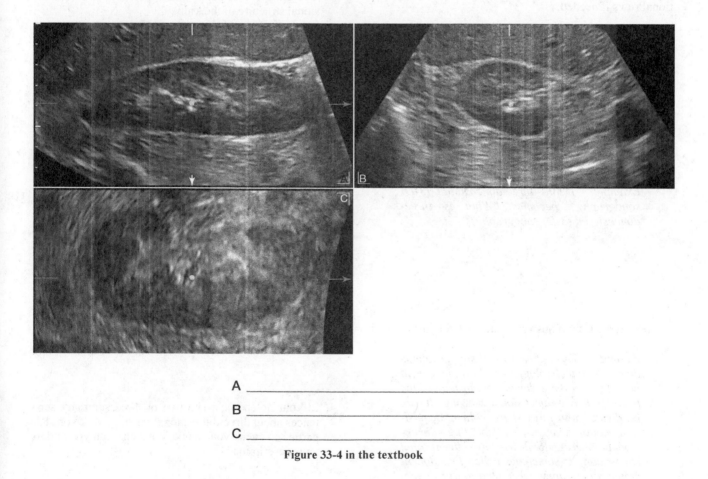

A _____

B _____

C _____

Figure 33-4 in the textbook

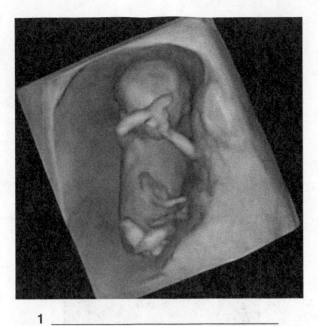

1 _____

Figure 33-10 in the textbook

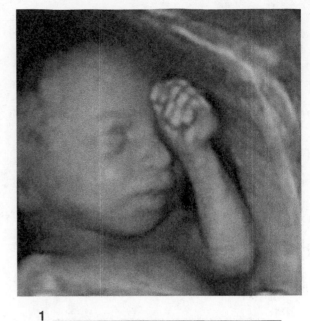

1 _____

Figure 33-20 in the textbook

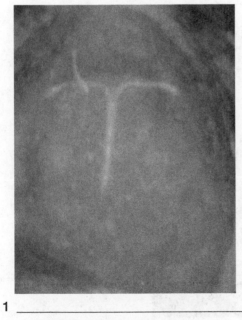

1 _____

Figure 33-21 in the textbook

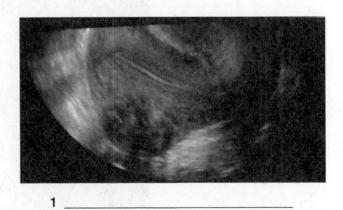

1 _____

Figure 33-25 in the textbook

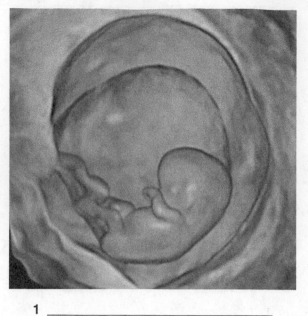

1 _____

Figure 33-26 in the textbook

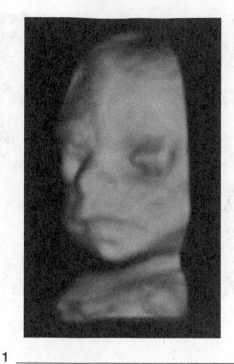

1 _____

Figure 33-27 in the textbook

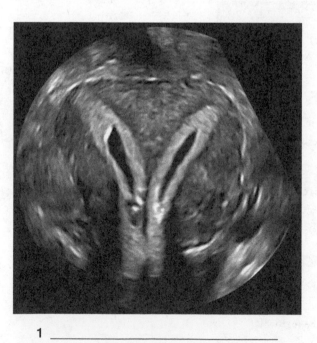

1 _____

Figure 33-29 in the textbook

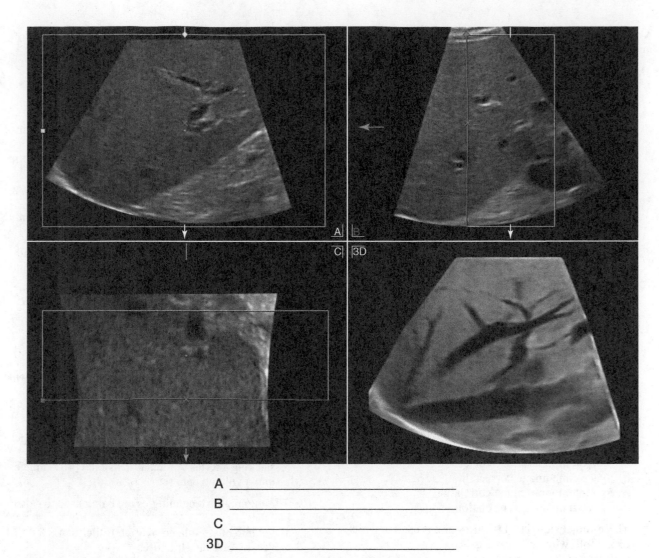

A _____

B _____

C _____

3D _____

Figure 33-30 in the textbook

V. CHAPTER SUBHEADINGS EXERCISE

Directions to Students:

1. Convert each chapter subheading into a question; for example, change "Sonographic Applications" to "What are the sonographic applications of 3-D/4-D sonography?" Briefly answer each question in a short paragraph in your notebook.

2. Exchange answers with your lab partner and check each other's work. Refer back to the textbook for further information and explanation.

3. What questions do you still have about the chapter? Write your questions in your notebook.

VI. CHAPTER EVALUATION EXERCISE

Directions to Students: Use a fresh sheet of notebook paper. Based on your work with the chapter and its accompanying laboratory assignments, identify three concepts you believe are the most important. You may draw from any of the assignments you've already completed in the previous pages, including learning objectives, anatomy and physiology, images, or chapter subheadings. Include a detailed rationale in your answers.

Answer the questions below. Refer to page 384 for the answers.

Multiple Choice

1. Which of the following is a rendering algorithm that displays anechoic structures as a solid object, giving the appearance of a cast or mold of the structure?
   a. STIC
   b. Thick-slice imaging
   c. Inversion mode
   d. Tomographic imaging

2. What is the first step of the Z-technique used to align 3-D/4-D volume data sets?
   a. Z-rotate the A-plane.
   b. Move the axis dot to the center of the anatomy of interest.
   c. Z-rotate the C-plane.
   d. Move the axis dot to a linear structure within the anatomy of interest.

3. Which of the following is true of 4-D sonography?
   a. It is also known as real-time 3-D sonography.
   b. It is useful when imaging the heart.
   c. It cannot be performed using manual acquisition techniques.
   d. All of the above.

4. What does STIC stand for?
   a. Spatiotemporal image correction
   b. Space-time image correction
   c. Spatiotemporal image correlation
   d. Space-time image correlation

5. Three-dimensional (3-D) ultrasound is used in which of the following applications?
   a. Imaging the coronal uterus
   b. STIC acquisitions of the fetal heart
   c. Neonatal head imaging
   d. A and C only
   e. All of the above

6. What are the three basic steps of 3-D/4-D sonography?
   a. Acquisition, manipulation, and display
   b. X-, Y-, Z-axis rotation
   c. A-, B-, and C-plane acquisition
   d. Orthogonal, axial, and coronal display

7. How can the volume acquisition time be reduced?
   a. Increase the quality and increase the volume angle.
   b. Decrease the quality and decrease the volume angle.
   c. Increase the quality and decrease the volume angle.
   d. Decrease the quality and increase the volume angle.

8. The _____ is used to simplify the manipulations necessary to align the orthogonal planes into standard imaging planes?
   a. A-plane
   b. Z-technique
   c. Y-rotation
   d. C-axis

9. Three-dimensional sonography is created by
   a. slowly moving the transducer back and forth across the anatomy of interest.
   b. rapidly moving the transducer back and forth across the anatomy of interest.
   c. stacking a series of two-dimensional (2-D) images into a volume data set.
   d. stacking a series of four-dimensional (4-D) images into a volume data set.

10. 3-D automation technologies are being used to calculate the
    a. volume of stimulated ovarian follicles.
    b. density of bone structures.
    c. flow rate of carotid stenosis.
    d. volumetric pressure of neonatal hydrocephalus.

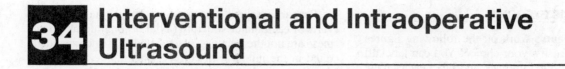

34 Interventional and Intraoperative Ultrasound

I. MEMORIZATION EXERCISE

Directions to Students: Write the key words in your notebook or on note cards. Write the words on one side of the notepaper and then write the definitions on the opposite side of the page or on the back of the paper. If using note cards, write the key word on the front and the definition on the back. *This step should be completed before the lab session begins.*

Memorize the key word definitions silently for 5 minutes, then work with a lab partner and identify the words you still need help with. List the words here. Add additional rows if needed.

II. COMPREHENSION EXERCISE

Directions to Students: Work with a lab partner to complete this exercise. You will need to write in your notebook. First, change the objective into a question.

> *Example: "Understand ultrasound-assisted interventional and intraoperative procedures" becomes "What are ultrasound-assisted interventional and intraoperative procedures?"*

Next, write a short answer to the question just created.

> *Example: "Interventional sonography is the use of sonographic procedures to assist the physician in completing an invasive procedure, such as an endoscopic examination of the pancreas."*

Highlight or circle any part of your answers about which you are unsure, and check the answers in your textbook. If you are still unsure of the answers, put a question mark next to the answer(s) for the review session of the lab.

III. APPLICATION OF ANATOMY AND PHYSIOLOGY EXERCISE

Directions to Students: Work on the following with your lab partner.
1. Write two or three summary sentences about interventional sonographic imaging and two or three summary sentences about intraoperative sonographic imaging. Include in your description the similarities and differences in procedures and applicable use. Ask your lab partner to check your work. What else can you add to your description?

IV. IMAGE ANALYSIS EXERCISE

Directions to Students: Work on the following figures with your lab partner. It's your choice! You can label all the sketches at once, then go back and label each image with your lab partner, or you can label an image and its accompanying sketch at the same time. Either way, the goal is to label correctly all of the sketches and carefully compare the sketch with the sonographic image.

For each sonographic image, write a brief observation that could be "presented" to your instructor, a clinical sonographer, or a sonologist. Your observation should be based on Chapter 7 in the textbook, which describes how to write a technical observation. Please go back and review that chapter if necessary.

For each image, your assessment should include (1) the view of each major structure (axial or longitudinal; note: these are not the scanning planes) and (2) structures identified in the image with correct sonographic appearance description and measurements if shown (see Chapter 7 in the textbook for information on how to write a technical observation).

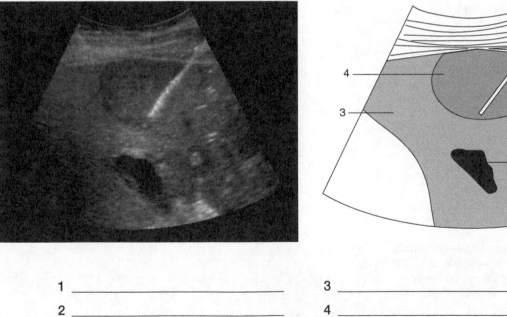

1 _____   3 _____

2 _____   4 _____

Figure 34-1 in the textbook

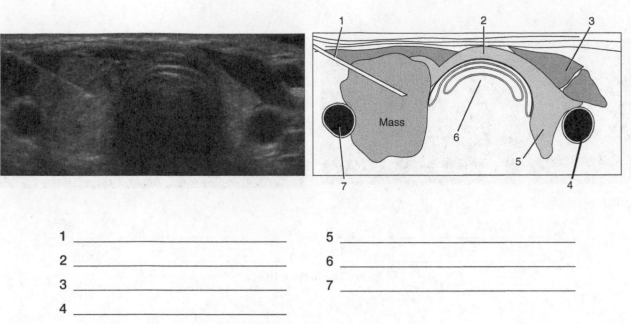

1 _____   5 _____

2 _____   6 _____

3 _____   7 _____

4 _____

Figure 34-2, top, in the textbook

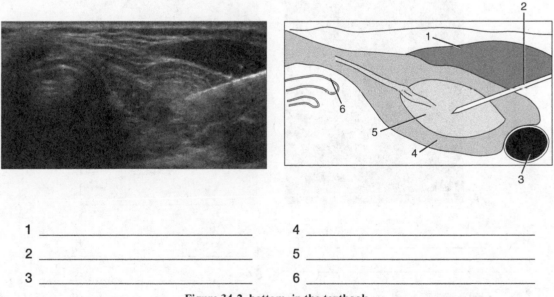

1 _____   4 _____

2 _____   5 _____

3 _____   6 _____

Figure 34-2, bottom, in the textbook

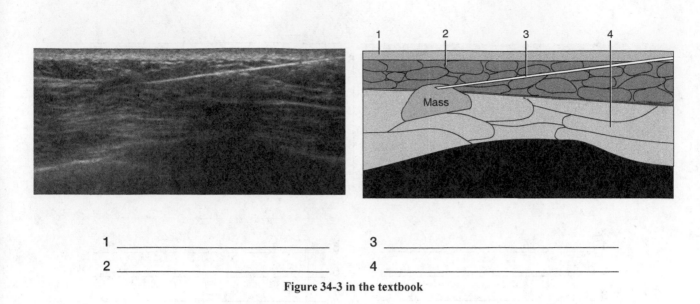

1 _____ 3 _____
2 _____ 4 _____

Figure 34-3 in the textbook

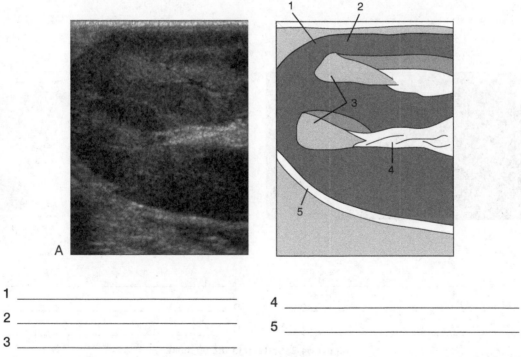

1 _____ 4 _____
2 _____ 5 _____
3 _____

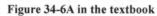

Figure 34-6A in the textbook

376

Chapter **34 Interventional and Intraoperative Ultrasound**

Copyright © 2017, Elsevier Inc. All rights reserved.

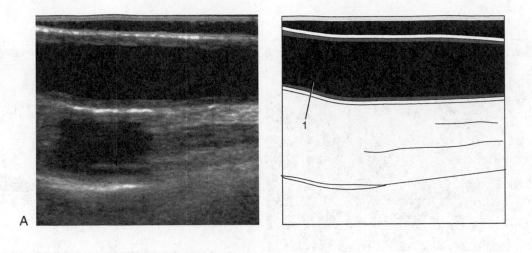

A

1 _____

Figure 34-7A in the textbook

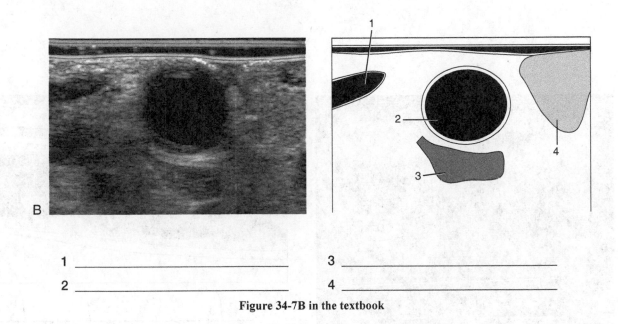

B

1 _____   3 _____

2 _____   4 _____

Figure 34-7B in the textbook

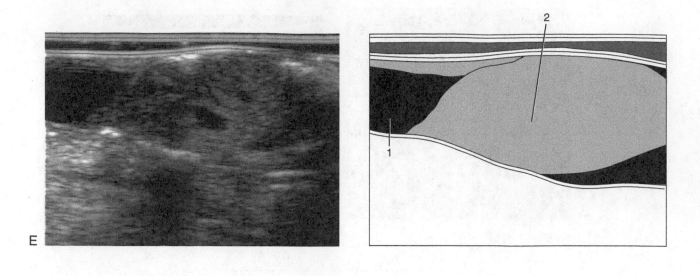

1 _____   2 _____

Figure 34-7E in the textbook

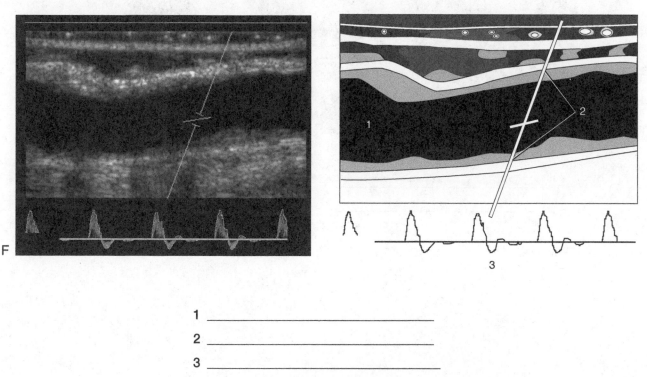

1 _____

2 _____

3 _____

Figure 34-7F in the textbook

V. CHAPTER SUBHEADINGS EXERCISE

Directions to Students:

1. Convert each chapter subheading into a question; for example, change "Intraoperative Ultrasound" to "What is intraoperative ultrasound?" Briefly answer each question in a short paragraph in your notebook.

2. Exchange answers with your lab partner and check each other's work. Refer back to the textbook for further information and explanation.

3. What questions do you still have about the chapter? Write your questions in your notebook.

VI. CHAPTER EVALUATION EXERCISE

Directions to Students: Use a fresh sheet of notebook paper. Based on your work with the chapter and its accompanying laboratory assignments, identify three concepts you believe are the most important. You may draw from any of the assignments you've already completed in the previous pages, including learning objectives, anatomy and physiology, images, or chapter subheadings. Include a detailed rationale in your answers.

Answer the questions below. Refer to page 384 for the answers.

Multiple Choice

1. Which of the following is an advantage of interventional and intraoperative procedures?
   a. Nonvisualization of needle placement
   b. Needle or tube tracking
   c. Need for ionizing radiation
   d. Limited to biopsies
2. Intraoperative ultrasound is NOT limited by
   a. air.
   b. fluid.
   c. the need for ionizing radiation.
   d. sterile fields.
3. A biopsy site is scanned before the biopsy to determine the best point of entry with the shortest distance and the
   a. smallest angle.
   b. largest angle.
   c. smallest track.
   d. clearest sterile field.
4. During an ultrasound-guided aspiration,
   a. chorionic villus sampling is performed.
   b. any change in the shape or size of a fluid-filled structure can be visualized.
   c. the transducer is endoluminal.
   d. a laparoscopic transducer is always used.
5. Ultrasound is used during _____ to determine accurate needle placement for tissue sampling.
   a. percutaneous aspiration
   b. percutaneous cholangiogram
   c. cyst aspiration
   d. percutaneous biopsies

True/False

6. The term percutaneous means "to sample." ___

7. Ultrasound-guided biopsies assist needle placement for fluid sampling. ___

8. An option for a sterile transducer sheath during interventional ultrasound is an alcohol bath. ___

9. Ultrasound-guided aspirations assist needle placement for small organ or stone extraction. ___

10. Chorionic villus sampling is limited to intraoperative surgical procedures. ___

Answer Key

CHAPTER 1

1. Assessment notes, lab test results, correlating image modality study reports
2. Descriptions of ultrasound findings based on echo pattern and size, origin or location, number
3. Origin or location, number, size, and composition of abnormal findings
4. physician
5. TO
6. CH
7. CH
8. TO
9. IR
10. IR

CHAPTER 2

1. c
2. c
3. a
4. d
5. a
6. b
7. d
8. b
9. c
10. a

CHAPTER 3

1. b
2. c
3. a
4. d
5. c
6. T
7. F
8. F
9. F
10. T

CHAPTER 4

1. d
2. d
3. b
4. e
5. b
6. c
7. T
8. T
9. T
10. F

CHAPTER 5

1. c
2. b
3. a
4. d
5. a
6. d
7. d
8. F
9. F
10. T

CHAPTER 6

1. T
2. F
3. F
4. F
5. T
6. T
7. F
8. T
9. T
10. F

CHAPTER 7

1. c
2. b
3. c
4. c
5. F
6. F
7. T
8. F
9. T
10. F

CHAPTER 8

1. d
2. c
3. b
4. c
5. d
6. c
7. b
8. a
9. c
10. d

CHAPTER 9

1. b
2. e
3. d
4. d
5. c
6. c and d
7. d
8. prostate
9. 50-75; 40-45
10. creatine

CHAPTER 10

1. b
2. c
3. F
4. F
5. T
6. T
7. T
8. F
9. F
10. T

CHAPTER 11

1. a
2. b
3. b
4. c
5. a
6. F
7. F
8. T
9. F
10. T

CHAPTER 12

1. F
2. T
3. F
4. F
5. IS
6. IS
7. LM
8. R
9. L
10. IS

CHAPTER 13

1. b
2. a
3. c
4. c

5. d
6. b
7. b
8. b
9. a
10. c

CHAPTER 14

1. d
2. a
3. c
4. d
5. d
6. b
7. a
8. c
9. a
10. d

CHAPTER 15

1. b
2. d
3. c
4. F
5. T
6. F
7. T
8. T
9. F
10. T

CHAPTER 16

1. c
2. b
3. a
4. a
5. d
6. 2.0-3.0 cm
7. 1.5-2.5 cm
8. 2.0-3.0 cm
9. 1.0-2.0 cm
10. 12.0-18 cm

CHAPTER 17

1. d
2. b
3. a
4. c
5. e
6. f
7. F
8. T
9. F
10. F

CHAPTER 18

1. c
2. d
3. E
4. F
5. C
6. A
7. H
8. G
9. D
10. B

CHAPTER 19

1. d
2. b
3. b
4. c
5. d
6. F
7. T
8. T
9. F
10. T

CHAPTER 20

1. b
2. c
3. a
4. c
5. d
6. T
7. F
8. T
9. F
10. F

CHAPTER 21

1. c
2. c
3. c
4. a
5. d
6. b
7. c
8. a
9. a
10. d

CHAPTER 22

1. d
2. b
3. d
4. b
5. b
6. b
7. d
8. d
9. d
10. c

CHAPTER 23

1. d
2. c
3. c
4. b
5. c
6. T
7. T
8. F
9. T
10. T

CHAPTER 24

1. b
2. a
3. c
4. b
5. 2
6. 2
7. 0
8. 2
9. 0
10. 2

CHAPTER 25

1. c
2. d
3. c
4. c
5. a
6. F
7. T
8. T
9. F
10. F

CHAPTER 26

1. c
2. c
3. b
4. a
5. c
6. b
7. b
8. b
9. b
10. a

CHAPTER 27

1. b
2. b
3. a
4. a
5. c
6. d
7. b
8. b
9. a
10. c

CHAPTER 28

1. E
2. G
3. H
4. F
5. A
6. J
7. C
8. D
9. B
10. I

CHAPTER 29

1. c
2. d
3. b
4. c
5. c
6. b
7. b
8. F
9. T
10. F

CHAPTER 30

1. a
2. d
3. a
4. d
5. a
6. interatrial septum
7. sinoatrial node
8. endocardium
9. foramen secundum
10. epicardium

CHAPTER 31

1. d
2. c
3. c
4. 60; 100
5. sinoatrial (SA)
6. systole
7. 4.0
8. 55-70%
9. embolus
10. anterior and posterior

CHAPTER 32

1. b
2. d
3. c
4. c
5. d
6. a
7. c
8. a
9. c
10. b

CHAPTER 33

1. c
2. d
3. d
4. c
5. d
6. a
7. b
8. b
9. c
10. a

CHAPTER 34

1. b
2. a
3. a
4. b
5. d
6. F
7. F
8. T
9. F
10. F